COVID-19 and Gastroenterology

Editor

MITCHELL S. CAPPELL

GASTROENTEROLOGY CLINICS OF NORTH AMERICA

www.gastro.theclinics.com

Consulting Editor
ALAN L. BUCHMAN

March 2023 • Volume 52 • Number 1

ELSEVIER

1600 John F. Kennedy Boulevard • Suite 1800 • Philadelphia, Pennsylvania, 19103-2899
http://www.theclinics.com

GASTROENTEROLOGY CLINICS OF NORTH AMERICA Volume 52, Number 1
March 2023 ISSN 0889-8553, ISBN-13: 978-0-443-18216-7

Editor: Kerry Holland
Developmental Editor: Hannah Almira Lopez

Gastroenterology Clinics of North America (ISSN 0889-8553) is published quarterly by Elsevier Inc., 360 Park Avenue South, New York, NY 10010-1710. Months of issue are March, June, September, and December. Business and Editorial Offices: 1600 John F. Kennedy Blvd., Suite 1800, Philadelphia, PA 19103-2899. Customer Service Office: 6277 Sea Harbor Drive, Orlando, FL 32887-4800. Periodicals postage paid at New York, NY and additional mailing offices. Subscription prices are $379.00 per year (US individuals), $100.00 per year (US students), $849.00 per year (US institutions), $407.00 per year (Canadian individuals), $100.00 per year (Canadian students), $1041.00 per year (Canadian institutions), $482.00 per year (international individuals), $220.00 per year (international students), and $1041.00 per year (international institutions). Foreign air speed delivery is included in all *Clinics* subscription prices. All prices are subject to change without notice. **POSTMASTER**: Send address changes to *Gastroenterology Clinics of North America*, Elsevier Health Sciences Division, Subscription Customer Service, 3251 Riverport Lane, Maryland Heights, MO 63043. **Telephone: 1-800-654-2452 (U.S. and Canada); 314-447-8871 (outside U.S. and Canada). Fax: 314-447-8029. E-mail: journalscustomerservice-usa@elsevier.com (for print support); journalsonlinesupport-usa@elsevier.com (for online support)**.

Reprints. For copies of 100 or more, of articles in this publication, please contact the Commercial Reprints Department, Elsevier Inc., 360 Part Avenue South, New York, New York 10010-1710. Tel. 212-633-3874, Fax: 212-633-3820, E-mail: reprints@elsevier.com.

Gastroenterology Clinics of North America is also published in Italian by Il Pensiero Scientifico Editore, Rome, Italy; and in Portuguese by Interlivros Edicoes Ltda., Rua Commandante Coelho 1085, 21250 Cordovil, Rio de Janeiro, Brazil.

Gastroenterology Clinics of North America is covered in *MEDLINE/PubMed (Index Medicus), Excerpta Medica, Current Contents/Clinical Medicine, Science Citation Index, ISI/BIOMED*, and *BIOSIS*.

Contributors

CONSULTING EDITOR

ALAN L. BUCHMAN, MD, MSPH, FACP, FACN, FACG, AGAF
Professor of Clinical Surgery, Medical Director, Intestinal Rehabilitation and Transplant Center, The University of Illinois at Chicago/UI Health, Chicago, Illinois, USA

EDITOR

MITCHELL S. CAPPELL, MD, PhD
Senior Gastroenterology Attending, Gastroenterology Service, Department of Medicine, Aleda E. Lutz Veterans Affairs Hospital, Saginaw, Michigan, USA

AUTHORS

ILARIA AMBROSINI, MD
Academic Radiology, Department of Translational Research, University of Pisa, Pisa, Italy

DIAS ARGANDYKOV, MD
Trauma, Emergency Surgery, and Surgical Critical Care, Massachusetts General Hospital, Harvard Medical School, Boston, Massachusetts, USA

PIERO BORASCHI, MD
2nd Unit of Radiology, Department of Diagnostic and Interventional Radiology, and Nuclear Medicine, Pisa University Hospital, Pisa, Italy

LUCIANA BRUNI, MD
Academic Radiology, Department of Translational Research, University of Pisa, Pisa, Italy

LIJUN CAI, MD
Department of Pathology, Zhongnan Hospital of Wuhan University, Wuhan, China

MITCHELL S. CAPPELL, MD, PhD
Senior Gastroenterology Attending, Gastroenterology Service, Department of Medicine, Aleda E. Lutz Veterans Affairs Hospital, Saginaw, Michigan, USA

TIAGO CORREIA DE SÁ, MD
General Surgery Department, Centro Hospitalar do Tâmega e Sousa, Penafiel, Portugal

JAMES M. CRAWFORD, MD, PhD
Professor and Chair, Department of Pathology and Laboratory Medicine, Donald and Barbara Zucker School of Medicine at Hofstra/Northwell, New Hyde Park, New York, USA

FRANCESCAMARIA DONATI, MD
2nd Unit of Radiology, Department of Diagnostic and Interventional Radiology, and Nuclear Medicine, Pisa University Hospital, Pisa, Italy

ANDER DORKEN-GALLASTEGI, MD
Division of Trauma, Emergency Surgery, and Surgical Critical Care, Massachusetts General Hospital, Harvard Medical School, Boston, Massachusetts, USA

SIRINA EKPANYAPONG, MD
Division of Gastroenterology and Hepatology, Department of Medicine, Huachiew General Hospital, Bangkok, Thailand; Division of Gastroenterology and Hepatology, Department of Medicine, University of Pennsylvania, Philadelphia, Pennsylvania, USA

DAVID M. FRIEDEL, MD
Division of Therapeutic Endoscopy, Division of Gastroenterology, Department of Medicine, NYU Langone Hospital, Mineola, New York, USA

ANTHONY GEBRAN, MD
Division of Trauma, Emergency Surgery, and Surgical Critical Care, Massachusetts General Hospital, Harvard Medical School, Boston, Massachusetts, USA

STEPHEN B. HANAUER, MD
Clifford Joseph Barborka Professor, Division of Gastroenterology and Hepatology, Department of Medicine, Northwestern University Feinberg School of Medicine, Chicago, Illinois, USA

HAYTHAM M.A. KAAFARANI, MD, MPH
Division of Trauma, Emergency Surgery, and Surgical Critical Care, Massachusetts General Hospital, Harvard Medical School, Boston, Massachusetts, USA

MARIA LETIZIA MAZZEO, MD
Academic Radiology, Department of Translational Research, University of Pisa, Pisa, Italy

SAURABH MEHANDRU, MD
Henry D. Janowitz Division of Gastroenterology, Department of Medicine, Precision Immunology Institute, Icahn School of Medicine at Mount Sinai, New York, New York, USA

HADAR MERINGER, MD
Henry D. Janowitz Division of Gastroenterology, Department of Medicine, Precision Immunology Institute, Icahn School of Medicine at Mount Sinai, New York, New York, USA

EMANUELE NERI, MD
Academic Radiology, Department of Translational Research, University of Pisa, Pisa, Italy

K. RAJENDER REDDY, MD
Founder's Professor of Medicine, Division of Gastroenterology and Hepatology, Department of Medicine, University of Pennsylvania, Philadelphia, Pennsylvania, USA

ANAM RIZVI, MD
Gastroenterology and Hepatology Fellow, Division of Gastroenterology, Donald and Barbara Zucker School of Medicine at Hofstra/Northwell, Northwell Health System, New Hyde Park, New York, USA

MÓNICA ROCHA, MD
Hepato-Pancreato-Biliary Unit, General Surgery Department, Centro Hospitalar do Tâmega e Sousa, Penafiel, Portugal

SHAHNAZ SULTAN, MD, MHSc
Professor of Medicine, Division of Gastroenterology, Hepatology and Nutrition, University of Minnesota, Minneapolis Veterans Affairs Health Care System, Minneapolis, Minnesota, USA

KEITH C. SUMMA, MD, PhD
Instructor, Division of Gastroenterology and Hepatology, Department of Medicine, Northwestern University Feinberg School of Medicine, Chicago, Illinois, USA

RACHELE TINTORI, MD
2nd Unit of Radiology, Department of Diagnostic and Interventional Radiology, and Nuclear Medicine, Pisa University Hospital, Pisa, Italy

MARTIN TOBI, MB, ChB
Department of Research and Development, John D. Dingell Veterans Affairs Medical Center, Detroit, Michigan, USA

MICHELE TONERINI, MD
Unit of Emergency Radiology, Department of Surgical, Medical, Molecular and Critical Area Pathology, Pisa University Hospital, Pisa, Italy

ARVIND J. TRINDADE, MD
Regional Director of Endoscopy, Northwell Health System (Central Region), Associate Professor of Medicine, Donald and Barbara Zucker School of Medicine at Hofstra/Northwell, Northwell Health System, New Hyde Park, New York, USA

ANDREW WANG
Henry D. Janowitz Division of Gastroenterology, Department of Medicine, Precision Immunology Institute, Icahn School of Medicine at Mount Sinai, New York, New York, USA

SHU-YUAN XIAO, MD
Department of Pathology, University of Chicago Medicine, Chicago, Illinois, USA

CHUNXIU YANG, PhD
Department of Pathology, Union Hospital, Tongji Medical College, Huazhong University of Science and Technology, Wuhan, China

YONATAN ZIV, MD
Gastroenterology and Hepatology Fellow, Division of Gastroenterology, Donald and Barbara Zucker School of Medicine at Hofstra/Northwell, Northwell Health System, New Hyde Park, New York, USA

Contents

The coronavirus disease 2019 (COVID-19), caused by the severe acute respiratory syndrome coronavirus 2, has quickly spread over the world since December 2019. COVID-19 is a systemic disease that can affect various organs throughout the body. Gastrointestinal (GI) symptoms have been reported in 16% to 33% of all patients with COVID-19 and in 75% of critically ill patients. This chapter reviews the GI manifestations of COVID-19 as well as their diagnostic and treatment modalities.

The global coronavirus disease-2019 (COVID-19) pandemic has caused significant morbidity and mortality, thoroughly affected daily living, and caused severe economic disruption throughout the world. Pulmonary symptoms predominate and account for most of the associated morbidity and mortality. However, extrapulmonary manifestations are common in COVID-19 infections, including gastrointestinal (GI) symptoms, such as diarrhea. Diarrhea affects approximately 10% to 20% of COVID-19 patients. Diarrhea can occasionally be the presenting and only COVID-19 symptom. Diarrhea in COVID-19 subjects is usually acute but is occasionally chronic. It is typically mild-to-moderate and nonbloody. It is usually much less clinically important than pulmonary or potential thrombotic disorders. Occasionally the diarrhea can be profuse and life-threatening. The entry receptor for COVID-19, angiotensin converting enzyme-2, is found throughout the GI tract, especially in the stomach and small intestine, which provides a pathophysiologic basis for local GI infection. COVID-19 virus has been documented in feces and in GI mucosa. Patients with preexisting diarrhea before contracting COVID-19 infection may have diarrhea exacerbation with COVID-19 infection, or alternatively the diarrhea may be incidental to COVID-19 infection. Treatment of COVID-19 infection, especially antibiotic therapy, is a common culprit, but secondary infections including bacteria, especially Clostridioides difficile, are sometimes implicated. Workup for diarrhea in hospitalized patients usually includes routine chemistries; basic metabolic panel; and a complete hemogram; sometimes stool studies, possibly including calprotectin or lactoferrin; and occasionally abdominal CT scan or colonoscopy. Treatment for the diarrhea is intravenous fluid infusion and electrolyte supplementation as necessary, and symptomatic antidiarrheal therapy, including Loperamide, kaolin-pectin, or possible alternatives. Superinfection with C difficile should be treated expeditiously. Diarrhea is prominent in post-COVID-19 (long COVID-19), and is occasionally noted after COVID-19 vaccination. The spectrum of diarrhea in COVID-19 patients is presently reviewed including the pathophysiology, clinical presentation, evaluation, and treatment.

COVID-19 infection is an ongoing catastrophic global pandemic with significant morbidity and mortality that affects most of the world population.

Respiratory manifestations predominate and largely determine patient prognosis, but gastrointestinal (GI) manifestations also frequently contribute to patient morbidity and occasionally affect mortality. GI bleeding is usually noted after hospital admission and is often one aspect of this multisystem infectious disease. Although the theoretical risk of contracting COVID-19 from GI endoscopy performed on COVID-19-infected patients remains, the actual risk does not seem to be high. The literature concerning GI bleeding in COVID-19 patients is presently reviewed.

COVID-19 and Inflammatory Bowel Disease 103

Keith C. Summa and Stephen B. Hanauer

The COVID-19 pandemic caused by the SARS-CoV-2 virus represents an unprecedented global health crisis. Safe and effective vaccines were rapidly developed and deployed that reduced COVID-19-related severe disease, hospitalization, and death. Patients with inflammatory bowel disease are not at increased risk of severe disease or death from COVID-19, and data from large cohorts of patients with inflammatory bowel disease demonstrate that COVID-19 vaccination is safe and effective. Ongoing research is clarifying the long-term impact of SARS-CoV-2 infection on patients with inflammatory bowel disease, long-term immune responses to COVID-19 vaccination, and optimal timing for repeated COVID-19 vaccination doses.

The Impact of COVID-19 Infection on Miscellaneous Inflammatory Disorders of the Gastrointestinal Tract 115

Mitchell S. Cappell, Martin Tobi, and David M. Friedel

The novel coronavirus pandemic of COVID-19 has emerged as a highly significant recent threat to global health with about 600,000,000 known infections and more than 6,450,000 deaths worldwide since its emergence in late 2019. COVID-19 symptoms are predominantly respiratory, with mortality largely related to pulmonary manifestations, but the virus also potentially infects all parts of the gastrointestinal tract with related symptoms and manifestations that affect patient treatment and outcome. COVID-19 can directly infect the gastrointestinal tract because of the presence of widespread angiotensin-converting enzyme 2 receptors in the stomach and small intestine that can cause local COVID-19 infection and associated inflammation. This work reviews the pathopysiology, clinical manifestations, workup, and treatment of miscellaneous inflammatory disorders of the gastrointestinal tract other than inflammatory bowel disease.

Gastrointestinal and Hepatobiliary Symptoms and Disorders with Long (Chronic) COVID Infection 139

Anam Rizvi, Yonatan Ziv, James M. Crawford, and Arvind J. Trindade

Long COVID is a novel syndrome characterizing new or persistent symptoms weeks after COVID-19 infection and involving multiple organ systems. This review summarizes the gastrointestinal and hepatobiliary sequelae of long COVID syndrome. It describes potential biomolecular mechanisms, prevalence, preventative measures, potential therapies, and health care and economic impact of long COVID syndrome, particularly of its gastrointestinal (GI) and hepatobiliary manifestations.

Gastrointestinal Endoscopy in Patients with Coronavirus Disease 2019: Indications, Findings, and Safety **157**

Shahnaz Sultan

The coronavirus disease 2019 (COVID-19) pandemic has changed the practice of gastroenterology and how we perform endoscopy. As with any new or emerging pathogen, early in the pandemic, there was limited evidence and understanding of disease transmission, limited testing capability, and resource constraints, especially availability of personal protective equipment (PPE). As the COVID-19 pandemic progressed, enhanced protocols with particular emphasis on assessing the risk status of patients and proper use of PPE have been incorporated into routine patient care. The COVID-19 pandemic has taught us important lessons for the future of gastroenterology and endoscopy.

Surgical Implications of Coronavirus Disease-19 **173**

Ander Dorken-Gallastegi, Dias Argandykov, Anthony Gebran, and Haytham M.A. Kaafarani

As the coronavirus disease-19 (COVID-19) pandemic continues to evolve in 2022 with the surge of novel viral variants, it is important for physicians to understand and appreciate the surgical implications of the pandemic. This review provides an overview of the implications of the ongoing COVID-19 pandemic on surgical care and provides recommendations for perioperative management. Most observational studies suggest a higher risk for patients undergoing surgery with COVID-19 compared with risk-adjusted non-COVID-19 patients.

Diagnostic and Therapeutic Radiology of the GI Tract, Liver, and Pancreas in Patients with COVID **185**

Piero Boraschi, Francescamaria Donati, Ilaria Ambrosini, Luciana Bruni, Maria Letizia Mazzeo, Rachele Tintori, Michele Tonerini, and Emanuele Neri

Coronavirus disease 2019 (COVID-19) pulmonary involvement has been extensively reported in the literature. Current data highlight how COVID-19 is a systemic disease, affecting many other organs, including the gastrointestinal, hepatobiliary, and pancreatic organs. Recently, these organs have been investigated using imaging modalities of ultrasound and particularly computed tomography. Radiological findings of the gastrointestinal, hepatic, and pancreatic involvement in patients with COVID-19 are generally nonspecific but are nonetheless helpful to evaluate and manage COVID-19 patients with involvement of these organs.

Pathologic Characteristics of Digestive Tract and Liver in Patients with Coronavirus Disease 2019 **201**

Chunxiu Yang, Lijun Cai, and Shu-Yuan Xiao

With the high prevalence of coronavirus disease-2019 (COVID-19), there has been increasing understanding of the pathologic changes associated with the severe acute respiratory syndrome coronavirus 2 (SARS-CoV-2). This review summarizes the pathologic changes in the digestive system and liver associated with COVID-19, including the injuries induced by

SARS-CoV2 infection of GI epithelial cells and the systemic immune responses. The common digestive manifestations associated with COVID-19 include anorexia, nausea, vomiting, and diarrhea; the clearance of the viruses in COVID-19 patients with digestive symptoms is usually delayed. COVID-19-associated gastrointestinal histopathology is characterized by mucosal damage and lymphocytic infiltration. The most common hepatic changes are steatosis, mild lobular and portal inflammation, congestion/sinusoidal dilatation, lobular necrosis, and cholestasis.

Special Critical Review Articles

Critical Review Two-Years Thereafter of the Effectiveness of the Revolutionary Changes in a Gastroenterology Division at A Medical School Teaching Hospital in Response to the COVID-19 Pandemic Medical School, Residency, and Gastrointestinal Fellowship Education and Clinical Practice of Gastroenterology Attendings and Gastrointestinal Endoscopy **215**

Mitchell S. Cappell

AIM: Critically review two-years afterwards effectiveness of revolutionary changes in academic-gastroenterologydivision due to COVID-19 pandemic.HOSPITAL-SETTING: William-Beaumont-Hospital-Royal-Oak, primary teachinghospital, Oakland-University-Medical-School, 6 GI fellows, 36 GI attendings (reduced to 29 with resignations). COVID-19 epicenter, metropolitan Detroit (daily hospital census: 0-patients, March-2020, increased to 300-patients, April-2020). Review based on expert opinion: (GI chief/Program Director >14 years, >320 publications). ADVANAGEOUS-CHANGES: 1- Temporarily pulled GI fellows to supervise exclusively COVID-19 wards; 2- performed only emergency/urgent endoscopy during pandemic peak (reduction from 100 to 4 endoscopies/day at nadir); 3-Changed "live" to "virtual" lectures, conferences, interviews, and graduations; 4-initially used "canned" video talks which worked poorly, eventually changed to Google- Zoom/Microsoft-Teams which performed superbly; 5-medical students/GI fellows graduated on-time despite missing minor requirements due to pandemic; 6-GI clinic reduced 50%; 7-GI-fellowship-program-director contacted fellows twice weekly to monitor pandemic-induced emotional stress; 8-ACGME cancelled annual fellowship survey in 2020. DISADVANTAGEOUSCHANGES: Huge hospital revenue shortfall exacerbated by Hospital's $84.5-milion governmental fine for Stark-Law/antikickback violations. Employee terminations during pandemic: reduced GI-fellowship support staff and endoscopy nurses. Severe personnel shortages from changing long-term academic anesthesiology group to low-cost anesthesiology group and many nurse resignations (after hospital prevented nursing unionization) caused 50% reduction in endoscopies and long endoscopy delays. Hospital terminated without cause numerous, most senior, highly respected, and elderly hospital leaders (e.g., chief medical officer, multiple department chairs).CONCLUSION: Profound, pervasive, GI-Divisional changes maximized clinical resources devoted to pandemic and minimized risk of infection transmission. Massive cost-cutting degraded academic quality of hospital while offering hospital to about 100 hospital systems, until hospital eventually "sold" to Spectrum Health, without faculty input.

AIM: Critically review two-years afterward effectiveness of revolutionary changes in academic-gastroenterologydivision due to COVID-19 pandemic.HOSPITAL-SETTING: William-Beaumont-Hospital-Royal-Oak, primary teachinghospital, Oakland-University-Medical-School, 6 GI fellows, 36 GI attendings (reduced to 29 with resignations). COVID-19 epicenter, metropolitan Detroit (daily hospital census: 0-patients, March-2020, increased to 300-patients, April-2020). Review based on expert opinion: (GI chief/Program Director >14 years, >320 publications).ADVANAGEOUS-CHANGES: 1- Temporarily pulled GI fellows to supervise exclusively COVID-19 wards; 2- performed only emergency/urgent endoscopy during pandemic peak (reduction from 100 to 4 endoscopies/day at nadir); 3-Changed "live" to "virtual" lectures, conferences, interviews, and graduations; 4-initially used "canned" video talks which worked poorly, eventually changed to Google-Zoom/Microsoft-Teams which performed superbly; 5-medical students/GI fellows graduated on-time despite missing minor requirements due to pandemic; 6-GI clinic reduced 50%; 7-GI-fellowship-program-director contacted fellows twice weekly to monitor pandemic-induced emotional stress; 8-ACGME cancelled annual fellowship survey in 2020. DISADVANTAGEOUSCHANGES: Huge hospital revenue shortfall exacerbated by Hospital's $84.5-milion governmental fine for Stark-Law/antikickback violations. Employee terminations during pandemic: reduced GI-fellowship support staff and endoscopy nurses. Severe personnel shortages from changing long-term academic anesthesiology group to low-cost anesthesiology group and many nurse resignations (after hospital prevented nursing unionization) caused 50% reduction in endoscopies and long endoscopy delays. Hospital terminated without cause numerous, most senior, highly respected, and elderly hospital leaders (e.g., chief medical officer, multiple department chairs).CONCLUSION: Profound, pervasive, GI-Divisional changes maximized clinical resources devoted to pandemic and minimized risk of infection transmission. Massive cost-cutting degraded academic quality of hospital while offering hospital to about 100 hospital systems, until hospital eventually "sold" to Spectrum Health, without faculty input.

GASTROENTEROLOGY CLINICS OF NORTH AMERICA

FORTHCOMING ISSUES

June 2023
Management of Obesity, Part I: Overview and Basic Mechanisms
Lee M. Kaplan, *Editor*

September 2023
Management of Obesity, Part 2: Treatment Strategies
Lee M. Kaplan, *Editor*

December 2023
Pediatric Inflammatory Bowel Disease
Marla Dubinsky, *Editor*

RECENT ISSUES

December 2022
Psychogastroenterology
Laurie Keefer, *Editor*

September 2022
Diagnosis and Treatment of Gastrointestinal Cancers
Marta L. Davila and Raquel E. Davila, *Editors*

June 2022
Medical and Surgical Management of Crohn's Disease
Sunanda V. Kane, *Editor*

Dedication

I dedicate this issue to Dr Anthony Fauci, who despite his long, dedicated, distinguished, and selfless public service as Director of the National Institute of Allergy and Infectious Diseases and Chief Medical Advisor to the President, has been subjected to public vilification because of his advocating public vaccination for the COVID-19 pandemic, an endorsement which has been proven to have saved millions of American lives. I am pleased to offer this dedication to celebrate his official retirement from the National Institutes of Health.[1]

Mitchell S. Cappell, MD, PhD
Gastroenterology Service
Department of Medicine
Aleda E. Lutz VA Hospital
Saginaw, MI 48602, USA

E-mail address:
mitchell.cappell@va.gov

The Aleda E. Lutz Veterans Administration Hospital at Saginaw and the United States federal government have no opinion on this dedication.

REFERENCE

1. Manning S. Dr Fauci reflects on more than five decades at NIH ahead of retirement from government. WFTV November 14, 2022. Available at: https://news.yahoo.com/dr-fauci-reflects-more-five-223036776.html. Accessed December 16, 2022.

Gastroenterol Clin N Am 52 (2023) xv
https://doi.org/10.1016/j.gtc.2022.12.006
0889-8553/23/© 2022 Published by Elsevier Inc.

Preface
Gastrointestinal, Hepatic, and Pancreatic Manifestations of COVID-19 Infection

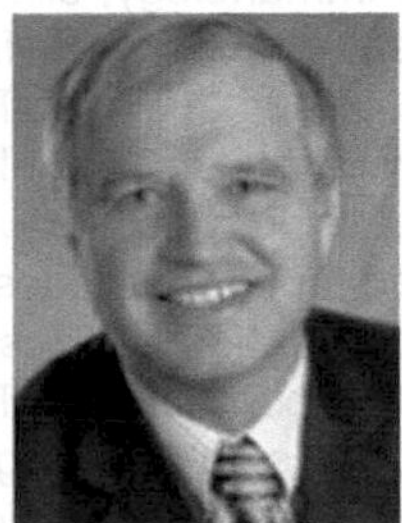

Mitchell S. Cappell, MD, PhD
Editor

We are living a false conceit that the world's health ineluctably improves and advances every year. For example, the average life expectancy of the population of Toronto was 50 years in 1900 and is currently 81.8 years.[1] Moreover, the average life expectancy increased appreciably every year for the last several generations.[2] We have assumed this wonderfully optimistic trend is preordained.

Then came the great COVID-19 pandemic!

And life expectancy in America precipitously declined in 2020 and in 2021, two years in a row, for the first time in generations.[3]

The pandemic, I believe, constitutes a cataclysmic warning: if we are not proactive, take proper precautions,institute preventive measures, and adapt infection control, another calamitous infectious disease can strike inevitably, hard, and soon. This Malthusian future may occur not by insufficient growth of the food supply as Malthus predicted, but from a novel virus crossing over to humans from bats or another animal host that is deadly, devastating, and annihilating to humans because humans lack any natural immunity to this novel virus. It is critical to increase investments by public health organizations, pharma, and medical institutions directed to virology, infectious diseases, and vaccine research to prevent and mitigate the next pending pandemic, which may be imminently jumping from bats to humans!

Consider our experience over the last three years with the COVID-19 pandemic as a roadmap on how to deal faster, more effectively, and more efficiently with the next global pandemic. Analysis of the history of this current pandemic response offers us the opportunity to critically analyze what we did, how we did it, what we did right, and what we did inefficiently to improve our response to the next inevitable pandemic. The worldwide response, greatly supported by the American government, National

Gastroenterol Clin N Am 52 (2023) xvii–xix
https://doi.org/10.1016/j.gtc.2022.12.005

Institutes of Health, and Food and Drug Administration, with notable contributions by Western democracies, institutions, and the World Health Organization, led the international effort. The current work provides an intense survey of the gastrointestinal (GI), hepatic, and pancreatic manifestations of COVID-19 infection. While the primary morbidity and mortality from COVID-19 are from pneumonia and respiratory decompensation, the GI tract is an important contributor to morbidity and an occasional contributor to mortality from COVID-19 infection, a connection reinforced by the presence of the angiotensin-converting enzyme-2 receptors in the GI tract,[4] and the passage of viral particles in stool.[5]

The current thorough study of the pathophysiology, virology, immunology, clinical manifestations, natural history, and treatment of GI tract disease represents the first comprehensive analysis of GI manifestations of COVID-19 in a journal issue. The venue of the *Gastroenterology Clinics of North America* is admirably suited to publish recent related advances quickly since it combines the quick turnaround typical of journals with the comprehensiveness of a book publication on related topics in a series of monographs, such as in *The Clinics* format. Indeed, the *Gastroenterology Clinics of North America* was published six months after I first recruited its contributors. The assembled senior article authors did a wonderful job on the articles as acknowledged national or international experts in the field of GI manifestations of COVID-19 infection, including Dr Saurabh Mehandru on the pathophysiology, immunology, and virology; Dr K. Rajender Reddy on liver and biliary manifestations of COVID-19 infection; Dr Tiago Correia de Sá on pancreatic manifestations; Dr H. Kaafarani on surgical aspects of GI disease; Dr David M. Friedel on diarrhea as a symptom of COVID-19 infection; Dr Mitchell S. Cappell on GI bleeding with COVID-19 infection; Dr Stephen B. Hanauer on inflammatory bowel disease with COVID-19 infection; Dr Mitchell S. Cappell on miscellaneous GI inflammatory disorders with COVID-19 infection; Dr Shahnaz Sultan on GI endoscopy with COVID-19 infection; Dr Piero Boraschi on diagnostic and interventional radiology for GI manifestations of COVID-19; Dr Arvind G. Trindade on GI manifestations of long (chronic) COVID-19 infection; and Dr Chuxiu Yang on GI pathology with COVID-19 infection. Beyond these contributors, I am also delighted to acknowledge the important contributions of the other article authors who substantively improved the articles for publication. The importance of these timely reviews is indicated by the huge number of articles published in peer-reviewed journals on GI and related infections associated with COVID-19 infection.[6]

The last two special articles are devoted to critical reviews two years thereafter of the revolutionary changes occurring at a medical school and teaching hospital due to the pandemic. These institutions are proposed as a microcosm of the revolutionary changes with a critical review offering the opportunity to critique these changes from the perspective of two years thereafter. These novel critical analyses provide an opportunity for performance improvement to prepare the next (and I believe inevitable) pandemic in terms of streamlining efficiency and improving the quality of the next pandemic response.

Finally, I thank Dr Alan Buchman for carefully supervising my selection of experts and the article topics for this issue. I am delighted to have worked and collaborated with Hannah Lopez and Kerry Holland for help inediting this journal issue. It was wonderful for me to collaborate with these highly talented individuals!

I believe this issue is my most important and clinically relevant editorship among the 12 issues of the *Medical Clinics of North America* and the *Gastroenterology Clinics of North America* that I have edited over the past 20 years because this work outlines a new discipline of GI manifestations of COVID-19 infection for the first time published in a book or monograph format. I believe this novel issue represents an important addition to this discipline.

Mitchell S. Cappell, MD, PhD
Gastroenterology Service
Department of Medicine
Aleda E. Lutz VA Hospital
Saginaw, MI 48602, USA

E-mail address:
mitchell.cappell@va.gov

The Aleda E. Lutz VA Hospital in Saginaw, Michigan and *the US government takes no opinion or position on this publication.*

REFERENCES

1. Edmiston J. Dead men walking: under 19th-century conditions, millions of Canadians would already be dead. National Post October 26, 2013. Available at: https://nationalpost.com/news/canada/dead-men-walking-under-19th-century-conditions-millions-of-canadians-would-already-be-dead#:~:text=In%20the%20year%201900%2C%20the%20average%20Canadian%20life,is%2081%2C%20an%20astonishing%2062%25%20increase%20Jake%20Edmiston. Accessed December 16, 2022.
2. Chart and table of Canada life expectancy from 1950 to 2022. Macrotrends: Life expectancy. Available at: https://www.macrotrends.net/countries/CAN/canada/life-expectancy. Accessed December 16, 2022.
3. Lipfert F. COVID and life expectancy: between 2019 and 2021, our national life expectancy, which is a measure of our overall health and lifespan, decreased by two years. It was the first such decline in over 50 years—and linked to COVID. As with all things COVID, those life losses were unevenly distributed. Available at: https://www.acsh.org/news/2022/10/31/covid-19-and-life-expectancy-16634. Accessed December 16, 2022.
4. Han-Yu L, Ying-He D, Kai N, et al. Potential effects of SARS-CoV-2 on the gastrointestinal tract and liver. Rev Biomed Pharmacother 2021;133:111064. https://doi.org/10.1016/j.biopha.2020.111064. PMID: 33378966.
5. Daou M, Kannout H, Khalili M, et al. Analysis of SARS-CoV-2 viral loads in stool samples and nasopharyngeal swabs from COVID-19 patients in the United Arab Emirates. PLoS One 2022;17(9):e0274961. https://doi.org/10.1371/journal.pone.0274961. Available at: https://www.bing.com/search?q=viral+partcles+COVID+and+stool&cvid=3f7eda8a5a834311849e59574c81d25a&aqs=edge..69i57.12269j0j4&FORM=ANAB01&PC=U531. Accessed December 16, 2022.
6. NCBI SARS-CoV-2 resources. National Institutes of Health, Library of Medicine, National Center for Biotechnology Information. SARS-CoV-2 data. Available at: https://www.ncbi.nlm.nih.gov/sars-cov-2/. Accessed December 16, 2022.

The Pathogenesis of Gastrointestinal, Hepatic, and Pancreatic Injury in Acute and Long Coronavirus Disease 2019 Infection

Hadar Meringer, MD[a,b], Andrew Wang, BS[a,b],
Saurabh Mehandru, MD[a,b,*]

KEYWORDS

• SARS-CoV-2 • Long COVID • Gastrointestinal • MAFLD • Insulin resistance

KEY POINTS

- Gastrointestinal (GI) and pancreatic tissues express high levels of angiotensin-converting enzyme-2 and are targeted during acute coronavirus disease 2019 (COVID-19) infection.
- A subset of patients with long COVID develops GI manifestations.
- Mechanisms underlying GI involvement in long COVID are complex and include viral persistence, mucosal and systemic immune dysregulation, microbial dysbiosis, insulin resistance, and metabolic abnormalities.
- Rigorous definitions and pathophysiology-based therapeutic approaches are needed to mitigate the morbidity associated with these disorders.

INTRODUCTION

Severe acute respiratory syndrome coronavirus 2 (SARS-CoV-2) and the resulting disease, coronavirus disease 2019 (COVID-19), first emerged in Wuhan, China, in 2019 and became a worldwide pandemic within months. The manifestations of COVID-19 infection range from asymptomatic infection to severe disease and death. Although respiratory failure and systemic inflammatory response syndrome (SIRS) are the hallmarks of severe disease, COVID-19 is clearly a multisystem disorder with postacute sequelae. Rigorous research focused on understanding the acute and chronic illness associated with COVID-19 remains a priority.

[a] Henry D. Janowitz Division of Gastroenterology, Department of Medicine; [b] Precision Immunology Institute, Icahn School of Medicine at Mount Sinai, 1425 Madison Avenue, Icahn Building 11-02, New York, NY 10029, USA

* Corresponding author. Precision Immunology Institute, Icahn School of Medicine at Mount Sinai, 1425 Madison Avenue, Icahn Building 11-02, New York, NY 10029.

E-mail address: saurabh.mehandru@mssm.edu

Gastroenterol Clin N Am 52 (2023) 1–11
https://doi.org/10.1016/j.gtc.2022.12.001

PATHOGENESIS OF ACUTE CORONAVIRUS DISEASE 2019 INFECTION

SARS-CoV-2 is a member of the Betacoronavirus genus,[1,2] which also includes severe acute respiratory syndrome coronavirus (SARS-CoV) and Middle East respiratory syndrome coronavirus (MERS-CoV). The virus is an enveloped virus with a positive-sense RNA-strand genome. The virion contains 4 main structural proteins—spike (S), envelope (E) and membrane (M) proteins in the viral membrane, with genomic RNA complexed with nucleocapsid (N) protein. Cellular entry is facilitated by interactions between the viral spike (S) glycoprotein and the host cell receptor, angiotensin-converting enzyme-2 (ACE2), leading to the fusion of viral and cellular membranes.[3] The transmembrane serine protease (TMPRSS2) is the main host cell protease, which cleaves the S protein of SARS-CoV-2 and facilitates viral entry into the cytoplasm of the host cell. Therefore, coexpression of ACE2 and TMPRSS2 is critical for host-cell entry by SARS-CoV-2. After entry, viral RNA is released and translated into viral polyproteins.[4] These polyproteins are cleaved by virus-encoded proteases to facilitate replication and produce full-length negative-strand RNA and subgenomic RNA. Subgenomic RNA is then translated into structural and accessory proteins and mature virions are exocytosed from the host cell.

The innate immune system serves as the first line of defense against SARS-CoV-2[5] by limiting viral entry, translation, replication, and assembly. Further, the innate immune system helps identify and remove infected cells, coordinates with and accelerates the development of adaptive immunity. The adaptive immune responses, driven by B cells and T cells,[6] are slower due to the intrinsic requirement of selecting and expanding virus-specific cells from the large pools of naïve cells. Viral Spike protein is targeted by SARS-CoV-2 neutralizing antibodies, with the receptor-binding domain of Spike being the target of greater than 90% of neutralizing antibodies. Further, SARS-CoV-2-specific $CD4^+$ and $CD8^+$ T cells are directed against a range of viral antigens that are significantly associated with reduced disease severity.

Evolution of SARS-CoV-2 and emergence of new variants has raised concerns that these variants (variants of concern [VOC]) could increase pathogenesis by escaping antiviral immune responses.[7] SARS-CoV-2 can specifically evade the innate immune system by encoding for several proteins that disrupt the retinoic acid-inducible gene I-like receptors sensing pathways, as well as the induction, signaling, or effector functions of interferons (IFNs). Mutations found in VOCs primarily cluster in the receptor binding motif, resulting in increased binding to ACE2 and escape from neutralizing antibodies. Furthermore, mutations and deletions in the N-terminal domain can change the domain structure and may account for differences in the induction of neutralizing antibodies. Understanding the mechanisms that new variants use to escape the immune system and their relation to altered disease pathogenesis is an active area of research.

Acute COVID-19 usually lasts for 4 weeks from symptoms onset. However, in a subset of individuals, postacute sequelae of COVID-19 (PASC) or "long COVID" are observed, although the natural history of long COVID and the inciting causes are not well understood. This review is focused on understanding the manifestations and mechanisms of long COVID, particularly because they relate to the gastrointestinal (GI) tract.

Pathogenesis of "Long Coronavirus Disease"

Persistent, prolonged, and often debilitating sequelae are increasingly recognized in COVID-convalescent individuals[8] and are termed "long COVID," "long-haul-COVID," or PASC. Although the definitions of this syndrome are inconsistent,[9] the WHO definition of long COVID includes prior "probable or confirmed" SARS-CoV-2 infection, with symptoms that last for at least 2 months and cannot be explained by an alternative diagnosis. However, the National Institute for Health and Care Excellence defines long COVID as a syndrome that develops during or after an infection consistent with COVID-19 continues for more than 12 weeks and is not explained by an alternative diagnosis.

The common manifestations of long COVID are systemic (fatigue and poor concentration), neuropsychiatric (sleep abnormalities, chronic headache, "brain fog," defects in memory, mood impairment, and pain syndromes), cardiac (palpitations, syncope, dysrhythmias, and postural symptoms), respiratory (dyspnea and cough), and GI (nausea, vomiting, anorexia, diarrhea, and/or abdominal pain).[8] Adopting accurate and consistent definitions of long COVID permits careful clinical evaluation of the symptoms, and distinguishes prolonged damage associated with acute illness from new symptoms that develop after the acute disease resolves.

Several hypotheses regarding the pathogenesis of long COVID have been proposed,[10] including the following: (1) delay in the resolution of infection and persistent inflammation, (2) persistence of virus or viral antigens in tissues, (3) triggering of autoimmunity, and (4) aberrant immune responses, including dysregulated cytokine production.

Among the studies that have defined the pathogenesis of long COVID, a prospective, case–control study of 31 patients with long COVID, matched with 31 convalescent individuals without long-COVID sequelae,[11] found elevated serum levels of proinflammatory cytokines (IFNβ, IFNλ1, IFNγ, CXCL9, CXCL10, IL-8, and soluble T cell immunoglobulin and mucin domain-containing protein 3 [Tim-3]) in both groups after 4 months of acute infection. However, at 8 months after infection, only the patients with long COVID had a persistent increase in levels of IFNβ and IFNλ1 in circulation and expansion of peripheral blood-associated $PD1^+$ or $TIM3^+CD8^+$ memory T cells, activated ($CD86^+CD38^+$) plasmacytoid dendritic cells, and $CD14^+CD16^+$ monocytes.[11] These data demonstrate that long COVID is associated with a sustained inflammatory response.

Long COVID was further studied longitudinally in a cohort of 309 patients with COVID-19 who were evaluated from the time of diagnosis to convalescence, 2 to 3 months postinfection.[12] Detailed multiomic investigation identified 4 parameters that anticipated the development of long COVID. These included type 2 diabetes mellitus, high initial SARS-CoV-2 viremia, reactivation of latent viruses (especially Epstein–Barr virus [EBV]), and the presence of specific autoantibodies during or preceding the acute stage of COVID-19 infection.[12] Notably, specific autoantibodies such as anti-IFNα2 were linked to inhibition of IFN-dependent B cell responses (evidenced by a negative correlation between anti-SARS-CoV-2 antibodies and anti-IFNα2 antibodies). Additionally, IFNα2 inhibition was linked to the upregulation of inflammatory cytokines that characterize long COVID. Furthermore, many aberrant immune cell populations were enriched in patients with long COVID. These included cytotoxic $CD4^+$ T cells, exhausted T cells and myeloid-derived suppressor cells.[12]

Another prospective, multicenter study of 215 individuals identified a distinct SARS-CoV-2-specific immunoglobulin signature during acute infection among those who subsequently developed long COVID.[13] This included reduced IgM and IgG3 titers during acute infection. Because IgM and, particularly, IgG3 secretion by B cells is induced by IFNs and antagonized by interleukin-4 (IL-4), this study suggested that the aberrant immunoglobulin signature associated with long COVID is related to reduced production of type I IFNs, resulting in a failure of antibody isotype switching.

In a recent cross-sectional study that included 101 individuals with long COVID, 41 convalescent individuals without long COVID (median times from acute disease of 432 days and 344 days, respectively) and 41 uninfected healthy controls, cellular and soluble immune parameters were examined.[14] In this study, when compared with individuals without long COVID, those with long COVID had a significant increase in levels of nonclassical monocytes ($CD14^{low}CD16^{hi}$), activated B cells ($CD86^{hi}HLA\text{-}DR^{hi}$), double-negative B cells ($IgD^{-}CD27^{-}CD24^{-}CD38^{-}$ cells), and exhausted ($PD\text{-}1^{+}/Tim\text{-}3^{+}$) $CD4^{+}$ T cells and $CD8^{+}$ T cells. Additionally, long COVID individuals had higher titers of anti-EBV antibodies, although the overall seroprevalence of EBV in long COVID individuals was not different from healthy or convalescent controls. Further, and perhaps a striking observation was that long COVID individuals had a persistently decreased cortisol production more than a year after acute infection when compared with healthy or convalescent controls. This high-dimensional profiling of the peripheral blood supports the hypothesis that there are significant and persistent biological differences in patients who develop long COVID that include persistence of antigen, reactivation of latent herpesviruses, and chronic inflammation.

TARGETING OF THE GASTROINTESTINAL TRACT BY SEVERE ACUTE RESPIRATORY SYNDROME CORONAVIRUS-2 DURING ACUTE CORONAVIRUS DISEASE 2019 INFECTION

GI symptoms including nausea, vomiting, anorexia, diarrhea, and/or abdominal pain are common extrapulmonary manifestations during acute COVID-19 infection.[15] The incidence of GI symptoms in patients with COVID-19 varies between different studies, ranging from 3% in the initial reports from Wuhan,[16] up to 61.3% in a multicenter cohort from the United States.[17] Based on a systematic review and meta-analysis of 47 studies and more than 10,000 patients, GI symptoms were observed in around 10% of patients with acute COVID-19.[18] An important clinical question is the association of GI symptoms with COVID-19 outcomes. To address this, we investigated a cohort of 634 patients with COVID-19 who were admitted to Mount Sinai Hospital. Patients presenting with GI symptoms had less severe disease than patients without GI symptoms ($P < .001$), and mortality was significantly lower in patients with GI symptoms (15.7%) than those without (31.0%; $P < .0001$).[19] These data were confirmed in an external validation cohort of 287 hospitalized patients from Milan, Italy,[19] and were consistent with 2 prior studies.[20,21] However, these findings contrast with early studies from Wuhan, China, where the presence of GI symptoms in patients with COVID-19 was associated with an unfavorable prognosis.[22,23] Possibly this discrepancy may arise from the inclusion of abnormal liver enzymes (which are associated with worse outcomes)[23] or iatrogenic confounders[22] in the Wuhan studies.

Robust and constitutive expression of ACE2, the receptor for SARS-CoV-2, on the brush border of small intestinal epithelium,[24] enables viral entry into intestinal cells. GI infection by SARS-CoV-2 is further supported by in vitro studies using human small intestinal organoids[25,26] and a high prevalence of viral shedding in stool, particularly after viral RNA negativity in respiratory specimens.[27] Endoscopic evaluation of the GI tract in patients with COVID-19 (in the acute, or immediate postacute stage of COVID-19) is usually unremarkable with a notably "normal" histological appearance of intestinal tissues, often with a scant neutrophilic infiltrate or mild increase in intraepithelial lymphocytes[19] in contrast to the dense inflammatory infiltrate that accompanies pulmonary infection with SARS-CoV-2. Further, detailed immunophenotyping of intestinal tissues in patients with COVID-19, reveals reduced frequencies of conventional dendritic cells ($CD206^{+}CD1c^{+}$ cDC2) and plasmacytoid dendritic cells with an increase in the frequency of effector T cells. Transcriptional signatures (using bulk RNAseq of intestinal biopsies) reveal a significant downregulation of pathways associated with inflammation and antigen presentation in the lamina propria with a concomitant activation of antiviral response signaling genes in the epithelial compartment.[19] Further, patients with COVID-19 with GI symptoms have reduced levels of circulating inflammatory cytokines (including IL-6, IL-8, IL-17, and CCL28) compared with patients with COVID-19 without GI symptoms.[19] Altogether, these data suggest that although the GI tract can be infected by SARS-CoV-2, when compared with the lungs, there appears to be an attenuated inflammatory response in the intestines in the acute stage. Although speculative, this raises the possibility that a "less than sterilizing" intestinal immune response to SARS-CoV-2 may allow for viral persistence in GI tissues as detailed below.

GASTROINTESTINAL INVOLVEMENT IN LONG CORONAVIRUS DISEASE

GI manifestations are well reported in patients with long COVID, although their frequency is not clearly defined.[10] Long COVID–associated GI symptoms include—loss of appetite, nausea, weight loss, abdominal pain, heartburn, dysphagia, altered bowel motility, and irritable bowel syndrome (IBS).[10] In a prospective cohort of 1783 COVID-19 recovered individuals (with 749 responders to survey questionnaires), 220 patients (29%) self-reported GI symptoms at 6 months that included diarrhea (10%), constipation (11%), abdominal pain (9%), nausea and/or vomiting (7%), and heartburn (16%).[28] In another study of 73,435 users of the Veterans Health Administration, motility disorders (including constipation and diarrhea) and esophageal disorders (including dysphagia) were reported as postacute sequalae of acute COVID.[29]

Unique characteristics of the GI mucosal immune compartment may underlie the pathophysiology of long COVID that include viral persistence, aberrant immune activation in the GI tract, intestinal dysbiosis, and maladaptive neuro-immune interactions as detailed below.

Viral Persistence in the Gastrointestinal Tract

We first reported on the persistence of SARS-CoV-2 antigens in the GI tract after an average of 4 months (range 2.8–5.7 months) post-COVID-19 infection.[30] Intestinal enterocyte-associated SARS-CoV-2 N protein was detected in 5 out of 14 individuals while in 3 out of the 14 participants, polymerase chain reaction (PCR) amplicons were sequence verified as SARS-CoV-2.[30] Viral detection in GI tissues, which was patchy and sporadic, likely truly underestimate viral persistence. Although none of the patients in the initial study suffered from long COVID, the data provided proof of the principle that SARS-CoV-2 can potentially persist in specific tissues in a manner consistent with the persistence of other nonretroviral RNA viruses. Goh and colleagues[31] established the presence of residual virus in GI tissue (appendix) and non-GI tissues (skin, and breast) in 2 patients who exhibited long COVID symptoms 163 and 426 days after symptom onset, respectively. In another cohort of 46 patients with inflammatory bowel disease, patients who tested negative for mucosal SARS-CoV-2 RNA (30%) did not experience persistent symptoms, whereas in patients who tested positive for SARS-CoV-2 RNA (70%), a majority (65.5%) experienced long COVID symptoms.[32] GI involvement in long COVID is associated with unique T cell clonal and transcriptome dynamics that include a significant enrichment of the cytotoxic T cells associated with bystander activation of CMV-specific cells.[12] Ongoing work in our group also identifies persistent lymphoid and myeloid cell abnormalities in the GI tract up to 10 months after initial infection.[33] Altogether, emerging data provide evidence of protracted viral antigen persistence and immune cell abnormalities in GI tissues. However, to-date, intact virions have not been cultured from patients with long COVID, and there is no evidence yet of viral evolution in intestinal tissues.

Microbial Dysbiosis Associated with Long Coronavirus Disease

Studies have also begun to dissect the association between the intestinal microbiome and long COVID. The composition of the fecal microbiome was examined using shotgun metagenomic sequencing in a prospective cohort of 106 patients who were followed from admission up to 6 months postinfection.[34] Although this study was skewed by a high representation of individuals with moderate-to-severe COVID-19 (73.5%) and a high prevalence of long COVID–associated symptoms (73.5%), reduced microbial diversity and higher levels of *Ruminococcus gnavus*, *Bacteroides vulgatus*, and lower levels of *Faecalibacterium prausnitzii* were associated with long COVID in this study.[34]

Alterations in the Gut–Brain Axis in Long Coronavirus Disease

In a survey of patients hospitalized with COVID-19 and followed-up for at least 6 months, persistent GI symptoms meeting the Rome IV criteria were found in 39% (44 out of 112) of patients.[35] A validated survey to determine the severity of IBS symptoms (the IBS severity scoring system IBS-SSS) reported a significant increase in severe IBS after COVID-19. Given the high frequency of motility-related disorders associated with GI long COVID, postinfectious neuro-immune related disorders should be considered in disease pathogenesis. Possible mechanisms involve microbial dysbiosis, increased intestinal permeability, and low-grade intestinal immune activation. Small animal model studies demonstrate that cross talk among gut-innervating specialized sensory neurons (nociceptors), microbes, and intestinal epithelial cells regulate the mucosal host defense.[36] Further, muscularis propria-resident macrophages, in close apposition with enteric neurons cell bodies, acquire tissue-protective phenotypes that prevent neuronal loss after infection.[37] Although there are no data at present, we anticipate that examination of intestinal neuro-immune cross talk in patients with long COVID will be illuminative.

HEPATIC INVOLVEMENT BY SEVERE ACUTE RESPIRATORY SYNDROME CORONAVIRUS-2

The mechanisms of hepatic dysfunction in long COVID patients are poorly understood. A subset of patients may manifest with abnormal liver function tests 6 months after COVID-19 resolution. In most such cases, patients receive the diagnosis of metabolic-associated fatty liver disease (MAFLD). However, it is unclear whether MAFLD is coincidental, or a consequence of persistent inflammation seen in some COVID-19 patients. A few other hypothesized mechanisms include SARS-CoV-2-induced direct injury or persistence within the liver, dysregulated gut–liver axis, or chronic and systemic inflammation.

Although hepatocytes exhibit a lower expression of ACE2 than enterocytes, scavenger receptor class B type 1, posited as a potential interactor with SARS-CoV-2, is highly expressed in the liver.[38] A study of hepatic autopsies demonstrated the presence of SARS-CoV-2 RNA and S proteins in liver tissue by reverse transcription-PCR, immunofluorescence, and confocal microscopy.[39] Furthermore, transcriptomic and proteomic data suggest similarities between infection with SARS-CoV-2 and known hepatotropic viruses such as HBV, HCV, and HIV.[39] Nonetheless, there are no data at present to suggest that SARS-CoV-2 persists in the liver or is directly causative of MAFLD.

The gut–liver axis serves as a bidirectional conduit that enables a complex regulatory control of both systems. As detailed previously, a subset of patients manifest with protracted shedding of SARS-CoV-2 RNA in the stool, beyond acute infection.[27] Persistence of viral antigens in the GI tract can potentially alter intestinal permeability, exposing the liver to luminal microflora, and accelerating hepatic injury due to the ensuing inflammatory responses. Furthermore, microbial dysbiosis post-COVID-19 could potentially affect not only the GI system but the gut–liver axis as well.[40,41] Notably, patients with long COVID when compared with non–long COVID convalescent individuals have a depletion of homeostatic, butyrate-producing bacteria and depletion of short-chain fatty acids.[42,43] Such perturbations are potentially associated with the establishment of a proinflammatory milieu in the liver, as demonstrated by elevated levels of proinflammatory cytokines including IFN-α, IFN-γ, IL-1β, IL-6, and TNF-α,[11,44,45] which can lead to MAFLD over time.[46] Additionally, dysregulation of oxidative and fatty acid metabolic pathways in patients with COVID-19,[47,48] and the resulting metabolic stress may result in hepatocyte apoptosis, lipid accumulation, and ultimately MAFLD.[44,49]

PANCREATIC INVOLVEMENT BY SEVERE ACUTE RESPIRATORY SYNDROME CORONAVIRUS-2

During acute COVID-19 infection, both endocrine and exocrine pancreatic dysfunction is described, characterized by new-onset diabetes and persistent hyperglycemia. It is plausible that patients with long COVID may develop new-onset diabetes through mechanisms that include direct cytotoxicity or pancreatic tropism, chronic inflammation, or both.

Pancreatic tissues express ACE2 and TMPRSS2 in ductal and β-islet cells at levels that are comparable to lung tissues.[50] In vitro studies utilizing induced pluripotent stem cell (iPSC)-derived pancreatic cultures as well as postmortem tissues demonstrate SARS-CoV-2 in pancreatic endocrine and exocrine cells and increased the expression of some pancreatic ductal stress response genes.[51,52] It was further suggested that β-cell infection could contribute to metabolic dysregulation observed in patients with COVID-19.[52] Detailed analysis of pancreatic autopsy tissue from patients with COVID-19 using immunofluorescence, immunohistochemistry, RNA scope, and electron microscopy reveals SARS-CoV-2 viral infiltration of beta-cells.[53,54] Notably, viral RNA within the pancreas, was detected in cells with weaker expression of ACE2 but a high expression of DPP4.[53] Moreover, SARS-CoV-2–induced local inflammation was associated with islet cell apoptosis.[53] In addition to direct cytotoxicity, β cell dysfunction may be attributed to the proinflammatory milieu associated with long COVID.

Altogether, based on existing data, both direct cytotoxicity of SARS-CoV-2, indirect inflammatory response within pancreatic tissue and the overall inflammatory milieu can lead to long-term pancreatic dysfunction in patients with long COVID.

SUMMARY

Gastrointestinal involvement is a recognized manifestation of long COVID. Underlying mechanisms are complex and may include viral persistence, immune dysregulation, reactivation of latent viruses, microbial dysbiosis, metabolic stress, and insulin resistance. Prospective studies with clearly defined patient populations and uniform definitions of the long COVID syndrome are required to better define the pathophysiology and to enable much needed therapeutic trials for this syndrome.

DISCLOSURE

This work was supported in part by PolyBio Research Foundation and Balvi Philanthropic Fund. S. Mehandru reports receiving research grants from Genentech, United States and Takeda, United States; receiving payment for lectures from Takeda, Genentech, Morphic; and receiving consulting fees from Takeda, Morphic, Ferring, and

Arena Pharmaceuticals. H. Meringer, A. Wang, and S. Mehandru do not declare any conflicts of interest relating to this study.

CLINICS CARE POINTS

- GI and pancreatic tissues are targeted during acute COVID-19 infection due to high levels of expression of ACE-2 in the physiological state.
- Common GI manifestations during acute COVID-19 include diarrhea, nausea, vomiting and abdominal pain.
- The common GI manifestations during long COVID are loss of appetite, nausea, weight loss, abdominal pain, heartburn, dysphagia, altered bowel motility, and irritable bowel syndrome.
- Several hypotheses regarding the pathogenesis of long COVID have been proposed. These include a) delay in the resolution of infection and persistent inflammation; b) persistence of virus or viral antigens in tissues; c) triggering of autoimmunity; and d) aberrant immune responses, including dysregulated cytokine production.
- A subset of patients who recover from acute COVID continue to demonstrate abnormal liver function tests up to 6 months post-infection that are related to metabolic associated fatty liver disease (MAFLD).
- Rigorous case definitions, longitudinal patient follow up and therapeutic clinical trials are urgently needed in patients with long COVID.

REFERENCES

1. Zhou P, Yang XL, Wang XG, et al. A pneumonia outbreak associated with a new coronavirus of probable bat origin. Nature 2020;579(7798):270–3.
2. Lu R, Zhao X, Li J, et al. Genomic characterisation and epidemiology of 2019 novel coronavirus: implications for virus origins and receptor binding. Lancet 22 2020;395(10224):565–74.
3. Hoffmann M, Kleine-Weber H, Schroeder S, et al. SARS-CoV-2 Cell Entry Depends on ACE2 and TMPRSS2 and Is Blocked by a Clinically Proven Protease Inhibitor. Cell 2020;181(2):271–80.e8.
4. Kim D, Lee JY, Yang JS, et al. The Architecture of SARS-CoV-2 Transcriptome. Cell 2020;181(4):914–21.e10.
5. Diamond MS, Kanneganti TD. Innate immunity: the first line of defense against SARS-CoV-2. Nat Immunol 2022;23(2):165–76.
6. Sette A, Crotty S. Adaptive immunity to SARS-CoV-2 and COVID-19. Cell 2021; 184(4):861–80.
7. Merad M, Blish CA, Sallusto F, et al. The immunology and immunopathology of COVID-19. Science 2022;375(6585):1122–7.
8. Mehandru S, Merad M. Pathological sequelae of long-haul COVID. Nat Immunol 2022;23(2):194–202.
9. Munblit D, O'Hara ME, Akrami A, et al. Long COVID: aiming for a consensus. Lancet Respir Med 2022;10(7):632–4.
10. Meringer H, Mehandru S. Gastrointestinal post-acute COVID-19 syndrome. Nat Rev Gastroenterol Hepatol 2022;19(6):345–6.
11. Phetsouphanh C, Darley DR, Wilson DB, et al. Immunological dysfunction persists for 8 months following initial mild-to-moderate SARS-CoV-2 infection. Nat Immunol 2022;23(2):210–6.

12. Su Y, Yuan D, Chen DG, et al. Multiple early factors anticipate post-acute COVID-19 sequelae. Cell 2022;185(5):881–95.e20.
13. Cervia C, Zurbuchen Y, Taeschler P, et al. Immunoglobulin signature predicts risk of post-acute COVID-19 syndrome. Nat Commun 2022;13(1):446.
14. Klein J, Wood J, Jaycox J, et al. Distinguishing features of Long COVID identified through immune profiling. medRxiv 2022. https://doi.org/10.1101/2022.08.09.22278592.
15. Gupta A, Madhavan MV, Sehgal K, et al. Extrapulmonary manifestations of COVID-19. Nat Med 2020;26(7):1017–32.
16. Chen N, Zhou M, Dong X, et al. Epidemiological and clinical characteristics of 99 cases of 2019 novel coronavirus pneumonia in Wuhan, China: a descriptive study. Lancet 2020;395(10223):507–13.
17. Redd WD, Zhou JC, Hathorn KE, et al. Prevalence and characteristics of gastrointestinal symptoms in patients with severe acute respiratory syndrome coronavirus 2 infection in the united states: a multicenter cohort study. Gastroenterology 2020;159(2):765–7.e2.
18. Sultan S, Altayar O, Siddique SM, et al. AGA Institute Rapid Review of the Gastrointestinal and Liver Manifestations of COVID-19, Meta-Analysis of International Data, and Recommendations for the Consultative Management of Patients with COVID-19. Gastroenterology 2020;159(1):320–34.e27.
19. Livanos AE, Jha D, Cossarini F, et al. Intestinal Host Response to SARS-CoV-2 Infection and COVID-19 Outcomes in Patients With Gastrointestinal Symptoms. Gastroenterology 2021;160(7):2435–50.e34.
20. Hajifathalian K, Krisko T, Mehta A, et al. Gastrointestinal and Hepatic Manifestations of 2019 Novel Coronavirus Disease in a Large Cohort of Infected Patients From New York: Clinical Implications. Gastroenterology 2020;159(3):1137–40.e2.
21. Borobia AM, Carcas AJ, Arnalich F, et al. A Cohort of Patients with COVID-19 in a Major Teaching Hospital in Europe. J Clin Med 2020;9(6). https://doi.org/10.3390/jcm9061733.
22. Chen R, Yu YL, Li W, et al. Gastrointestinal symptoms associated with unfavorable prognosis of COVID-19 patients: a retrospective study. Front Med (Lausanne) 2020;7:608259.
23. Mao R, Qiu Y, He JS, et al. Manifestations and prognosis of gastrointestinal and liver involvement in patients with COVID-19: a systematic review and meta-analysis. Lancet Gastroenterol Hepatol 2020;5(7):667–78.
24. Suárez-Fariñas M, Tokuyama M, Wei G, et al. Intestinal Inflammation Modulates the Expression of ACE2 and TMPRSS2 and Potentially Overlaps With the Pathogenesis of SARS-CoV-2-related Disease. Gastroenterology 2021;160(1):287–301.e20.
25. Lamers MM, Beumer J, van der Vaart J, et al. SARS-CoV-2 productively infects human gut enterocytes. Science 2020;369(6499):50–4.
26. Zang R, Gomez Castro MF, McCune BT, et al. TMPRSS2 and TMPRSS4 promote SARS-CoV-2 infection of human small intestinal enterocytes. Sci Immunol 2020;5(47). https://doi.org/10.1126/sciimmunol.abc3582.
27. Cheung KS, Hung IFN, Chan PPY, et al. Gastrointestinal Manifestations of SARS-CoV-2 Infection and Virus Load in Fecal Samples From a Hong Kong Cohort: Systematic Review and Meta-analysis. Gastroenterology 2020;159(1):81–95.
28. Blackett JW, Wainberg M, Elkind MSV, et al. Potential Long Coronavirus Disease 2019 Gastrointestinal Symptoms 6 Months After Coronavirus Infection Are Associated With Mental Health Symptoms. Gastroenterology 2022;162(2):648–50.e2.

29. Al-Aly Z, Xie Y, Bowe B. High-dimensional characterization of post-acute sequelae of COVID-19. Nature 2021;594(7862):259–64.
30. Gaebler C, Wang Z, Lorenzi JCC, et al. Evolution of antibody immunity to SARS-CoV-2. Nature 2021;591(7851):639–44.
31. Goh D, Lim JCT, Fernaíndez SB, et al. Case report: persistence of residual antigen and RNA of the SARS-CoV-2 virus in tissues of two patients with long COVID. Front Immunol 2022;13:939989.
32. Zollner A, Koch R, Jukic A, et al. Postacute COVID-19 is Characterized by Gut Viral Antigen Persistence in Inflammatory Bowel Diseases. Gastroenterology 2022;163(2):495–506.e8.
33. Meringer H, Tokuyama M, Tankelevich M, et al. 1161: Persistent immune cell abnormalities in the intestinal mucosa of patients after recovery from COVID-19 infection. Gastroenterology 2022;162(7):S-277.
34. Liu Q, Mak JWY, Su Q, et al. Gut microbiota dynamics in a prospective cohort of patients with post-acute COVID-19 syndrome. Gut 2022;71(3):544–52.
35. Blackett JW, Li J, Jodorkovsky D, et al. Prevalence and risk factors for gastrointestinal symptoms after recovery from COVID-19. Neurogastroenterol Motil 2022; 34(3):e14251.
36. Lai NY, Musser MA, Pinho-Ribeiro FA, et al. Gut-Innervating Nociceptor Neurons Regulate Peyer's Patch Microfold Cells and SFB Levels to Mediate Salmonella Host Defense. Cell 2020;180(1):33–49.e22.
37. Ahrends T, Aydin B, Matheis F, et al. Enteric pathogens induce tissue tolerance and prevent neuronal loss from subsequent infections. Cell 2021;184(23): 5715–27.e12.
38. Wei C, Wan L, Yan Q, et al. HDL-scavenger receptor B type 1 facilitates SARS-CoV-2 entry. Nat Metab 2020;2(12):1391–400.
39. Wanner N, Andrieux G, Badia IMP, et al. Molecular consequences of SARS-CoV-2 liver tropism. Nat Metab 2022;4(3):310–9.
40. Wang B, Zhang L, Wang Y, et al. Alterations in microbiota of patients with COVID-19: potential mechanisms and therapeutic interventions. Signal Transduct Target Ther 2022;7(1):143.
41. Ferreira-Junior AS, Borgonovi TF, De Salis LVV, et al. Detection of Intestinal Dysbiosis in Post-COVID-19 Patients One to Eight Months after Acute Disease Resolution. Int J Environ Res Public Health 2022;19(16). https://doi.org/10.3390/ijerph191610189.
42. Clerbaux LA, Fillipovska J, Muñoz A, et al. Mechanisms Leading to Gut Dysbiosis in COVID-19: Current Evidence and Uncertainties Based on Adverse Outcome Pathways. J Clin Med 2022;11(18). https://doi.org/10.3390/jcm11185400.
43. Dang AT, Marsland BJ. Microbes, metabolites, and the gut-lung axis. Mucosal Immunol 2019;12(4):843–50.
44. Luci C, Bourinet M, Leclère PS, et al. Chronic Inflammation in Non-Alcoholic Steatohepatitis: Molecular Mechanisms and Therapeutic Strategies. Front Endocrinol (Lausanne) 2020;11:597648.
45. Queiroz MAF, Neves P, Lima SS, et al. Cytokine Profiles Associated With Acute COVID-19 and Long COVID-19 Syndrome. Front Cell Infect Microbiol 2022;12: 922422.
46. Song Q, Zhang X. The Role of Gut-Liver Axis in Gut Microbiome Dysbiosis Associated NAFLD and NAFLD-HCC. Biomedicines 2022;10(3). https://doi.org/10.3390/biomedicines10030524.

47. Pérez-Torres I, Guarner-Lans V, Soria-Castro E, et al. Alteration in the Lipid Profile and the Desaturases Activity in Patients With Severe Pneumonia by SARS-CoV-2. Front Physiol 2021;12:667024.
48. Nie X, Qian L, Sun R, et al. Multi-organ proteomic landscape of COVID-19 autopsies. Cell 2021;184(3):775–91.e14.
49. Petrescu M, Vlaicu SI, Ciumărnean L, et al. Chronic Inflammation-A Link between Nonalcoholic Fatty Liver Disease (NAFLD) and Dysfunctional Adipose Tissue. Medicina (Kaunas) 2022;58(5). https://doi.org/10.3390/medicina58050641.
50. Fignani D, Licata G, Brusco N, et al. SARS-CoV-2 Receptor Angiotensin I-Converting Enzyme Type 2 (ACE2) Is Expressed in Human Pancreatic β-Cells and in the Human Pancreas Microvasculature. Front Endocrinol (Lausanne) 2020; 11:596898.
51. Shaharuddin SH, Wang V, Santos RS, et al. Deleterious Effects of SARS-CoV-2 Infection on Human Pancreatic Cells. Front Cell Infect Microbiol 2021;11:678482.
52. Müller JA, Groß R, Conzelmann C, et al. SARS-CoV-2 infects and replicates in cells of the human endocrine and exocrine pancreas. Nat Metab 2021;3(2):149–65.
53. Steenblock C, Richter S, Berger I, et al. Viral infiltration of pancreatic islets in patients with COVID-19. Nat Commun 2021;12(1):3534.
54. Ji N, Zhang M, Ren L, et al. SARS-CoV-2 in the pancreas and the impaired islet function in COVID-19 patients. Emerg Microbes Infect 2022;11(1):1115–25.

Liver and Biliary Tract Disease in Patients with Coronavirus disease-2019 Infection

Sirina Ekpanyapong, MD[a,b], K. Rajender Reddy, MD[b,*]

KEYWORDS

- COVID-19 • SARS-CoV-2 • Cirrhosis • Chronic liver disease • Acute liver disease • Abnormal liver biochemistries • Liver transplantation • Vaccination

KEY POINTS

- Hepatic biochemical test abnormalities in patients with Coronavirus disease-2019 (COVID-19) can be encountered in up to 50% of infected individuals; the pattern of liver injury is mostly hepatocellular, whereas the mechanism of liver injury is thought to be multifactorial. Chronic hepatobiliary manifestation of cholangiopathy is being increasingly recognized.
- Underlying chronic liver disease is not uncommon in patients with COVID-19 infection, and such patients with cirrhosis have higher and increasing mortality with liver disease severity as assessed by Child-Pugh class.
- Because of the high rate of hepatic decompensation in patients with cirrhosis following COVID-19 infection, early diagnosis and early admission should be emphasized.
- Although response to the severe acute respiratory syndrome coronavirus 2 (SARS-CoV-2) vaccination may be suboptimal in immunosuppressed and immunocompromised patients, patients with cirrhosis receiving SARS-CoV-2 vaccination can result in a reduction of COVID-19 infection, COVID-19–related hospitalization, and mortality; thus, patients with chronic liver disease and particularly patients with cirrhosis, liver-transplant candidates and liver transplant recipients are strongly recommended for COVID-19 vaccination.

INTRODUCTION

Coronavirus disease-2019 (COVID-19), the disease caused by the severe acute respiratory syndrome coronavirus 2 (SARS-CoV-2), was first reported in Wuhan, China, in December 2019, and has become a global pandemic since March

[a] Division of Gastroenterology and Hepatology, Department of Medicine, Huachiew General Hospital, 665 Bumroongmueang Road, Khlong Mahanak, Bangkok 10100, Thailand; [b] Division of Gastroenterology and Hepatology, Department of Medicine, University of Pennsylvania, 2 Dulles, Liver Transplant Office, HUP3400 Spruce Street, Philadelphia, PA 19104, USA
* Corresponding author.
E-mail address: ReddyR@pennmedicine.upenn.edu

Gastroenterol Clin N Am 52 (2023) 13–36
https://doi.org/10.1016/j.gtc.2022.09.001
gastro.theclinics.com

2020, leading to significant morbidity and mortality in humans. Although, it most commonly presents with pulmonary manifestations, hepatic abnormalities can be encountered in up to 50% of infected individuals, which can vary in severity from asymptomatic to severe liver injury.[1] Chronic liver disease (CLD) is not uncommon in the background of patients hospitalized with COVID-19 infection, which is, in itself, associated with more severe COVID-19 disease and higher mortality,[2] especially in patients with cirrhosis.[3] This review summarizes hepatic manifestations in patients with COVID-19 infection and outcome in those with CLD and addresses vaccination and management of patients with CLD during the ongoing COVID-19 pandemic.

Prevalence of Liver Dysfunction and Hepatobiliary Manifestation in SARS-CoV-2–Infected Patients

The incidence of elevated liver biochemistries in hospitalized COVID-19 infected patients ranges from 14% to 83%.[2] More commonly, an elevation of aspartate transaminase (AST) has been reported in 8% to 83%, and an elevation of alanine transaminase (ALT) in 10% to 61%; however, mild elevation of bilirubin has been reported in 3% to 23%, of ALP in 1% to 22%, and of gamma-glutamyl transferase in 13% to 54% of patients with COVID-19 infection.[4–25] Abnormalities in liver biochemistries are reported with similar frequencies regardless of the presence of preexisting liver disease.[26] The pattern of liver injury is mostly hepatocellular rather than cholestatic.[1] Mild AST and ALT elevations of 1 to 2 times the upper limit of normal (ULN) are commonly observed early in the disease course. AST is usually higher than ALT, and this may increase with COVID-19-associated-disease severity and mortality, which could possibly reflect nonhepatic injury.[2,27] One retrospective cohort of patients with COVID-19 infection from the United States (n = 3381) noted mild liver injury in 45%, moderate in 21%, and severe acute liver injury in 6.4% of hospitalized patients with COVID-19.[28] Usually the hepatic biochemical test abnormalities return to normal values within 2 to 3 weeks without specific treatment.[18] Liver injury is more commonly observed in severe COVID-19 cases than in mild cases, and COVID-19 infection in patients with elevated liver biochemistries (especially with AST and ALT elevation greater than 5 times ULN) was associated with higher mortality.[29] Hypoalbuminemia at hospital admission has also been a marker of COVID-19 severity.[30–32] When assessing COVID-19 patients with elevated hepatic biochemical tests, other causes unrelated to COVID-19 such as viral hepatitis should be considered.[2] Further, pregnant patients with COVID-19 infection have also been reported to have AST or ALT elevation in up to 21% to 22%, suggesting that appropriate monitoring of hepatic biochemical tests is needed in this population.[33] Notably, a recent study reported that patients with COVID-19 had underlying CLD in around 2% to 11%.[14] Patients with more advanced liver disease had higher mortality after COVID-19 infection, with the highest mortality among patients with cirrhosis and with the rate increasing with more severe liver disease, as assessed by Child-Pugh class.[2,34]

Mechanisms of Liver Injury from Coronavirus Disease-2019 Infection

SARS-CoV-2 is a single, positive-stranded RNA virus that replicates using a virally encoded RNA-dependent RNA polymerase.[2] There are several potential mechanisms and causes of liver injury in patients with COVID-19 infection, some of which may be virus specific and others nonspecific. Liver histologic findings at autopsy[35] have noted one or more features of microvesicular/macrovesicular steatosis, mixed lobular necroinflammation and portal inflammation, focal necrosis, and porto-venous/sinusoidal microthrombosis (**Fig. 1**).

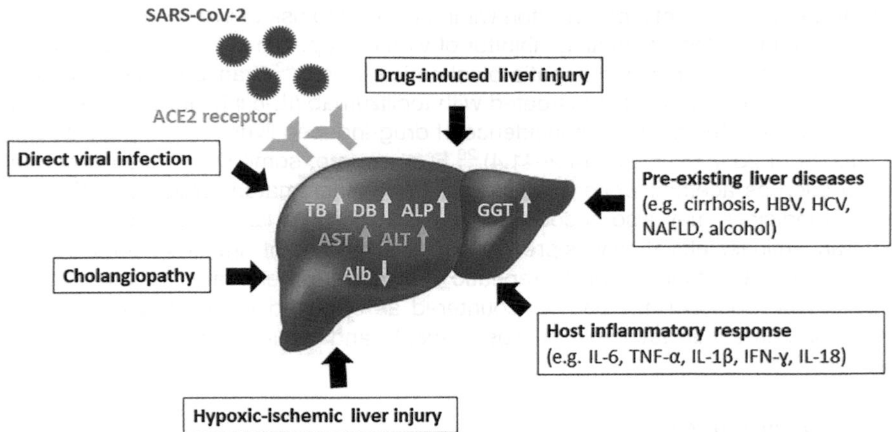

Fig. 1. Proposed mechanisms of liver injury from SARS-CoV-2 infection.

Direct hepatic infection by SARS-CoV-2

SARS-CoV-2 binds to target cells through angiotensin-converting enzyme 2 (ACE2) entry receptors. ACE2 is present in both hepatocytes and cholangiocytes; therefore, liver is a potential target for infection and may be the pathogenesis of SARS-CoV-2–related liver injury. ACE2 expression in healthy liver is found in the cholangiocytes (59.7%), and this rate is much higher than in the hepatocytes (2.6%)[36]; thus, liver injury may result from direct viral damage to bile duct epithelial cells, which has been known to be significant in liver regeneration and immune response,[37] although the exact mechanism is still unclear. Multiple levels of evidence, using autopsy samples, suggest SARS-CoV-2 liver tropism, including the detection of SARS-CoV-2 viral RNA by PCR in up to 55% to 69% of liver samples,[38,39] successful isolation of infectious SARS-CoV-2 particles, and identification of transcription-based, proteomic-based, and transcription factor-based activity profiles in hepatic autopsy samples.[39] For example, transcriptomic profiling confirmed the expression of known SARS-CoV-2 entry receptors and proteins that included ACE2, transmembrane protease serine 2 (TMPRSS2), procathepsin L (CTSL), Ras-related protein Rab-7a (RAB7A), and the high-density lipoprotein scavenger receptor B type 1 (SR-B1)[39] and with relative upregulation of type-I, type-II, and type-III interferons (IFNs), JAK/STAT (Janus kinase/signal transducerik and activator of transcription) and metabolic signaling in the RT-PCR-positive livers.[40]

Host inflammatory response to SARS-CoV-2

Following SARS-CoV-2 infection, the host immune response can be triggered, which can cause excessive release of inflammatory mediators such as IL-6, IL-10, IL-2, and IFN gamma in parallel with disease severity and which in turn may lead to a cytokine storm.[41] To support this hypothesis, studies have noted that COVID-19 patients in an ICU setting with multiorgan failure have features of severe hepatic dysfunction associated with higher inflammatory markers.[6,18] Global proteomic profiling in hepatic tissues has noted significant upregulation of type I and II IFN responses after SARS-CoV-2 infection.[39]

Drug-induced liver injury

Medications used during treatment of COVID-19 include antibiotics, antiviral agents, corticosteroids, and immunomodulators, which can variably cause liver injury. Cai Q reported that the use of lopinavir/ritonavir increased the risk of liver injury by 4-fold.[17] Remdesivir (a nucleoside analog inhibitor of viral RNA polymerase) has been associated with a 23% increase in hepatic biochemical levels.[42] Transaminase elevations have been observed in patients treated with tocilizumab (IL-6 inhibitors).[43] A systematic review reported the pooled incidence of drug-induced liver injury in patients with COVID-19 at 25.4% (95%CI 14.2–41.4).[29] Furthermore, some drugs used in combination such as acetaminophen, nonsteroidal anti-inflammatory drugs, and Chinese herbal medicines may also account for hepatotoxicity. A large global series noted that transaminase elevation was preferentially caused by antiviral drugs administered empirically due to their known therapeutic efficacy for other viral infections. Often a hepatocellular pattern has been encountered as opposed to cholestatic or mixed injury. Outcome was favorable in most patients and fatality attributable to a drug was rare.[2,14]

Preexisting liver diseases

About 2% to 11% of patients with COVID-19 have underlying CLD.[14] Data on preexisting liver diseases in COVID-19 from 2 international registries (SECURE-Cirrhosis and COVID-Hep; n = 745) reported causes including nonalcoholic fatty liver disease (NAFLD) 43%, alcohol-related liver disease (ALD) 24%, chronic hepatitis B (HBV) infection 12%, and chronic hepatitis C (HCV) infection 13%. In this cohort, 48% had CLD without cirrhosis and 52% had cirrhosis.[3] Corticosteroids or other immunosuppressive agents for COVID-19 treatment may facilitate HBV reactivation in patients with occult or chronic HBV infection.[35] Further, patients with more advanced liver disease may be at increased risk of infection due to cirrhosis-associated immune dysfunction.[44]

Cholangiopathy/secondary sclerosing cholangitis

Several case series have reported delayed-onset and progressive cholestasis as a unique clinical entity in patients following severe COVID-19 infection.[45–48] Cholestasis is present early in the disease course and cholangiopathy occurs later. A retrospective study from a single US center[45] reported 12 patients who experienced progressive biliary injury after recovering from severe COVID-19, characterized by marked elevation in serum ALP accompanied by evidence of biliary tree abnormalities on imaging. Median time from COVID-19 diagnosis to onset of cholangiopathy was 118 days. Magnetic resonance cholangiopancreatography (MRCP) findings included beading of intrahepatic ducts, multifocal strictures, and dilation of the biliary tree. Liver biopsy has noted features of acute and/or chronic bile duct obstruction without ductopenia. The pathogenesis is still unclear. These manifestations may represent changes due to biliary tree ischemia, which may reflect a continuum of secondary sclerosing cholangitis in critically ill patients (SSC-CIP), and/or may also be a consequence of direct infection of SARS-CoV-2 of the liver and biliary tract.[46,49] Furthermore, this complication may be more frequently encountered in patients with preexisting CLD.[48]

Hypoxic-ischemic liver injury

In critically ill patients, hemodynamic instability may cause liver injury from a hypoxic-ischemic process, which causes an increase in aminotransferases in the setting of shock or cardiac failure.[41] Ischemic hepatitis and hepatic congestion related to cardiomyopathy is a common consequence of COVID-19 infection, occurring in 33% of individuals in 1 US series.[22] Further, venous and arterial thromboses are currently recognized as a feature of COVID-19, including hepatic involvement.[50]

COVID-19 and Patients with Chronic Liver Diseases

In a cohort of 2780 multicenter US patients with COVID-19 (CLD 9%), CLD was associated with significantly higher mortality (RR = 2.8, 95%CI 1.9–4.0). Mortality was higher in patients with cirrhosis (RR = 4.6, 95%CI 2.6–8.3). Fatty liver disease and nonalcoholic steatohepatitis (NASH) were the most common causes among the patients with CLD, and the mortality was independent of risk factors of body mass index, hypertension, and diabetes.[26] Another large cohort from an International Registry (SECURE-Cirrhosis and COVID-Hep) in patients with CLD and cirrhosis (n = 745) noted 32% mortality in patients with cirrhosis versus 8% in those without cirrhosis ($P < .001$); and mortality in patients with cirrhosis increased according to liver disease severity based on Child-Pugh classification.[3] Studies on COVID-19 outcome and mortality in patients with CLD and cirrhosis are described in **Table 1**.

Viral Hepatitis

A retrospective cohort from Hong Kong (n = 5639, 6.3% current HBV infection, 6.4% past HBV infection) demonstrated that current or past HBV infection was not associated with more severe liver injury or mortality from COVID-19.[51] Similarly, a large retrospective cohort from China (n = 2073 patients with COVID-19) found that HBV infection was not associated with the risk of poor COVID-19 outcomes.[52] Notably an appropriate use of antiviral therapy for HBV during corticosteroid therapy for COVID-19 should be considered to minimize the risk of HBV reactivation. In parallel, data from the Electronically Retrieved Cohort of HCV infected Veterans (ERCHIVES; including 975 HCV-positive and 975 propensity score matched HCV-negative persons with SARS-CoV-2 infection) demonstrated similar mortality in patients with versus without HCV infection.[53]

Autoimmune Liver Diseases

De novo autoimmune hepatitis may rarely occur following SARS-CoV-2 infection.[49] Data on patients with autoimmune hepatitis (AIH) and SARS-CoV-2 infection from 3 international registries (ERN RARE-LIVER/COVID-Hep/SECURE-Cirrhosis; n = 932 CLD with SARS-CoV-2, including 70 with AIH) demonstrated that patients with AIH were not at increased risk of adverse outcomes and mortality despite receiving immunosuppressants.[54] Another retrospective study on patients with AIH and COVID-19 from an international multicenter study (110 patients with AIH) revealed that patients with AIH were not at risk for worse outcomes following COVID-19. Cirrhosis was an independent predictor of severe COVID-19 in patients with AIH (odds ratio [OR] = 17.46; 95%CI 4.22–72.13, $P < .001$), and maintenance of immunosuppression during COVID-19 was not associated with an increased risk of severe COVID-19 but could lower the risk of new-onset liver injury.[55] This finding should reassure clinicians not to routinely reduce immunosuppression in such patients following COVID-19 infection.

Nonalcoholic Fatty Liver Disease

Patients with NAFLD are at increased overall risk of developing severe COVID-19, which may be contributed by the presence of other high-risk comorbidities such as obesity, diabetes mellitus, and hypertension.[49] A retrospective study from China (202 patients with COVID-19, including 37.6% with NAFLD, demonstrated that NAFLD was associated with COVID-19 progression (OR = 6.4, 95%CI 1.5–31.2), and patients with NAFLD had a longer viral shedding time (17.5 ± 5.2 days vs 12.1 ± 4.4 days, $P < .0001$) compared with patients without NAFLD.[56] Patients with NAFLD are more

Table 1
Studies on coronavirus disease-2019 outcome and mortality in patients with chronic liver disease and cirrhosis

Study	Number	Country	Pre-Existing Liver Diseases	Findings
Yadav DK, et al.,[86] 2020 (meta-analysis)	2115	China	4% (mostly cirrhosis and HBV)	• High prevalence of liver injury (27%) • Patients with liver injury had more severe COVID infection (OR = 2.57, P = .01), and higher mortality (OR = 1.66, P = .03) • Overall mortality in patients with COVID-19 infection with liver injury is 23.5%
Sarin SK, et al,[87] 2020 (The APCOLIS study)	228	13 Asian countries	185 CLD patients including 43 with cirrhosis (NAFLD in 55%, and viral hepatitis in 30%)	• Mortality in CLD patients with COVID-19 vs cirrhosis with COVID-19 (2.7% vs 16.3%, P = .002) • 43% of CLD presented with acute liver injury, 20% of patients with cirrhosis presented with either ACLF (11.6%) or acute decompensation (9%) • A Child-Turcotte Pugh score $\geq$ 9 at presentation predicted high mortality (HR = 19.2 [95% CI 2.3–163.3], $P < .001$)
Mallet V, et al,[68] 2020	15,476 COVID-19 patients with chronic liver disease	France	Chronic liver disease (alcohol-induced 23%, HBV 5%, HCV 4.6%, HCC 4.6%, LT 2.1%)	• 30-d post-COVID mortality with chronic liver disease 19% • Chronic liver disease increased risk of COVID-19–related death • Patients with alcohol use disorders, decompensated cirrhosis, or primary liver cancer had an increased risk of COVID-19-related mortality
Butt AA, et al,[53] 2021 (ERCHIVES database)	SARS-CoV-2 with HCV = 975 SARS-CoV-2 without HCV = 975	United States	HCV	• HCV infected persons with SARS-CoV-2 are more likely to be admitted to a hospital • Mortality was not different between those with vs without HCV infection

Verhelst X, et al,[88] 2021	110	Belgium	Autoimmune hepatitis	• Low COVID-19 infection rate (1.2%), survival 100%, liver decompensation 0%, hospitalization 3.5% • Supports not stopping immunosuppressive treatment during COVID-19 infection
Di Giorgio A, et al,[89] 2020	148	Italy	Autoimmune liver diseases (AILD)	• Confirmed cases of COVID-19 3%, survival 99%, mortality 1% • Patients with AILD were not more susceptible to COVID-19 than the general population. Tapering or withdrawal of immunosuppression was not required
Marjot T, et al,[54] 2021(ERN RARE-LIVER/COVID-Hep/ SECURE-Cirrhosis)	932 patients with CLD and COVID-19 (70 with AIH)	International registry	Autoimmune hepatitis	• No differences in major outcomes between patients with AIH and non-AIH CLD, including hospitalization (76% vs 85%; $P = .06$), ICU admission (29% vs 23%; $P = .240$), and death (23% vs 20%; $P = .64$) • Factors associated with mortality within the AIH cohort included old age, and Child-Pugh class B and C cirrhosis but not use of immunosuppression
Younossi ZM, et al,[90] 2021	4835 patients with COVID-19 (NAFLD = 553)	United States	NAFLD	• 3.9% of patients with NAFLD and COVID-19 infection experienced acute liver injury • Crude inpatient mortality in the NAFLD group was 11% • Independent predictors of mortality included higher FIB-4 and multimorbidity scores, morbid obesity, older age, and hypoxemia on admission

(*continued on next page*)

Table 1
(*continued*)

Study	Number	Country	Pre-Existing Liver Diseases	Findings
Kim D, et al,[67] 2021 (The COLD study)	867 CLD = 620 (71.5%) Cirrhosis = 227 (26.2%) ALD = 94 NAFLD = 456 HBV = 62 HCV = 190 HCC = 22	US multicenter	Chronic liver disease and cirrhosis	• The overall all-cause mortality was 14% • Independent risk factors for overall mortality were ALD (HR = 2.42, 95%CI 1.29–4.55), decompensated cirrhosis (HR = 2.91, 95%CI 1.70–5.00) and HCC (HR = 3.31, 95%CI 1.53–7.16)
Jin Ge, et al,[91] 2021 (The National COVID Cohort Collaborative (N3C) study)	220,727 patients with CLD and known SARS-CoV-2 test status: 58% noncirrhosis/negative, 13% noncirrhosis/positive, 24% cirrhosis/negative 4% cirrhosis/positive SARS-CoV-2 test	United States	Chronic liver disease and cirrhosis	• SARS-CoV-2 infection was associated with 2.38 times hazard ratio of all-cause mortality within 30 d among patients with cirrhosis
Marjot T, et al,[3] 2021 (SECURE -cirrhosis and COVID-Hep)	745 ALD = 179 NAFLD = 322 HBV = 96 HCV = 92 HCC = 48	International registry	Chronic liver disease and cirrhosis	• Mortality in patients with cirrhosis 32% vs mortality in chronic liver disease 8% • Mortality according to Child-Pugh classes was class A (19%), B (35%), and C (51%) • ALD was an independent risk factor for death (OR = 1.79, 95%CI 1.03–3.13) • In the CLD cohort, mortality increased following hospitalization, admission to ICU, and invasive ventilation • After adjusting for baseline characteristics, NAFLD, viral hepatitis, and HCC were not independently associated with death

Lavarone M, et al,[92] 2020	50	Italy	Cirrhosis	• Overall 30-d mortality was 34% • COVID-19 was associated with liver function deterioration and mortality in cirrhosis • Severity of lung and liver diseases (according to CLIF-C ACLF, CLIF-OF and MELD scores) independently predicted mortality • No major adverse events were related to thromboprophylaxis (heparin administered to 80% of patients) or antiviral treatments
Clift AK, et al,[93] 2020 (population-based cohort study)	11,865 patients with cirrhosis (0.2% of total cohort)	United Kingdom	Cirrhosis	• Increased hazard ratio for COVID-19-related mortality in patients with cirrhosis • Male cirrhosis (HR = 1.29, 95%CI 0.83–2.02), Female cirrhosis (HR = 1.85,95%CI 1.15–2.99)
Bajaj JS, et al,[62] 2021	• Patients with cirrhosis and COVID-19 (n = 37) • Patients with COVID-19 (n = 108) • Patients with cirrhosis (n = 127)	North America and Canada	Cirrhosis	• Patients with cirrhosis and COVID-19 had higher mortality compared with patients with COVID-19 (30% vs 13%, $P = .03$) but not between patients with COVID-19 and those with cirrhosis alone (30% vs 20%, $P = .16$)
Ioannou GN, et al,[94] 2021 (Veterans Affairs national healthcare system)	305 cirrhosis with SARS-CoV-2	United States	Cirrhosis	• SARS-CoV-2 infection was associated with a 3.5-fold increase in mortality in patients with cirrhosis • 30-d mortality for patients with cirrhosis and SARS-CoV-2 infection was 18% • The most important predictors of mortality were advanced age, decompensated cirrhosis, and high MELD score

Abbreviations: AIH, autoimmune hepatitis; FIB-4, fibrosis-4; HBV, hepatitis B virus; HCV, hepatitis C virus; HR, hazard ratio; LT, liver transplant; MELD, Model for End-Stage Liver Disease.

likely to develop liver injury when having COVID-19 infection but no patient developed severe liver-related complications during hospitalization in one cohort from China (280 COVID-19 patients including 30% with NAFLD).[57] Moreover, patients with NAFLD, with noninvasive fibrosis scores (fibrosis-4 index and NAFLD fibrosis score) seemed to correlate with a higher likelihood of developing severe COVID-19, irrespective of metabolic comorbidities.[58] A large US multicenter study (n = 363, NAFLD 15.2%) demonstrated that NAFLD was independently associated with ICU admission (OR = 2.30, 95%CI 1.27–4.17) and mechanical ventilation (OR = 2.15, 95%CI 1.18–3.91); and presence of cirrhosis was an independent predictor of mortality (OR = 12.5, 95%CI 2.16–72.5).[59] Additionally, a systematic review and meta-analysis on clinical outcomes in NAFLD patients with COVID-19 (14 studies including 1851 NAFLD patients) found an increased risk of severe COVID-19 and admission to ICU due to COVID-19 in patients with underlying NAFLD; however, no difference in mortality was observed between NAFLD versus non-NAFLD patients.[60]

Alcohol-Related Liver Disease

ALD has been reported as an independent risk factor for mortality (OR = 1.79, 95%CI 1.03–3.13) in CLD patients with COVID-19.[3] The frequency of ALD has rapidly increased since the beginning of COVID-19 pandemic. Data from United Network for Organ Sharing (UNOS) demonstrated a significant increase in ALD listing (+7.26%; $P < .001$) during the COVID-19 pandemic, and ALD (40.1%) accounted for more listings than those due to HCV (12.4%) and NASH (23.4%) combined.[61] The greatest increase in ALD listing has been among young adults aged 18 to 34 years and aged 35 to 50 years (plus 35%) and among patients with severe alcohol-associated hepatitis (plus 50%). This increase in alcoholism may be due to COVID-19–related stressors, such as unemployment or increased health risks due to the pandemic.

Cirrhosis

Patient with cirrhosis have high rates of hepatic decompensation, acute-on-chronic liver failure (ACLF), and death from respiratory failure following SARS-CoV-2 infection.[50] Data from an International Registry (SECURE-Cirrhosis and COVID-Hep) on COVID-19–infected patients with CLD and cirrhosis (n = 745, including 386 patients with cirrhosis, 359 with noncirrhotic CLD from 21 countries in 4 continents reported mortality in COVID-19-infected patients with cirrhosis at 32% versus mortality in CLD without cirrhosis at 8% ($P < .001$). Mortality increased according to Child-Pugh class (mortality in classes A [19%], B [35%], and C [51%]) in patients with cirrhosis with respiratory failure being the main cause of death (71%). In this study, there was also an increase in mortality following hospitalization, admission to ICU, and invasive ventilation, with Child-Pugh class C patients having 90% mortality in those requiring mechanical ventilation (**Fig. 2**).[3] Acute hepatic decompensation occurred in 46% and half of these patients had ACLF, and around 21% of patients with cirrhosis infected with SARS-CoV-2 lacked respiratory symptoms; hence, patients with new onset of hepatic decompensation or ACLF should be tested for SARS-CoV-2 even in the absence of respiratory symptoms. This large cohort also demonstrated that age, baseline liver disease stage (especially Child-Pugh classes B and C), and ALD were independent risk factors for mortality from COVID-19.[3] The possible pathogenesis linking cirrhosis and severe COVID-19 lung disease is likely multifactorial and likely related to factors such as increased systemic inflammation, cirrhosis-associated immune dysfunction, coagulopathy, and intestinal dysbiosis.[50] A multicenter-matched cohort study from North America compared mortality in those

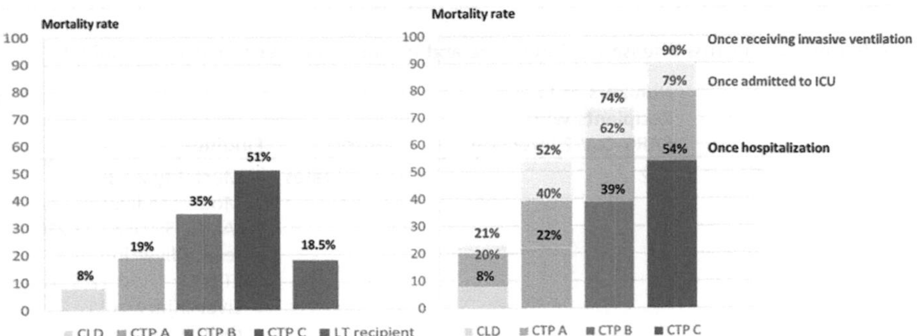

Fig. 2. Mortality in patients with COVID-19 infection in chronic liver disease, cirrhosis (Child-Turcotte-Pugh classes A, B, and C) and liver-transplant recipients, and stepwise increment of mortality in patients with chronic liver disease and cirrhosis following hospitalization, admission to ICU and invasive ventilation. *(Data from* Marjot T, Moon AM, Cook JA, et al. Outcomes following SARS-CoV-2 infection in patients with chronic liver disease: An international registry study. Journal of hepatology. 2021;74(3):567-577; and Webb GJ, Marjot T, Cook JA, et al. Outcomes following SARS-CoV-2 infection in liver transplant recipients: an international registry study. The Lancet Gastroenterology & Hepatology. 2020;5(11):1008-1016.)

with cirrhosis and COVID-19 (n = 37) versus cirrhosis alone (n = 127) versus COVID-19 alone (n = 108) and reported that patients with cirrhosis and COVID-19 had higher mortality compared with COVID-19 alone (30% vs 13%, $P = .03$) but comparable to cirrhosis alone (30% vs 20%, $P = .16$); in those with ACLF, the mortality was similar regardless of COVID-19 (55% vs 36%, $P = .25$).[62] Recent meta-analysis of 63 studies revealed a pooled OR for all-cause mortality of 2.48 (95% CI: 2.02–3.04) in patients with cirrhosis and COVID-19.[63] Accordingly, patients with cirrhosis infected with SARS-CoV-2 should have their COVID-19 vaccination prioritized due to their high mortality.

Postliver Transplant

As opposed to patients with cirrhosis, liver-transplant recipients do not seem to have an increased mortality following SARS-CoV-2 infection compared with the matched general population.[50] A prospective nationwide study conducted by the Spanish Society of Liver Transplantation (SETH) reported the incidence of COVID-19 to be higher in LT patients but mortality (around 18%) was lower than in the matched general population; in this cohort, mycophenolate was associated with a risk of developing severe COVID-19 in a dose-dependent manner.[64] Another large multicenter study from 2 international registries (COVID-Hep and SECURE-Cirrhosis), including 151 LT recipients with COVID-19 infection, found that LT was not associated with increased mortality (rate = 18.5%; see **Fig. 2**), whereas increased age and presence of comorbidities (such as elevated creatinine level and nonliver cancer) were associated with mortality among LT-recipients.[65] Such data are consistent with data from the European Liver and Intestine Transplantation Association (ELITA)/the European Liver Transplant Registry (ELTR) multicenter COVID-19 registry (149 LT centers, 243 COVID-19-infected LT recipients) where the mortality was 20%, with mortality being higher in patients aged older than 70 years and with comorbidities (such as impaired renal function or diabetes mellitus); contrariwise, tacrolimus use was associated with an improved survival.[66] Studies on COVID-19 outcomes in patients with postliver transplantation are reported in **Table 2**.

Table 2
Studies on coronavirus disease-2019 outcome and mortality in liver transplant recipients

Study	Numbers of LT Recipients with SARS-CoV-2 Infection	Country	Findings
Rabiee A, et al,[95] 2020	112	United States	• Mortality 22.3% • Moderate liver injury (ALT 2-5x ULN) 22.2%, severe liver injury (ALT > 5× ULN) 12.3% • Liver injury in LT recipients was associated with mortality (*P* = .007; OR = 6.91) and ICU admission (*P* = .007; OR = 7.93) • Reduction of immunosuppression during COVID-19 was not associated with mortality (*P* = .084)
Colmenero J, et al,[64] 2021 (SETH registry)	111	Spain	• Mortality 18%, severe COVID-19 31.5% • LT patients had an increased risk of acquiring COVID-19 but their mortality was lower than the matched general population • Mycophenolate may increase the risk of severe COVID-19 in a dose-dependent manner
Kates OS, et al,[96] 2021	73	United States	• The 28-d mortality among solid organ transplant cohort (n = 482 hospitalized with COVID-19) was 20.5% • LT was not associated with increased 28-d mortality (*P* = .36)

(*continued on next page*)

Table 2
(continued)

Study	Numbers of LT Recipients with SARS-CoV-2 Infection	Country	Findings
Ravanan R, et al,[97] 2020 (UK National Health Service Blood and Transplant registry)	64	England	• SOT recipients with SARS-CoV-2 infection had a higher all-cause mortality compared with wait-listed patients (25.8% vs 10.2%) • LT recipients had a lower SARS-CoV-2 infection rate than other SOT recipients (OR = 0.53, 95%CI 0.40–0.70)
Webb GJ, et al,[65] 2020 (SECURE-cirrhosis and COVID-Hep)	151	International registry	• Overall mortality was 18.5% • LT did not significantly increase the risk of death • Age, high creatinine level, and nonliver cancer were associated with mortality among LT recipients
Belli LS, et al,[66] 2021 (ELITA/ELTR COVID-19 registry)	243	Europe	• Mortality 20.2%, respiratory failure was the major cause of death • Older age, diabetes, and chronic kidney disease were associated with mortality • Tacrolimus use (HR = 0.55, 95%CI 0.31–0.99) had a positive independent effect on survival
Polak WG, et al,[98] 2020 (ELITA/ELTR COVID-19 registry)	57 SARS-CoV-2–infected LT candidates 272 SARS-CoV-2–infected LT recipients	Europe	• Incidence of COVID-19 among LT candidates was 1.05% and LT recipients 0.34% • Mortality was 18% among LT candidates and 15% among LT recipients

Abbreviations: HR, hazard ratio; LT, liver transplant; N, number of patients; SOT, solid organ transplant.

Hepatocellular Carcinoma

In a US multicenter study of adult patients with CLD and COVID-19 (n = 867), hepatocellular carcinoma (HCC) was found to be a factor associated with higher overall mortality (hazard ratio = 3.31, 95%CI 1.53–7.16) independent of ALD and decompensated cirrhosis.[67] Concomitantly, in another study from France on COVID-19 patients with CLD (15,476 CLD patients with COVID-19), 30-day mortality was associated with primary liver cancer (OR = 1.38, 95%CI 1.17–1.62, $P < .001$), CLD (OR = 1.79, 95%CI 1.71–1.87, $P < .001$), decompensated cirrhosis (OR = 2.21, 95%CI 1.94–2.51, $P < .001$), and alcohol use disorders (OR = 1.11, 95%CI 1.05–1.17, $P < .001$).[68] HCC is often associated with liver cirrhosis, suggesting that impaired immunity may increase the risk of developing severe COVID-19.[69]

Notably, COVID-19 may exacerbate preexisting liver disease and thus complicate HCC management.[70] An experience from a multicenter study from France in patients with HCC (n = 670, 293 with SARS-CoV-2 infection and 377 without infection) demonstrated fewer patients with HCC presenting to the multidisciplinary tumor board, especially with their initial HCC diagnosis. Treatment strategy was modified in 13.1% of patients, and patients experienced significant treatment delay (≥1 month) in 2020 compared with 2019 (21.5% vs 9.5%, $P < .001$). Around 7.1% of HCC patients had a diagnosis of active COVID-19 infection (52.4% hospitalized, 19.1% mortality).[71] Summaries of recommendations from the AASLD Expert Panel Consensus Statement[1] and the EASL-ESCMID position article[34,72] on the management of patients with CLDs during COVID-19 era are reported in **Table 3.**

COVID-19 Vaccination in Patients with Chronic Liver Disease and Liver-Transplant Recipients

Adult CLD patients, particularly those with cirrhosis, are strongly recommended to receive COVID-19 vaccination.[73] A large cohort study of patients with cirrhosis from the Veterans Administration on the clinical outcome of mRNA vaccines compared with unvaccinated patients reported that patients with CLD who received at least one dose of an mRNA vaccine (n = 20,037) had a 64.8% reduction in SARS-CoV-2 infections and 100% protection against hospitalization or death at 28 days after the initial dose.[74] The rate of reduction of SARS-CoV-2 infection after the first dose in those with decompensated cirrhosis was 50.3% and in those with compensated cirrhosis was 66.8%. Receiving a second dose of the vaccine was associated with a 78.6% reduction in COVID-19 infection and 100% reduction in COVID-19–related hospitalization or death after 7 days.[74] Another retrospective study among US veterans demonstrated that some patients with cirrhosis developed breakthrough COVID-19 infection after full or partial vaccination; however, these infections were associated with reduced mortality compared with those without vaccination.[75]

A case series (n = 40, including 21 with CLD and 19 with LT) from the SECURE-Cirrhosis and COVID-Hep international registries reported that vaccination against SARS-CoV-2 seems to result in favorable outcomes, as demonstrated by the absence of the need for mechanical ventilation, the need for ICU care, or death among fully vaccinated patients.[76] Risk factors for lower serologic response to immunization included older age, use of antimetabolite drugs, time from transplantation, and use of B cell–depleting therapies.[73] A study on immunogenicity of the first and second doses of the mRNA SARS-CoV-2 vaccine among solid organ transplant recipients demonstrated low levels of detectable antibody around 17% at 20 days after the first dose[77] and 54% at a median of 29 days after the second dose.[78] The French National Authority for Health recommends administration of a third dose of vaccine in

Table 3
Guideline recommendations for patients with chronic liver diseases during coronavirus disease-2019 pandemic

Chronic Liver Diseases	AASLD recommendation[1] and EASL-ESCMID Position article[34,49,72]
Chronic viral hepatitis (HBV and HCV)	• Continue treatment of hepatitis B or C if patient already receiving treatment • HBsAg and anti-HBc should be tested before initiating corticosteroid therapy, JAK 1/2 inhibitor, and tocilizumab therapy • Initiating hepatitis B treatment should be considered if hepatitis B flare is clinically suspected or when initiating immunosuppressive therapy, corticosteroids, or IL-6 monoclonal antibody therapy • Initiating hepatitis C treatment should be delayed until after resolution of COVID-19 infection
Autoimmune liver diseases	Without COVID-19 infection • Continue the same dosage of immunosuppressive agents to prevent a disease flare • Vaccination for *Streptococcus pneumoniae* and influenza should be emphasized With COVID-19 infection • In case of worsening pneumonia attributed to COVID-19 infection, lowering the overall level of immunosuppressive therapy should be considered (individualized adjustment) • If active AIH, initiating immunosuppressive therapy is recommended despite COVID-19 infection • In AIH patients with active COVID-19 infection and elevated liver biochemistries, do not presume flare of AIH without biopsy confirmation
NAFLD	• Preventing liver disease progression by intensive lifestyle modifications, including weight loss advice and diabetes control • Early admission should be considered for all patients with NAFLD who become infected with SARS-CoV-2
ALD	• Encourage alcohol cessation • Clinicians should weigh the risk of susceptibility for severe COVID-19 when initiating corticosteroids in patients with severe alcoholic hepatitis
Cirrhosis	• Prophylaxis for spontaneous bacterial peritonitis (SBP), gastrointestinal hemorrhage, and hepatic encephalopathy should be maintained to prevent hospitalization due to portal hypertension-related complications • Patients with new onset of hepatic decompensation or ACLF should be tested for SARS-CoV-2 even in the absence of respiratory symptoms • Early admission is recommended if COVID-19 is diagnosed • All patients should receive vaccination for *S pneumoniae* and influenza
Liver transplant recipients	Without COVID-19 infection • No reduction of immunosuppression to prevent acute rejection • Emphasize importance of vaccination for *S pneumoniae* and influenza With COVID-19 infection • Early admission is recommended • Do not assume acute cellular rejection without biopsy confirmation in LT recipients in the presence of active

(*continued on next page*)

Table 3
(*continued*)

Chronic Liver Diseases	AASLD recommendation[1] and EASL-ESCMID Position article[34,49,72]
	COVID-19 infection and elevated liver biochemistries • Minimizing dosage of immunosuppressive therapy should be considered case-by-case under specialist consultation based on severity of COVID-19 and risk of graft rejection • Lower the overall level of immunosuppression (eg, azathioprine or mycophenolate) to decrease the risks of superinfection, especially with antimetabolite therapies • Closely monitor calcineurin inhibitor levels, for features of acute kidney injury, and potential drug–drug interactions • Anti-IL-6 therapeutics have not been shown to increase the risk of acute cellular rejection
HCC	Without COVID-19 infection • Continue to perform surveillance in patients at risk for HCC as close to schedule as possible. Delay of schedule for 2 mo is reasonable • For HCC patients, care should be maintained according to guidelines, including continuing systemic treatments and evaluation for LT With COVID-19 infection • HCC surveillance can be deferred until after recovery • For HCC patients, early admission is recommended. Locoregional therapies should be postponed and immune-checkpoint inhibitors should be temporarily withdrawn

Abbreviations: AIH, autoimmune hepatitis; HBV, hepatitis B virus; HCV, hepatitis C virus; IL, interleukin; JAK, Janus kinase; LT, liver transplant.

immunosuppressed patients based on the data on 3 doses of the BNT162b2 mRNA COVID-19 vaccine (manufactured by Pfizer-BioNTech) in solid organ transplant recipients (n = 101) that reports significant improvement in anti-SARS-CoV-2 antibody response (up to 68% at 4 weeks after the third dose).[79] A fourth dose of SARS-CoV-2 vaccine was associated with slightly improved humoral response among patients with a weak response after 3 doses but no improvement among those with no response after 3 doses, although, no breakthrough infections were observed during follow-up.[80]

Additionally, a prospective cohort study that compared the SARS-CoV-2-specific humoral and T-cell immune response after the second mRNA vaccination in patients with cirrhosis and in LT recipients (n = 194 including 141 LT and 53 cirrhosis Child-Pugh classes A–C) demonstrated that after the second dose, seroconversion was achieved in 63% of LT recipients and 100% of patients with cirrhosis and controls using the anti-S trimer assay ($P < .001$).[81] Spike-specific T-cell response rates were 36.6%, 65.4%, and 100% in LT recipients, cirrhosis, and controls, respectively. Around 28% of LT recipients did not develop both humoral and T-cell responses after the second vaccination. These data, therefore, support the potential role for a third vaccine dose, especially in LT recipients with low or absent prior vaccine responses. In this cohort, predictors of absent or low humoral response were age greater than 65 years (OR = 4.57, 95%CI 1.48–14.05) and arterial hypertension (OR = 2.50, 95%CI 1.10–5.68). In contrast, failure was less likely with calcineurin inhibitor monotherapy versus other immunosuppressive regimens (OR = 0.36, 95%CI 0.13–0.99).[81] Guideline recommendations for COVID-19 vaccination in CLD and liver-transplant recipients[73,82,83] are described in **Box 1**. The

Box 1
Guideline recommendations for coronavirus disease-2019 vaccination in chronic liver disease and liver transplant recipients

Guideline recommendations for COVID-19 vaccination in CLD

- Patients with CLD who are receiving antiviral treatment of HBV or HCV or medical treatment of PBC or AIH should continue their medications while receiving the COVID-19 vaccines
- Patients with HCC undergoing locoregional or systemic therapy should be considered for vaccination without treatment interruption
- An additional third dose of an mRNA vaccine is recommended at least 28 d after the second dose of an mRNA COVID-19 vaccine in all immunosuppressed patients, HCC, and CLD patients receiving prednisone, antimetabolites, or biological therapies with a booster 3 mo after the third dose
- It is not recommended to withhold immunosuppression before or after COVID-19 vaccine

Guideline recommendations for COVID-19 vaccination in liver-transplant recipients

- COVID-19 vaccination is recommended for all LT recipients.
- LT candidates should receive a COVID-19 vaccine before transplantation whenever possible, if not, the optimal time to administer the COVID-19 vaccine is $\geq$ 3 mo post-LT. However, immunization may be initiated as early as 4 wk posttransplant, especially for high-risk individuals
- A reduction in immunosuppression is not recommended in LT recipients when receiving COVID-19 vaccine due to the risk of ACR
- COVID-19 vaccination should be avoided in LT recipients with active ACR
- Potential live liver donors and recipients should be vaccinated $\geq$2 weeks before transplantation if feasible
- Family members and caregivers of LT recipients should also be vaccinated against SARS-CoV-2
- LT recipients who recover from COVID-19 infection should still complete COVID-19 vaccine series

Abbreviations: ACR, acute cellular rejection; AIH, autoimmune hepatitis; HBV, hepatitis B virus; HCV, hepatitis C virus; LT, liver transplant; PBC, primary biliary cholangitis.

Data from Refs.[73,82,83]

Centers for Disease Control recommendations on vaccinations are periodically updated and can be accessed by the link of https://www.cdc.gov/coronavirus/2019-ncov/vaccines/index.html.

Acute Liver Injury after Coronavirus Disease-2019 Vaccination

A large epidemiologic study from Europe reported no increment in new AIH cases diagnosed during the widespread use of COVID-19 vaccination, and these data do not support the assumption that COVID-19 vaccination induces AIH.[84] However, de novo AIH-like liver injury occurring after COVID-19 vaccination has been reported in case series in which data from 18 countries demonstrated liver injury after SARS-CoV-2 vaccination (n = 87, 63% women).[85] Liver injury was diagnosed at a median of 15 (range 3–65) days after vaccination, attributed to the Pfizer-BioNTech (BNT162b2) vaccine in 59%, the Oxford-AstraZeneca (ChAdOX1 nCoV-19) vaccine in 23%, and the Moderna (mRNA-1273) vaccine in 18%. The liver injury was predominantly hepatocellular (84%) and 57% of patients had features of immune-mediated hepatitis (positive autoantibodies and elevated immunoglobulin G levels). Corticosteroids were administered to 53% of patients and resulted in complete biochemical resolution without a relapse after corticosteroid withdrawal. Outcome was generally favorable, except for one patient who developed fulminant liver failure.[85] Of note, the mechanisms leading to acute liver injury after COVID-19 vaccination have not been fully elucidated, and it is difficult to establish a definite causal relationship between COVID-19 vaccination and hepatitis. Furthermore, these events are extremely rare and respond well to corticosteroid treatment, and the overall benefits of vaccination outweigh the risks of liver injury; thus, this side effect should not represent a barrier to SARS-CoV-2 vaccination.[49]

SUMMARY

COVID-19 infection has had a major impact on people across the world since December 2019, causing up to 6.5 million deaths globally until now in 2022. Patients with CLD, especially cirrhosis, and liver-transplant recipients are particularly vulnerable to severe COVID-19. These populations are, therefore, strongly recommended to receive COVID-19 vaccination to reduce their morbidity and mortality. Data on vaccine safety and efficacy is emerging but several issues remain unresolved, such as prevalence of breakthrough infection after vaccinations and adequate doses and timing of vaccination in those receiving immunosuppressants or in transplant recipients. Management of immunosuppressive agents in post-LT patients with severe COVID-19 infection requires further study. Because the COVID-19 pandemic rapidly evolves in different regions due to the emergence of mutant strains, early diagnosis and treatment of COVID-19 in patients with advanced liver disease deserves a special focus to minimize the risk of hepatic decompensation. The pandemic has been further associated with increased alcohol consumption, unhealthy eating behaviors, and interruptions of hepatology care, which may lead to an increase in severity of liver disease; therefore, clinicians should strongly recommend alcohol cessation and provide health education to their patients with liver diseases.

CLINICS CARE POINTS

- Early admission in patients with cirrhosis and COVID-19 infection is recommended due to high rate of hepatic decompensation.
- SARS-CoV-2 vaccination is strongly recommended for all patients with chronic liver disease including those with cirrhosis, liver-transplant candidates and recipients.
- Areduction of immunosuppression in patients with autoimmune hepatitis and liver-transplant recipients without evidence of COVID-19 infection, is not recommended.
- Treatment should not be interrupted in those with HCC and without COVID-19 infection, while similarly liver transplantation should be pursued as needed.

DISCLOSURE

The authors declare no conflicts of interest relevant to this publication.

REFERENCES

1. Fix OK, Hameed B, Fontana RJ, et al. Clinical Best Practice Advice for Hepatology and Liver Transplant Providers During the COVID-19 Pandemic: AASLD Expert Panel Consensus Statement. Hepatology 2020;72(1):287–304.
2. Clinical best practice advice for hepatology and liver transplant providers during the covid-19 pandemic: Aasld Expert Panel Consensus Statement. Available

at: https://www.aasld.org/sites/default/files/2021-11/AASLD%20COVID-19%20Expert%20Panel%20Consensus%20Statement%20Update%2011.02.2021.pdf. Accessed November 2, 2021.
3. Marjot T, Moon AM, Cook JA, et al. Outcomes following SARS-CoV-2 infection in patients with chronic liver disease: An international registry study. J Hepatol 2021; 74(3):567–77.
4. Chen N, Zhou M, Dong X, et al. Epidemiological and clinical characteristics of 99 cases of 2019 novel coronavirus pneumonia in Wuhan, China: a descriptive study. The Lancet 2020;395(10223):507–13.
5. Guan WJ, Ni ZY, Hu Y, et al. Clinical Characteristics of Coronavirus Disease 2019 in China. N Engl J Med 2020;382(18):1708–20.
6. Huang C, Wang Y, Li X, et al. Clinical features of patients infected with 2019 novel coronavirus in Wuhan, China. The Lancet 2020;395(10223):497–506.
7. Shi H, Han X, Jiang N, et al. Radiological findings from 81 patients with COVID-19 pneumonia in Wuhan, China: a descriptive study. Lancet Infect Dis 2020;20(4): 425–34.
8. Xu X-W, Wu X-X, Jiang X-G, et al. Clinical findings in a group of patients infected with the 2019 novel coronavirus (SARS-Cov-2) outside of Wuhan, China: retrospective case series. BMJ (Clinical research ed) 2020;368:m606.
9. Yang X, Yu Y, Xu J, et al. Clinical course and outcomes of critically ill patients with SARS-CoV-2 pneumonia in Wuhan, China: a single-centered, retrospective, observational study. Lancet Respir Med 2020;8(5):475–81.
10. Cai Q, Huang D, Ou P, et al. COVID-19 in a designated infectious diseases hospital outside Hubei Province, China. Allergy 2020;75(7):1742–52.
11. Cao B, Wang Y, Wen D, et al. A Trial of Lopinavir-Ritonavir in Adults Hospitalized with Severe Covid-19. N Engl J Med 2020;382(19):1787–99.
12. Fan Z, Chen L, Li J, et al. Clinical Features of COVID-19-Related Liver Functional Abnormality. Clin Gastroenterol Hepatol 2020;18(7):1561–6.
13. Fan Z, Chen L, Li J, et al. Clinical features of COVID-19 related liver damage. medRxiv 2020;2020:2026, 20026971.
14. Zhang C, Shi L, Wang F-S. Liver injury in COVID-19: management and challenges. Lancet Gastroenterol Hepatol 2020;5(5):428–30.
15. Huang Y, Yang R, Xu Y, et al. Clinical characteristics of 36 non-survivors with COVID-19 in Wuhan, China. medRxiv 2020;2020. 2002.2027.20029009.
16. Cao M, Zhang D, Wang Y, et al. Clinical Features of Patients Infected with the 2019 Novel Coronavirus (COVID-19) in Shanghai, China. medRxiv 2020;2020. 2003.2004.20030395.
17. Cai Q, Huang D, Yu H, et al. COVID-19: Abnormal liver function tests. J Hepatol 2020;73(3):566–74.
18. Zhang Y, Zheng L, Liu L, et al. Liver impairment in COVID-19 patients: A retrospective analysis of 115 cases from a single centre in Wuhan city, China. Liver Int 2020;40(9):2095–103.
19. Vespa E, Pugliese N, Piovani D, et al. Liver tests abnormalities in COVID-19: trick or treat? J Hepatol 2020;73(5):1275–6.
20. Grasselli G, Zangrillo A, Zanella A, et al. Baseline characteristics and outcomes of 1591 patients infected with sars-cov-2 admitted to ICUs of the Lombardy Region, Italy. JAMA 2020;323(16):1574–81.
21. Cholankeril G, Podboy A, Aivaliotis VI, et al. High Prevalence of Concurrent Gastrointestinal Manifestations in Patients With Severe Acute Respiratory Syndrome Coronavirus 2: Early Experience From California. Gastroenterology 2020;159(2):775–7.

22. Arentz M, Yim E, Klaff L, et al. Characteristics and Outcomes of 21 Critically Ill Patients With COVID-19 in Washington State. JAMA 2020;323(16):1612–4.
23. Richardson S, Hirsch JS, Narasimhan M, et al. Presenting Characteristics, Comorbidities, and Outcomes Among 5700 Patients Hospitalized With COVID-19 in the New York City Area. jama 2020;323(20):2052–9.
24. Tang C, Zhang K, Wang W, et al. Clinical Characteristics of 20,662 Patients with COVID-19 in mainland China: A Systemic Review and Meta-analysis. medRxiv 2020;2020. 2004.2018.20070565.
25. Hundt MA, Deng Y, Ciarleglio MM, et al. Abnormal Liver Tests in COVID-19: A Retrospective Observational Cohort Study of 1,827 Patients in a Major U.S. Hospital Network. Hepatol 2020;72(4):1169–76.
26. Singh S, Khan A. Clinical Characteristics and Outcomes of Coronavirus Disease 2019 Among Patients With Preexisting Liver Disease in the United States: A Multicenter Research Network Study. Gastroenterology 2020;159(2):768–71.e763.
27. Lei F, Liu YM, Zhou F, et al. Longitudinal Association Between Markers of Liver Injury and Mortality in COVID-19 in China. Hepatology 2020;72(2):389–98.
28. Phipps MM, Barraza LH, LaSota ED, et al. Acute Liver Injury in COVID-19: Prevalence and Association with Clinical Outcomes in a Large U.S. Cohort. Hepatology 2020;72(3):807–17.
29. Kulkarni AV, Kumar P, Tevethia HV, et al. Systematic review with meta-analysis: liver manifestations and outcomes in COVID-19. Aliment Pharmacol Ther 2020; 52(4):584–99.
30. Liu W, Tao ZW, Wang L, et al. Analysis of factors associated with disease outcomes in hospitalized patients with 2019 novel coronavirus disease. Chin Med J 2020;133(9):1032–8.
31. Pereira MR, Mohan S, Cohen DJ, et al. COVID-19 in solid organ transplant recipients: Initial report from the US epicenter. Am J Transplant 2020;20(7):1800–8.
32. Xu L, Liu J, Lu M, et al. Liver injury during highly pathogenic human coronavirus infections. Liver Int 2020;40(5):998–1004.
33. Chen L, Li Q, Zheng D, et al. Clinical Characteristics of Pregnant Women with Covid-19 in Wuhan, China. N Engl J Med 2020;382(25):e100.
34. Boettler T, Marjot T, Newsome PN, et al. Impact of COVID-19 on the care of patients with liver disease: EASL-ESCMID position paper after 6 months of the pandemic. JHEP Rep 2020;2(5):100169.
35. Li Y, Xiao S-Y. Hepatic involvement in COVID-19 patients: Pathology, pathogenesis, and clinical implications. J Med Virol 2020;92(9):1491–4.
36. Chai X, Hu L, Zhang Y, et al. Specific ACE2 Expression in Cholangiocytes May Cause Liver Damage After 2019-nCoV Infection. bioRxiv 2020;2020:931766.
37. Banales JM, Huebert RC, Karlsen T, et al. Cholangiocyte pathobiology. Nat Rev Gastroenterol Hepatol 2019;16(5):269–81.
38. Lagana SM, Kudose S, Iuga AC, et al. Hepatic pathology in patients dying of COVID-19: a series of 40 cases including clinical, histologic, and virologic data. Mod Pathol 2020;33(11):2147–55.
39. Wanner N, Andrieux G, Badia-i-Mompel P, et al. Molecular consequences of SARS-CoV-2 liver tropism. Nat Metab 2022;4(3):310–9.
40. Barnes E. Infection of liver hepatocytes with SARS-CoV-2. Nat Metab 2022;4(3): 301–2.
41. Bertolini A, van de Peppel IP, Bodewes FAJA, et al. Abnormal Liver Function Tests in Patients With COVID-19: Relevance and Potential Pathogenesis. Hepatology 2020;72(5):1864–72.

42. Grein J, Ohmagari N, Shin D, et al. Compassionate Use of Remdesivir for Patients with Severe Covid-19. N Engl J Med 2020;382(24):2327–36.
43. Marra F, Smolders EJ, El-Sherif O, et al. Recommendations for Dosing of Repurposed COVID-19 Medications in Patients with Renal and Hepatic Impairment. Drugs R D 2021;21(1):9–27.
44. Bajaj JS, Kamath PS, Reddy KR. The Evolving Challenge of Infections in Cirrhosis. N Engl J Med 2021;384(24):2317–30.
45. Faruqui S, Okoli FC, Olsen SK, et al. Cholangiopathy After Severe COVID-19: Clinical Features and Prognostic Implications. Am J Gastroenterol 2021;116(7): 1414–25.
46. Roth NC, Kim A, Vitkovski T, et al. Post-COVID-19 Cholangiopathy: A Novel Entity. Am J Gastroenterol 2021;116(5):1077–82.
47. Bütikofer S, Lenggenhager D, Wendel Garcia PD, et al. Secondary sclerosing cholangitis as cause of persistent jaundice in patients with severe COVID-19. Liver Int 2021;41(10):2404–17.
48. Hartl L, Haslinger K, Angerer M, et al. Progressive cholestasis and associated sclerosing cholangitis are frequent complications of COVID-19 in patients with chronic liver disease. Hepatology 2022. https://doi.org/10.1002/hep.32582.
49. Marjot T, Eberhardt CS, Boettler T, et al. Impact of COVID-19 on the liver and on the care of patients with chronic liver disease, hepatobiliary cancer, and liver transplantation: an updated EASL position paper. J Hepatol 2022;77(4):1161–97.
50. Marjot T, Webb GJ, Barritt ASt, et al. COVID-19 and liver disease: mechanistic and clinical perspectives. Nat Rev Gastroenterol Hepatol 2021;18(5):348–64.
51. Yip TC, Wong VW, Lui GC, et al. Current and Past Infections of HBV Do Not Increase Mortality in Patients With COVID-19. Hepatology 2021;74(4):1750–65.
52. Ding ZY, Li GX, Chen L, et al. Association of liver abnormalities with in-hospital mortality in patients with COVID-19. J Hepatol 2021;74(6):1295–302.
53. Butt AA, Yan P, Chotani RA, et al. Mortality is not increased in SARS-CoV-2 infected persons with hepatitis C virus infection. Liver Int 2021;41(8):1824–31.
54. Marjot T, Buescher G, Sebode M, et al. SARS-CoV-2 infection in patients with autoimmune hepatitis. J Hepatol 2021;74(6):1335–43.
55. Efe C, Dhanasekaran R, Lammert C, et al. Outcome of COVID-19 in Patients With Autoimmune Hepatitis: An International Multicenter Study. Hepatology 2021; 73(6):2099–109.
56. Ji D, Qin E, Xu J, et al. Non-alcoholic fatty liver diseases in patients with COVID-19: A retrospective study. J Hepatol 2020;73(2):451–3.
57. Huang R, Zhu L, Wang J, et al. Clinical Features of Patients With COVID-19 With Nonalcoholic Fatty Liver Disease. Hepatol Commun 2020;4(12):1758–68.
58. Targher G, Mantovani A, Byrne CD, et al. Risk of severe illness from COVID-19 in patients with metabolic dysfunction-associated fatty liver disease and increased fibrosis scores. Gut 2020;69(8):1545–7.
59. Hashemi N, Viveiros K, Redd WD, et al. Impact of chronic liver disease on outcomes of hospitalized patients with COVID-19: A multicentre United States experience. Liver Int 2020;40(10):2515–21.
60. Singh A, Hussain S, Antony B. Non-alcoholic fatty liver disease and clinical outcomes in patients with COVID-19: A comprehensive systematic review and meta-analysis. Diabetes Metab Syndr 2021;15(3):813–22.
61. Cholankeril G, Goli K, Rana A, et al. Impact of COVID-19 Pandemic on Liver Transplantation and Alcohol-Associated Liver Disease in the USA. Hepatology 2021;74(6):3316–29.

62. Bajaj JS, Garcia-Tsao G, Biggins SW, et al. Comparison of mortality risk in patients with cirrhosis and COVID-19 compared with patients with cirrhosis alone and COVID-19 alone: multicentre matched cohort. Gut 2021;70(3):531–6.
63. Middleton P, Hsu C, Lythgoe MP. Clinical outcomes in COVID-19 and cirrhosis: a systematic review and meta-analysis of observational studies. BMJ open Gastroenterol 2021;8(1):e000739.
64. Colmenero J, Rodriguez-Peralvarez M, Salcedo M, et al. Epidemiological pattern, incidence, and outcomes of COVID-19 in liver transplant patients. J Hepatol 2021;74(1):148–55.
65. Webb GJ, Marjot T, Cook JA, et al. Outcomes following SARS-CoV-2 infection in liver transplant recipients: an international registry study. Lancet Gastroenterol Hepatol 2020;5(11):1008–16.
66. Belli LS, Fondevila C, Cortesi PA, et al. Protective Role of Tacrolimus, Deleterious Role of Age and Comorbidities in Liver Transplant Recipients With Covid-19: Results From the ELITA/ELTR Multi-center European Study. Gastroenterology 2021; 160(4):1151–63.e1153.
67. Kim D, Adeniji N, Latt N, et al. Predictors of Outcomes of COVID-19 in Patients With Chronic Liver Disease: US Multi-center Study. Clin Gastroenterol Hepatol 2021;19(7):1469–79.e1419.
68. Mallet V, Beeker N, Bouam S, et al. Prognosis of French COVID-19 patients with chronic liver disease: A national retrospective cohort study for 2020. J Hepatol 2021;75(4):848–55.
69. Kudo M, Kurosaki M, Ikeda M, et al. Treatment of hepatocellular carcinoma during the COVID-19 outbreak: The Working Group report of JAMTT-HCC. Hepatol Res 2020;50(9):1004–14.
70. Chan SL, Kudo M. Impacts of COVID-19 on Liver Cancers: During and after the Pandemic. Liver Cancer 2020;9(5):491–502.
71. Amaddeo G, Brustia R, Allaire M, et al. Impact of COVID-19 on the management of hepatocellular carcinoma in a high-prevalence area. JHEP Rep 2021;3(1): 100199.
72. Boettler T, Newsome PN, Mondelli MU, et al. Care of patients with liver disease during the COVID-19 pandemic: EASL-ESCMID position paper. JHEP Rep 2020;2(3):100113.
73. AASLD expert panel consensus statement: vaccines to prevent covid-19 in patients with liver disease. Available at: https://www.aasld.org/sites/default/files/2022-03/AASLD%20COVID-19%20Vaccine%20Document%20Update%203.28.2022.1%20FINAL.pdf. Accessed March 28, 2022.
74. John BV, Deng Y, Scheinberg A, et al. Association of BNT162b2 mRNA and mRNA-1273 Vaccines With COVID-19 Infection and Hospitalization Among Patients With Cirrhosis. JAMA Intern Med 2021;181(10):1306–14.
75. John BV, Deng Y, Schwartz KB, et al. Postvaccination COVID-19 infection is associated with reduced mortality in patients with cirrhosis. Hepatology 2022;76(1): 126–38.
76. Moon AM, Webb GJ, García-Juárez I, et al. SARS-CoV-2 Infections Among Patients With Liver Disease and Liver Transplantation Who Received COVID-19 Vaccination. Hepatol Commun 2022;6(4):889–97.
77. Boyarsky BJ, Werbel WA, Avery RK, et al. Immunogenicity of a Single Dose of SARS-CoV-2 Messenger RNA Vaccine in Solid Organ Transplant Recipients. JAMA 2021;325(17):1784–6.

78. Boyarsky BJ, Werbel WA, Avery RK, et al. Antibody Response to 2-Dose SARS-CoV-2 mRNA Vaccine Series in Solid Organ Transplant Recipients. JAMA 2021; 325(21):2204–6.
79. Kamar N, Abravanel F, Marion O, et al. Three Doses of an mRNA Covid-19 Vaccine in Solid-Organ Transplant Recipients. N Engl J Med 2021;385(7):661–2.
80. Kamar N, Abravanel F, Marion O, et al. Assessment of 4 Doses of SARS-CoV-2 Messenger RNA–Based Vaccine in Recipients of a Solid Organ Transplant. JAMA Netw Open 2021;4(11):e2136030.
81. Ruether DF, Schaub GM, Duengelhoef PM, et al. SARS-CoV2-specific Humoral and T-cell Immune Response After Second Vaccination in Liver Cirrhosis and Transplant Patients. Clin Gastroenterol Hepatol 2022;20(1):162–72.e169.
82. Centers for Disease Control and Prevention. Vaccines for COVID-19. Available at: https://www.cdc.gov/coronavirus/2019-ncov/vaccines/index.html. Accessed August 11, 2022.
83. Fix OK, Blumberg EA, Chang K-M, et al. American Association for the Study of Liver Diseases Expert Panel Consensus Statement: Vaccines to Prevent Coronavirus Disease 2019 Infection in Patients With Liver Disease. Hepatology 2021; 74(2):1049–64.
84. Rüther DF, Weltzsch JP, Schramm C, et al. Autoimmune hepatitis and COVID-19: No increased risk for AIH after vaccination but reduced care. J Hepatol 2022; 77(1):250–1.
85. Efe C, Kulkarni AV, Terziroli Beretta-Piccoli B, et al. Liver injury after SARS-CoV-2 vaccination: Features of immune-mediated hepatitis, role of corticosteroid therapy and outcome. Hepatology 2022.
86. Yadav DK, Singh A, Zhang Q, et al. Involvement of liver in COVID-19: systematic review and meta-analysis. Gut 2020;70(4):807–9.
87. Sarin SK, Choudhury A, Lau GK, et al. Pre-existing liver disease is associated with poor outcome in patients with SARS CoV2 infection; The APCOLIS Study (APASL COVID-19 Liver Injury Spectrum Study). Hepatol Int 2020;14(5):690–700.
88. Verhelst X, Somers N, Geerts A, et al. Health status of patients with autoimmune hepatitis is not affected by the SARS-CoV-2 outbreak in Flanders, Belgium. J Hepatol 2021;74(1):240–1.
89. Di Giorgio A, Nicastro E, Speziani C, et al. Health status of patients with autoimmune liver disease during SARS-CoV-2 outbreak in northern Italy. J Hepatol 2020; 73(3):702–5.
90. Younossi ZM, Stepanova M, Lam B, et al. Independent Predictors of Mortality Among Patients With NAFLD Hospitalized With COVID-19 Infection. Hepatol Commun 2021. n/a(n/a.
91. Ge J, Pletcher MJ, Lai JC, et al. Outcomes of SARS-CoV-2 Infection in Patients With Chronic Liver Disease and Cirrhosis: A National COVID Cohort Collaborative Study. Gastroenterology 2021;161(5):1487–501.e1485.
92. Iavarone M, D'Ambrosio R, Soria A, et al. High rates of 30-day mortality in patients with cirrhosis and COVID-19. J Hepatol 2020;73(5):1063–71.
93. Clift AK, Coupland CAC, Keogh RH, et al. Living risk prediction algorithm (QCOVID) for risk of hospital admission and mortality from coronavirus 19 in adults: national derivation and validation cohort study. BMJ (Clinical research ed) 2020; 371:m3731.
94. Ioannou GN, Liang PS, Locke E, et al. Cirrhosis and Severe Acute Respiratory Syndrome Coronavirus 2 Infection in US Veterans: Risk of Infection, Hospitalization, Ventilation, and Mortality. Hepatology 2021;74(1):322–35.

95. Rabiee A, Sadowski B, Adeniji N, et al. Liver Injury in Liver Transplant Recipients With Coronavirus Disease 2019 (COVID-19): U.S. Multicenter Experience. Hepatology 2020;72(6):1900–11.
96. Kates OS, Haydel BM, Florman SS, et al. Coronavirus Disease 2019 in Solid Organ Transplant: A Multicenter Cohort Study. Clin Infect Dis 2021;73(11):e4090–9.
97. Ravanan R, Callaghan CJ, Mumford L, et al. SARS-CoV-2 infection and early mortality of waitlisted and solid organ transplant recipients in England: A national cohort study. Am J Transplant 2020;20(11):3008–18.
98. Polak WG, Fondevila C, Karam V, et al. Impact of COVID-19 on liver transplantation in Europe: alert from an early survey of European Liver and Intestine Transplantation Association and European Liver Transplant Registry. Transpl Int 2020;33(10):1244–52.

The Pancreas in Coronavirus Disease 2019 Infection

Tiago Correia de Sá, MD[a,*], Mónica Rocha, MD[b]

KEYWORDS

• Acute pancreatitis • COVID-19 • SARS-CoV-2 • Pancreatic cancer
• Chronic pancreatitis

KEY POINTS

- Many similarities between severe acute respiratory syndrome coronavirus-2 infection and acute pancreatitis (AP) are described but there is still a paucity of evidence to establish coronavirus disease 2019 (COVID-19) as a cause of AP.
- Patients with both COVID-19 and AP should be carefully managed because evidence indicates they may have a worse outcome.
- Careful attention to etiologic workup, patients comorbidities and chronic medications, disease management and diagnosis, and publishing guidelines should guide future case reports.
- COVID-19 vaccination has indisputable advantages but a few cases of AP have been reported after vaccination, which should alert and turn physicians to abdominal pain development after inoculation.
- Pancreas cancer diagnosis and management have been deeply influenced by the pandemic. Expert consensus and international and local guidelines should be implemented to allow safe management pathways to be resumed and improved.

INTRODUCTION

Severe acute respiratory syndrome coronavirus-2 (SARS-CoV-2) is responsible for the pandemic of coronavirus disease 2019 (COVID-19) that has caused more than 600 million infections and 6.5 million deaths worldwide, involving more than 200 countries.[1]

Initially considered a respiratory disease, the gastrointestinal tract has been described as playing a key role in the route of infection, clinical manifestations, and disease outcomes.[2] Pancreatic involvement was also found and several cases of pancreatic enzyme elevation and acute pancreatitis (AP) have been reported. However,

[a] General Surgery Department, Centro Hospitalar do Tâmega e Sousa, Avenida do Hospital Padre Américo 210, 4564-007 Penafiel, Portugal; [b] Hepato-Pancreato-Biliary Unit, General Surgery Department, Centro Hospitalar do Tâmega e Sousa, Avenida do Hospital Padre Américo 210, 4564-007 Penafiel, Portugal
* Corresponding author.
E-mail address: tiago.rc.sa@gmail.com

Gastroenterol Clin N Am 52 (2023) 37–48
https://doi.org/10.1016/j.gtc.2022.12.002

the available data are difficult to interpret, and COVID-19 has not been definitively associated with AP, leaving several questions open.[3]

In this review, we aim to examine mechanisms of pancreatic involvement by SARS-CoV-2, the link between COVID-19 and AP, the influence of COVID-19 on chronic pancreatitis (CP), and the impact of COVID-19 on pancreatic cancer treatment, prognosis, and pancreatic surgery.

MATERIALS AND METHODS

A review of the literature was conducted using PubMed and EMBASE databases on September 26, 2022, for publications on COVID-19 and acute and CP and pancreatic cancer. A grey literature search using the same keywords was performed using Google Scholar to increase the search sensitivity. Articles on pediatric patients and pregnant women were excluded. References of eligible articles were also screened for additional articles. The literature search was restricted to articles published in English.

MECHANISMS OF PANCREATIC INJURY

Several studies have examined possible mechanisms of pancreatic injury by SARS-CoV-2.

SARS-CoV-2 enters human cells through angiotensin converting enzyme (ACE2) receptors, with transmembrane serine protease 2 (TMPRSS2) priming, which are highly expressed in human gastrointestinal cells.[4] After viral entry, virus-specific RNA and proteins are synthesized in the cytoplasm of host cells to assemble new virions, which are then released to the gastrointestinal tract and detected in stool, confirming fecal–oral transmission.[4]

ACE2 is also highly expressed in pancreatic ductal, acinar, and islet cells,[5] and the virus could thereby spread from the duodenal epithelium to the pancreatic cells. Furthermore, SARS-CoV-2 has been associated with endotheliitis and microischemic disease, which could occur in the pancreas.[6]

Histopathological studies in patients who died from severe COVID-19 infection report findings of pancreatitis and of SARS-CoV-2 identified in pancreatic pseudocyst fluid samples in patients who did not develop AP, showing SARS-CoV-2 tropism for pancreatic cells.[7–9]

SARS-CoV-2 has been reported to result in insulin deficiency and the development of type 1 diabetes mellitus.[10] Although an increase of type 1 diabetes mellitus was observed in children, it is still unknown whether β cell injury is permanent or transient.[10,11] Long-term results of the COVIDPAN study did not show an increased frequency of long-term diabetes.[12] In patients already diagnosed with diabetes, SARS-CoV-2 induced β cell dysfunction may cause an uncontrolled hyperglycemic state, which in turn may contribute to COVID-19 increased severity and mortality.[10,13] Derangements of Na^+/H^+ exchange and lactate pathway are other potential mechanisms of glucose metabolism dysregulation from SARS-CoV-2 infection.[14]

A broad-spectrum of proinflammatory cytokines, including interleukin-2 (IL-2), IL-6, IL-8, IL-10, CXCL12, interferon (IFN)-γ, and tumor-necrosis factor-α, are released during COVID-19 infection, which may result from SARS-CoV-2 binding to ACE2 receptors in pancreatic cells[15,16] but can also cause direct damage to surrounding dendritic cells and naïve T-cell activation in genetically predisposed individuals.[17] It is also hypothesized that pancreatic lipase increases lipolysis and plasma levels of unsaturated fatty acids, which can in turn damage mitochondria and contribute to proinflammatory cytokine release.[18,19] In both COVID-19 and AP, the cytokine storm is responsible for the disease severity, specifically elevated IL-6 levels, which are related to the development of the acute respiratory distress syndrome and cause increased mortality in AP.[20,21] Moreover, immune-response pathways are severely impacted by antibody production during SARS-CoV-2 infection, which may potentially cause increased IL-6 production.[22] The cytokine storm is also directly involved in the coagulation cascade deregulation, which may in turn increase AP severity.[23]

Several drugs used in the treatment of COVID-19, including corticosteroids, azithromycin, remdesivir, lopinavir/ritonavir, and IFN-β, have been implicated in the development of AP and hyperglycemia.[13,24–27] Nevertheless, prednisolone is recommended for the treatment of specific preexisting conditions in patients with COVID-19, including cases of autoimmune AP.[28]

Acute Pancreatitis and Coronavirus Disease 2019

AP seems an infrequent complication of COVID-19 and large retrospective studies found no increased incidence of AP during the pandemic.[29–31] In fact, some centers have reported a decreased number of admissions for AP, probably due to patient reluctance to present to the emergency department during the pandemic but also because of reluctance of emergency room physicians to admit patients with mild AP.[32,33] However, idiopathic AP was diagnosed in a greater proportion of patients with COVID-19, implicating SARS-CoV-2 in a causative role.[29,34]

The diagnosis of AP should rely on the Atlanta criteria, and isolated elevations of amylase and lipase should not be misdiagnosed as AP.[35] In fact, SARS-CoV-2 can directly cause increased amylase and/or lipase levels and can also cause several complications that can increase the levels of these enzymes, including renal failure, acidosis, and diabetes. Up to 23% of patients may exhibit increased amylase levels but only a minority has AP according to the Atlanta Criteria.[36–38] High lipasemia without AP can be detected in up to one-third of patients with COVID-19.[39–41] Many case reports and case series have been published linking COVID-19 to AP development. However, most reports have a paucity of clinical information and a lack of adherence to CARE guidelines on publishing. Moreover, the temporal gap between COVID-19 diagnosis and AP is very heterogeneous making it difficult to establish a causal link between these entities in some cases. Complete etiological workup according to current evidence, including MRI and endoscopic ultrasonography, was pursued in a minority of patients, rendering the attribution of SARS-CoV-2 as the causative agent of AP doubtful in some cases.[42] COVID-19 also causes immune dysregulation that may favor other infections, including cytomegalovirus (CMV), which in turn could cause AP.[43]

Multivariate regression analysis revealed that elevated amylase and lipase levels were significantly associated with the severity of COVID-19, ICU admission, and mortality in hospitalized patients with COVID-19.[36–38,44,45] Moreover, in patients without AP, elevations of pancreatic enzymes may be indicators of overall disease severity and poor prognostic indicators.[46–50] Lipase/lymphocyte ratio was also found to be a predictor of mortality in AP patients with COVID-19.[51] Single-cell sequencing data have identified a subgroup of neutrophils with high expression of IFN and a proinflammatory phenotype in COVID-19, which may be involved in AP severity.[52] A low T-cell count has also been suggested as a surrogate for poor clinical outcomes.[53]

Imaging findings suggestive of AP, including peripancreatic stranding and fluid collections, were more frequent in patients with COVID-19 and considering with elevations of pancreatic enzymes may aid in the diagnosis of AP, specifically in severe cases, when patients are frequently intubated.[54] However, computerized tomography of the abdomen is not strictly indicated in patients with elevated pancreatic enzymes levels because most frequently elevated amylase levels may be a nonspecific manifestation of shock/critical illness.[55]

The temporal relation between AP and COVID-19 infection is very variable. AP may be more severe in patients with COVID-19 but not necessarily linked to the SARS-CoV-2 viral load, as suggested by the COVIDPAN study.[3]

Several studies found that patients with COVID-19 infection had significantly AP mortality[32,56–60] and significantly increased the risk of severe AP,[56,58,61] necrotizing AP,[56] ICU admission,[32,57,60,61] need for mechanical ventilation[29] and longer length of hospital stay,[29,56–58,62] compared with COVID-negative patients. Thus, AP may have a poor prognosis in patients with COVID-19. However, patients with previous inflammatory insults to the pancreas were found at greater risk of severe COVID-19 infection and mortality.[63]

PANCREATITIS AFTER CORONAVIRUS DISEASE 2019 VACCINATION

The benefits of COVID-19 vaccination are indisputable. Only 2 cases of AP were reported in almost 38,000 patients during a phase 2/3 clinical trial of COVID-19 mRNA vaccine.[64] However, physicians should be aware of emerging side-effects, including severe abdominal pain after vaccination, which could indicate AP. The exact mechanisms of vaccine-induced AP are unclear but may be related to molecular mimicry. To our knowledge, only 6 cases of AP attributed to COVID-19 vaccination have been published.[65–70]

Alcohol-Induced Acute Pancreatitis During Coronavirus Disease 2019 Outbreak

COVID-19 lockdowns dramatically influenced the population's social behavior. Several studies have shown an increase in alcohol consumption in the general population during COVID-19 lockdowns. An increase in hospital admissions for alcohol-induced AP has been observed in some hospitals during these periods, which have decreased after the restrictions were eased.[71,72] However, this "shadow pandemic" of alcohol-related illnesses was not observed at all centers and all locations.[33]

Chronic Pancreatitis and Coronavirus Disease 2019

There is a paucity of data about CP during the pandemic. Most cases have an attributable cause, thus making it difficult to link SARS-CoV-2 to either an aggravation of an existing CP or a new diagnosis of CP.

Recommendations on CP surgery have been made. A large international survey on pancreatic surgery agreed that CP surgery should be postponed, unless the patient is experiencing lifethreatening complications.[73]

Pancreas Cancer and Pancreatic Surgery During the Pandemic

The pandemic has deeply affected the diagnostic, management, and referral pathways of pancreatic cancer worldwide, with significant geographic variability,[74] including suspension of patient visits, imaging and endoscopic examinations, and delays and changes of elective cancer therapies and surgeries. These changes inevitably affect short-term and long-term patient care and prognosis and possibly decrease overall survival, although the specific influence on patients' outcomes is still unknown.[75–83] In Italy, a reduction of 9.9% in new diagnosis of pancreatic cancer in 2020 compared with 2019 was reported.[84] More patients presented with more advanced pancreatic cancers in 2020 compared with 2019,[80,81] and the pandemic caused considerable emotional and social distress among these patients, suggesting the need for a psychological support network.[85,86] A third-level referral center in Italy recorded a 20% reduction in pancreatic resections during 2020 and a global survey from 267 centers in 37 countries reported a reduction in weekly pancreatic resections from 3 to 1.[73,87] Efforts should be made to reschedule pancreatic cancer surveillance programs and improve the staging and workup pathways to improve oncological outcomes.[88,89] In a large multicenter prospective cohort study on pancreas and liver surgery outcomes during the pandemic, patients without SARS-CoV-2 infection had acceptable morbidity and mortality, highlighting the need to protect patients and continue to evaluate them for pancreatic cancer surgery.[90]

Moreover, patients diagnosed with cancer require frequent hospital visits. They were found to have a 2-fold increase of COVID-19 infection, as compared with the general population.[91] Immunosuppression as a cancer treatment effect, elevated cytokine levels, altered expression of receptors for SARS-CoV-2, and a prothrombotic state in patients with various cancers may exacerbate the effects of COVID-19. SARS-CoV-2 infection was associated with a significant increase in perioperative morbidity and mortality.[90]

The optimal timing for surgery for pancreatic cancer is controversial, and no published guidelines exist on the timing for surgery for patients undergoing primary resection. The National Comprehensive Cancer Network (NCCN) guidelines recommend surgery at 4 to 8 weeks after completing neoadjuvant therapy.[92] Based on the finding that no differences in mortality were found among stage I patients with pancreatic adenocarcinoma who received neoadjuvant and adjuvant therapy, the Society of Surgical Oncology recommended the administration of neoadjuvant therapy to all patients with resectable pancreatic cancer. Other recommendations included the extension of neoadjuvant therapy or radiation therapy.[93,94]

The American College of Surgeons proposed an Elective Case Triage Guidelines for Surgical Care and categorized the growing severity of the COVID-19 pandemic in hospitals into 3 phases based on the availability of medical resources. Subsequently, a specific tier system for pancreatic surgery was proposed to guide pancreatic surgery for different pancreatic cancers according to patients' comorbidities, tumor malignant potential, and COVID-19 phase.[95] The European Society for Medical Oncology also developed specific guidelines for pancreatic cancer, defining priority grades for outpatient visits, imaging examinations, image-guided surgical procedures, and medical therapies to ensure the continuity of the oncological treatments during the pandemic.[96] An international survey on pancreatic surgery during COVID-19 also reached consensus on 13 statements and moderate agreement on 5 statements to guide pancreatic surgery.[73] National societies and expert centers developed consensus statements and analyzed the impact of COVID-19 on pancreas surgery to ensure optimal resource utilization and define treatment prioritization.[97–102]

Recommendations for the prophylaxis of venous thromboembolism (VTE) and for the treatment of established VTE for patients with cancer are similar, regardless of whether they have COVID-19. As such, patients with cancer and COVID-19 should be assessed for VTE risk similar to any other patient. Pharmacological prophylaxis should be given in the same dose and with the same anticoagulant but primary prophylaxis of VTE is not recommended in ambulatory patients with COVID-19 with cancer.[103]

New technologies, including telemedicine, have a role in the management of pancreatic cancer during the COVID-19 pandemic, and may gain increasing relevance in the future.[104]

SUMMARY

SARS-CoV-2 infection and AP share several pathophysiologic similarities but there is still a paucity of evidence to establish COVID-19 as a cause of AP. Complete etiological workup and attention to patients' comorbidities, chronic medications, and social habits, along with rigorous publishing guidelines, should guide future case reports.

COVID-19 also caused major challenges to pancreas cancer diagnosis and management, interrupting established management pathways. Several international and national concensus should be implemented as soon as possible to resume cancer treatments, including surgery, and minimize the negative pandemic effect on patient outcomes.

CLINICS CARE POINTS

- SARS-CoV-2 can cause pancreatic injury by several mechanisms, but it is yet to established as a cause of AP.
- Etiologic workup is of major importance in establishing AP cause, especially in CIOVID-19 positive patients.
- International and national guidelines and norms shloud be put in practice to minimize the effects of the pandemic in pancreatic cancer diagnosis and management.

DISCLOSURE

The authors have nothing to disclose.

REFERENCES

1. WHO. WHO Coronavirus Disease (COVID-19) Dashboard 2022, Available at: https://covid19.who.int/?adgroupsurvey=%7Badgroupsurvey%7D&gclid=EAIaIQobChMInp-Px8Le-QIVRpNmAh3-Xww9EAAYASABEgLA7PD_BwE. Accessed September 7, 2022.
2. Kariyawasam JC, Jayarajah U, Riza R, et al. Gastrointestinal manifestations in COVID-19. Trans R Soc Trop Med Hyg 2021;115(12):1362–88.
3. de-Madaria E, Capurso G. COVID-19 and acute pancreatitis: examining the causality. Nat Rev Gastroenterol Hepatol 2021;18(1):3–4.
4. Xiao F, Tang M, Zheng X, et al. Evidence for Gastrointestinal infection of SARS-CoV-2. Gastroenterology 2020;158(6):1831–3.e3.
5. Liu F, Long X, Zhang B, et al. ACE2 Expression in pancreas may cause pancreatic damage after SARS-CoV-2 infection. Clin Gastroenterol Hepatol 2020;18(9):2128–30.e2.
6. Pons S, Fodil S, Azoulay E, et al. The vascular endothelium: the cornerstone of organ dysfunction in severe SARS-CoV-2 infection. Crit Care 2020;24(1):353.
7. Schepis T, Larghi A, Papa A, et al. SARS-CoV2 RNA detection in a pancreatic pseudocyst sample. Pancreatology 2020;20(5):1011–2.
8. Hinojosa V, Gamboa E, Varon J. Pancreatic pseudocysts as a late manifestation of COVID-19. Cureus 2022;14(2):e22181.
9. Hanley B, Naresh KN, Roufosse C, et al. Histopathological findings and viral tropism in UK patients with severe fatal COVID-19: a post-mortem study. Lancet Microbe 2020;1(6):e245–53.
10. Boddu SK, Aurangabadkar G, Kuchay MS. New onset diabetes, type 1 diabetes and COVID-19. Diabetes Metab Syndr 2020;14(6):2211–7.
11. Unsworth R, Wallace S, Oliver NS, et al. New-onset Type 1 diabetes in children during COVID-19: Multicenter Regional Findings in the U.K. Diabetes Care 2020;43(11):e170–1.

12. Nayar M, Varghese C, Kanwar A, et al. SARS-CoV-2 infection is associated with an increased risk of idiopathic acute pancreatitis but not pancreatic exocrine insufficiency or diabetes: long-term results of the COVIDPAN study. Gut 2022; 71(7):1444–7.
13. Abramczyk U, Nowaczyński M, Słomczyński A, et al. Consequences of COVID-19 for the pancreas. Int J Mol Sci 2022;23(2).
14. Cure E, Cumhur Cure M. COVID-19 may affect the endocrine pancreas by activating Na+/H+ exchanger 2 and increasing lactate levels. J Endocrinol Invest 2020;43(8):1167–8.
15. Mehta P, McAuley DF, Brown M, et al. COVID-19: consider cytokine storm syndromes and immunosuppression. The Lancet 2020;395(10229):1033–4.
16. Shaharuddin SH, Wang V, Santos RS, et al. Deleterious effects of SARS-CoV-2 infection on human pancreatic cells. Front Cell Infect Microbiol 2021;11:678482.
17. Caruso P, Longo M, Esposito K, et al. Type 1 diabetes triggered by covid-19 pandemic: A potential outbreak? Diabetes Res Clin Pract 2020;164:108219.
18. Hegyi P, Szakács Z, Sahin-Tóth M. Lipotoxicity and cytokine storm in severe acute pancreatitis and COVID-19. Gastroenterology 2020;159(3):824–7.
19. Tang Q, Gao L, Tong Z, et al. Hyperlipidemia, COVID-19 and acute pancreatitis: a tale of three entities. Am J Med Sci 2022;364(3):257–63.
20. Liu B, Li M, Zhou Z, et al. Can we use interleukin-6 (IL-6) blockade for coronavirus disease 2019 (COVID-19)-induced cytokine release syndrome (CRS)? J Autoimmun 2020;111:102452.
21. Rao SA, Kunte AR. Interleukin-6: An early predictive marker for severity of acute pancreatitis. Indian J Crit Care Med 2017;21(7):424–8.
22. Iwasaki A, Yang Y. The potential danger of suboptimal antibody responses in COVID-19. Nat Rev Immunol 2020;20(6):339–41.
23. Wang D, Hu B, Hu C, et al. Clinical characteristics of 138 hospitalized patients with 2019 novel coronavirus-infected pneumonia in Wuhan, China. JAMA 2020; 323(11):1061–9.
24. Yamamoto K, Oka K, Sakae H, et al. Acute pancreatitis related to COVID-19 infection. Intern Med 2021;60(13):2159–60.
25. Khadka S, Williams K, Solanki S. Remdesivir-associated pancreatitis. Am J Ther 2022;29(4):e444–6.
26. Miyazaki K, Yoshimura Y, Miyata N, et al. Acute pancreatitis or severe increase in pancreatic enzyme levels following remdesivir administration in COVID-19 patients: an observational study. Sci Rep 2022;12(1):5323.
27. Kuraoka N, Hashimoto S, Matsui S. Remdesivir-induced pancreatitis in a patient with coronavirus disease 2019. Pancreas 2022;51(6):e88–9.
28. Liaquat H, Shupp B, Kapoor S, et al. High-dose prednisone for treatment of autoimmune pancreatitis in a patient with coronavirus disease 2019 (COVID-19) due to infection with severe acute respiratory syndrome coronavirus 2 (SARS-CoV-2). Am J Case Rep 2020;21:e926475.
29. Inamdar S, Benias PC, Liu Y, et al. Prevalence, risk factors, and outcomes of hospitalized patients with coronavirus disease 2019 presenting as acute pancreatitis. Gastroenterology 2020;159(6):2226–8.e2.
30. Ò Miró, Llorens P, Jiménez S, et al. Frequency of five unusual presentations in patients with COVID-19: results of the UMC-19-S(1). Epidemiol Infect 2020; 148:e189.
31. Ò Miró, Llorens P, Jiménez S, et al. A case-control emergency department-based analysis of acute pancreatitis in Covid-19: Results of the UMC-19-S(6). J Hepatobiliary Pancreat Sci 2021;28(11):953–66.

32. Çolak E. and Çiftci A.B., Acute biliary pancreatitis management during the coronavirus disease 2019 pandemic, *Healthcare (Basel)*, 10 (7), 2022, 1284.
33. Ramsey ML, Patel A, Sobotka LA, et al. Hospital trends of acute pancreatitis during the coronavirus disease 2019 pandemic. Pancreas 2022;51(5):422–6.
34. Ebib B, Bacaksiz F, Ekin N. Does COVID-19 cause pancreatitis? Arq Gastroenterol 2022;59(1):71–4.
35. Pezzilli R, Centanni S, Mondoni M, et al. Patients with coronavirus disease 2019 interstitial pneumonia exhibit pancreatic hyperenzymemia and not acute pancreatitis. Pancreas 2021;50(5):732–5.
36. Bacaksız F, Ebik B, Ekin N, et al. Pancreatic damage in COVID-19: Why? How? Int J Clin Pract 2021;75(10):e14692.
37. Troncone E, Salvatori S, Sena G, et al. Low frequency of acute pancreatitis in hospitalized COVID-19 patients. Pancreas 2021;50(3):393–8.
38. Ding P, Song B, Liu X, et al. Elevated pancreatic enzymes in ICU patients with COVID-19 in Wuhan, China: A retrospective study. Front Med (Lausanne) 2021; 8:663646.
39. Rasch S, Herner A, Schmid RM, et al. High lipasemia is frequent in Covid-19 associated acute respiratory distress syndrome. Pancreatology 2021;21(1): 306–11.
40. McNabb-Baltar J, Jin DX, Grover AS, et al. Lipase elevation in patients with COVID-19. Am J Gastroenterol 2020;115(8):1286–8.
41. Caruso S, Aloisio E, Dolci A, et al. Lipase elevation in serum of COVID-19 patients: frequency, extent of increase and clinical value. Clin Chem Lab Med 2022;60(1):135–42.
42. Juhász MF, Ocskay K, Kiss S, et al. Insufficient etiological workup of COVID-19-associated acute pancreatitis: A systematic review. World J Gastroenterol 2020; 26(40):6270–8.
43. Marchi G, Vianello A, Crisafulli E, et al. Cytomegalovirus-induced gastrointestinal bleeding and pancreatitis complicating severe Covid-19 pneumonia: A paradigmatic Case. Mediterr J Hematol Infect Dis 2020;12(1):e2020060.
44. Mitrovic M, Tadic B, Jankovic A, et al. Fatal gastrointestinal bleeding associated with acute pancreatitis as a complication of Covid-19: a case report. J Int Med Res 2022;50(5). 3000605221098179.
45. Goyal H, Sachdeva S, Perisetti A, et al. Hyperlipasemia and potential pancreatic injury patterns in COVID-19: A marker of severity or innocent bystander? Gastroenterology 2021;160(3):946–8.e2.
46. Benias PC, Inamdar S, Wee D, et al. Analysis of outcomes in COVID-19 patients with varying degrees of hyperlipasemia. Pancreas 2021;50(9):1310–3.
47. Li G, Liu T, Jin G, et al. Serum amylase elevation is associated with adverse clinical outcomes in patients with coronavirus disease 2019. Aging (Albany NY) 2021;13(20):23442–58.
48. Ramsey ML, Elmunzer BJ, Krishna SG. Serum lipase elevations in COVID-19 patients reflect critical illness and not acute pancreatitis. Clin Gastroenterol Hepatol 2021;19(9):1982–7.
49. Kiyak M, Düzenli T. Lipase elevation on admission predicts worse clinical outcomes in patients with COVID-19. Pancreatology 2022;22(5):665–70.
50. Singh RR, Chhabra P, Kumta NA. Does hyperlipasemia predict worse clinical outcomes in COVID-19? A multicenter retrospective cohort study. J Clin Gastroenterol 2022;56(3):e227–31.

51. Haydar FG, Otal Y, Avcioglu G. Evaluation of patients with acute pancreatitis associated with SARS-CoV-2 (COVID-19); The importance of lipase/lymphocyte ratio in predicting mortality. Bratisl Lek Listy 2022;123(6):428–34.
52. Zhang D, Wang M, Zhang Y, et al. Novel insight on marker genes and pathogenic peripheral neutrophil subtypes in acute pancreatitis. Front Immunol 2022;13:964622.
53. Wang K, Luo J, Tan F, et al. Acute pancreatitis as the initial manifestation in 2 cases of COVID-19 in Wuhan, China. Open Forum Infect Dis 2020;7(9):ofaa324.
54. Grusova G, Bruha R, Bircakova B, et al. Pancreatic injury in patients with SARS-Cov-2 (COVID-19) infection: a retrospective analysis of CT findings. Gastroenterol Res Pract 2021;2021:5390337.
55. Stephens JR, Wong JLC, Broomhead R, et al. Raised serum amylase in patients with COVID-19 may not be associated with pancreatitis. Br J Surg 2021;108(4): e152–3.
56. Mutneja HR, Bhurwal A, Arora S, et al. Acute pancreatitis in patients with COVID-19 is more severe and lethal: a systematic review and meta-analysis. Scand J Gastroenterol 2021;56(12):1467–72.
57. Annie FH, Chumbe J, Searls L, et al. Acute pancreatitis due to COVID-19 active infection. Cureus 2021;13(12):e20410.
58. Pandanaboyana S, Moir J, Leeds JS, et al. SARS-CoV-2 infection in acute pancreatitis increases disease severity and 30-day mortality: COVID PAN collaborative study. Gut 2021;70(6):1061–9.
59. Samanta J, Mahapatra SJ, Kumar N, et al. Virus related acute pancreatitis and virus superinfection in the 'Dual disease' model of acute pancreatitis and SARS-Co-V2 infection: a multicentre prospective study. Pancreatology 2022;22(3): 339–47.
60. Ahmed A, Fisher JC, Pochapin MB, et al. Hyperlipasemia in absence of acute pancreatitis is associated with elevated D-dimer and adverse outcomes in COVID 19 disease. Pancreatology 2021;21(4):698–703.
61. Karaali R, Topal F. Evaluating the effect of SARS-Cov-2 infection on prognosis and mortality in patients with acute pancreatitis. Am J Emerg Med 2021;49: 378–84.
62. Meric S, Aktokmakyan TV, Tokocin M, et al. COVID-19 and acute biliary pancreatitis: comparative analysis between the normal period and COVID-19 pandemic. Ann Ital Chir 2021;92:728–31.
63. Huang BZ, Sidell MA, Wu BU, et al. Pre-Existing pancreatitis and elevated risks of COVID-19 severity and mortality. Gastroenterology 2022;162(6):1758–60.e3.
64. Document VB. Pfizer-BioNTech COVID-19 Vaccine VRBPAC Briefing Document. In: Administration UFaD, editor. 2020. Available at: https://www.fda.gov/media/144246/download. Accessed December 10, 2020.
65. Parkash O, Sharko A, Farooqi A, et al. Acute pancreatitis: A possible side effect of COVID-19 vaccine. Cureus 2021;13(4):e14741.
66. Cieślewicz A., Dudek M., Krela-Kaźmierczak I., et al., Pancreatic injury after COVID-19 vaccine-A case report, *Vaccines (Basel)*, 9 (6), 2021, 576.
67. Ozaka S, Kodera T, Ariki S, et al. Acute pancreatitis soon after COVID-19 vaccination: a case report. Medicine (Baltimore) 2022;101(2):e28471.
68. Cacdac R, Jamali A, Jamali R, et al. Acute pancreatitis as an adverse effect of COVID-19 vaccination. SAGE Open Med Case Rep 2022;10. 2050313x221131169.

69. Patel AH, Amin R, Lalos AT. Acute liver injury and IgG4-related autoimmune pancreatitis following mRNA-based COVID-19 vaccination. Hepatol Forum 2022;3(3):97–9.
70. Walter T, Connor S, Stedman C, et al. A case of acute necrotising pancreatitis following the second dose of Pfizer-BioNTech COVID-19 mRNA vaccine. Br J Clin Pharmacol 2022;88(3):1385–6.
71. Mak WK, Di Mauro D, Pearce E, et al. Hospital admissions from alcohol-related acute pancreatitis during the COVID-19 pandemic: A single-centre study. World J Clin Cases 2022;10(25):8837–43.
72. Itoshima H, Shin JH, Takada D, et al. The impact of the COVID-19 epidemic on hospital admissions for alcohol-related liver disease and pancreatitis in Japan. Sci Rep 2021;11(1):14054.
73. Oba A, Stoop TF, Löhr M, et al. Global survey on pancreatic surgery during the COVID-19 pandemic. Ann Surg 2020;272(2):e87–93.
74. Kajiwara Saito M, Morishima T, Ma C, et al. Diagnosis and treatment of digestive cancers during COVID-19 in Japan: a cancer Registry-based Study on the Impact of COVID-19 on Cancer Care in Osaka (CanReCO). PLoS One 2022; 17(9):e0274918.
75. Kuzuu K, Misawa N, Ashikari K, et al. Gastrointestinal cancer stage at diagnosis before and during the COVID-19 pandemic in Japan. JAMA Netw Open 2021; 4(9):e2126334.
76. McKay SC, Pathak S, Wilkin RJW, et al. Impact of SARS-CoV-2 pandemic on pancreatic cancer services and treatment pathways: United Kingdom experience. HPB (Oxford) 2021;23(11):1656–65.
77. Katona BW, Mahmud N, Dbouk M, et al. COVID-19 related pancreatic cancer surveillance disruptions amongst high-risk individuals. Pancreatology 2021; 21(6):1048–51.
78. Tejedor-Tejada J, Gómez-Díez C, Robles Gaitero S, et al. Impact of the SARS-CoV-2 pandemic on pancreatic cancer: diagnosis and short-term survival. Rev Esp Enferm Dig 2022;114(8):509–10.
79. Peacock HM, Tambuyzer T, Verdoodt F, et al. Decline and incomplete recovery in cancer diagnoses during the COVID-19 pandemic in Belgium: a year-long, population-level analysis. ESMO Open 2021;6(4):100197.
80. Paluri R, Laursen A, Gaeta J, et al. Impact of the COVID-19 pandemic on management of patients with metastatic pancreatic ductal adenocarcinoma in the United States. Oncologist 2022;27(6):e518–23.
81. Brugel M, Letrillart L, Evrard C, et al. Impact of the COVID-19 pandemic on disease stage and treatment for patients with pancreatic adenocarcinoma: A French comprehensive multicentre ambispective observational cohort study (CAPANCOVID). Eur J Cancer 2022;166:8–20.
82. Madge O., Brodey A., Bowen J., et al., The COVID-19 pandemic is associated with reduced survival after pancreatic ductal adenocarcinoma diagnosis: A single-centre retrospective analysis, *J Clin Med*, 11 (9), 2022, 2574.
83. Balakrishnan A, Lesurtel M, Siriwardena AK, et al. Delivery of hepato-pancreato-biliary surgery during the COVID-19 pandemic: an European-African Hepato-Pancreato-Biliary Association (E-AHPBA) cross-sectional survey. HPB (Oxford) 2020;22(8):1128–34.
84. Buscarini E, Benedetti A, Monica F, et al. Changes in digestive cancer diagnosis during the SARS-CoV-2 pandemic in Italy: A nationwide survey. Dig Liver Dis 2021;53(6):682–8.

85. Brito M, Laranjo A, Sabino J, et al. Digestive oncology in the COVID-19 pandemic era. GE Port J Gastroenterol 2021;579(5):1–8.
86. Alexander A., Fung S., Eichler M., et al., Quality of life in patients with pancreatic cancer before and during the COVID-19 pandemic, *Int J Environ Res Public Health*, 19 (6), 2022, 3731.
87. Marchegiani G, Perri G, Bianchi B, et al. Pancreatic surgery during COVID-19 pandemic: major activity disruption of a third-level referral center during 2020. Updates Surg 2022;74(3):953–61.
88. Moslim MA, Hall MJ, Meyer JE, et al. Pancreatic cancer in the era of COVID-19 pandemic: Which one is the lesser of two evils? World J Clin Oncol 2021;12(2): 54–60.
89. Pergolini I, Demir IE, Stöss C, et al. Effects of COVID-19 pandemic on the treatment of pancreatic cancer: A perspective from Central Europe. Dig Surg 2021; 38(2):158–65.
90. McKay SC. Outcomes of patients undergoing elective liver and pancreas cancer surgery during the SARS-CoV-2 pandemic: an international, multicentre, prospective cohort study. HPB (Oxford) 2022;24(10):1668–78.
91. Yu J, Ouyang W, Chua MLK, et al. SARS-CoV-2 Transmission in patients with cancer at a tertiary care hospital in Wuhan, China. JAMA Oncol 2020;6(7): 1108–10.
92. Tempero MA, Malafa MP, Al-Hawary M, et al. Pancreatic Adenocarcinoma, Version 2.2017, NCCN Clinical Practice Guidelines in Oncology. J Natl Compr Cancer Netw J Natl Compr Canc Netw 2017;15(8):1028–61.
93. Datta SK, Belini G, Singh M, et al. Survival outcomes between surgery with adjuvant therapy compared to neoadjuvant therapy with surgery in stage I pancreatic adenocarcinoma: Results from a large national cancer database. J Clin Oncol 2019;37(4_suppl):335.
94. Fligor SC, Wang S, Allar BG, et al. Gastrointestinal malignancies and the COVID-19 pandemic: Evidence-based triage to surgery. J Gastrointest Surg 2020;24(10):2357–73.
95. Kato H, Asano Y, Arakawa S, et al. Surgery for pancreatic tumors in the midst of COVID-19 pandemic. World J Clin Cases 2021;9(18):4460–6.
96. Catanese S, Pentheroudakis G, Douillard JY, et al. ESMO Management and treatment adapted recommendations in the COVID-19 era: Pancreatic Cancer. ESMO Open 2020;5(Suppl 3):e000804.
97. Jones CM, Radhakrishna G, Aitken K, et al. Considerations for the treatment of pancreatic cancer during the COVID-19 pandemic: the UK consensus position. Br J Cancer 2020;123(5):709–13.
98. Kędzierska-Kapuza K, Witkowski G, Baumgart-Gryn K, et al. Impact of COVID-19 on pancreatic cancer surgery: A high-volume Polish center experience. Adv Clin Exp Med 2022;31(4):389–98.
99. Rodriguez-Freixinos V, Capdevila J, Pavel M, et al. Practical recommendations for the management of patients with gastroenteropancreatic and thoracic (carcinoid) neuroendocrine neoplasms in the COVID-19 era. Eur J Cancer 2021;144: 200–14.
100. Marchegiani G, Paiella S, Malleo G, et al. Love (Pancreatic Surgery) in the time of cholera (COVID-19). Dig Surg 2020;37(6):524–6.
101. Doyle JP, Patel PH, Doran SLF, et al. The cancer hub approach for upper gastrointestinal surgery during COVID-19 pandemic: Outcomes from a UK cancer centre. Ann Surg Oncol 2022;1–10. https://doi.org/10.1245/s10434-022-12571-4.

102. Pietrantonio F, Morano F, Niger M, et al. Systemic treatment of patients with gastrointestinal cancers during the COVID-19 outbreak: COVID-19-adapted Recommendations of the National Cancer Institute of Milan. Clin Colorectal Cancer 2020;19(3):156–64.
103. Farge D, Frere C, Connors JM, et al. 2022 international clinical practice guidelines for the treatment and prophylaxis of venous thromboembolism in patients with cancer, including patients with COVID-19. Lancet Oncol 2022;23(7):e334–47.
104. Tripepi M, Pizzocaro E, Giardino A, et al. Telemedicine and pancreatic cancer: a systematic review. Telemed J E Health 2022. https://doi.org/10.1089/tmj.2022.0140.

A Surgical Perspective of Gastrointestinal Manifestations and Complications of COVID-19 Infection

Anthony Gebran, MD[1], Ander Dorken-Gallastegi, MD[1], Haytham M.A. Kaafarani, MD, MPH*

KEYWORDS

• COVID-19 • Mesenteric ischemia • Pancreatitis • Cholecystitis • GI surgery

INTRODUCTION

The coronavirus disease 2019 (COVID-19), caused by the severe acute respiratory syndrome coronavirus 2 (SARS-CoV-2), has quickly spread over the world since December 2019. The most common symptoms of COVID-19 disease include fever, cough, dyspnea, fatigue, and myalgia. However, COVID-19 is a systemic disease that can affect various organs throughout the body. Gastrointestinal (GI) symptoms have been reported in 16% to 33% of all COVID-19 patients and in 75% of critically ill patients.[1,2]

This chapter reviews the GI manifestations of COVID-19 as well as their diagnostic and treatment modalities from a surgical perspective.

GASTROINTESTINAL MANIFESTATIONS

The most common presenting GI symptoms of COVID-19 disease include nausea, vomiting, diarrhea, and abdominal pain.[3] More severe GI complications ranging from ileus to life-threatening mesenteric ischemia arise in 74% to 86% of critically ill patients with COVID-19 during their frequently lengthy hospitalization.[2,4] These complications might be preceded by warning signs such as increasing abdominal distension and new or increasing vasopressor requirements.

Division of Trauma, Emergency Surgery, and Surgical Critical Care, Massachusetts General Hospital, Boston, MA, USA

[1] Present address: Division of Trauma, Emergency Surgery and Surgical Critical Care, Massachusetts General Hospital, 165 Cambridge Street, Suite 810, Boston, MA 02114.

* Corresponding author. Division of Trauma, Emergency Surgery and Surgical Critical Care, Massachusetts General Hospital, 165 Cambridge Street, Suite 810, Boston, MA 02114.

E-mail address: hkaafarani@mgh.harvard.edu

Gastroenterol Clin N Am 52 (2023) 49–58
https://doi.org/10.1016/j.gtc.2022.10.001

Acute Cholecystitis

Acute cholecystitis refers to acute inflammation of the gallbladder, either due to obstruction of the cystic duct by a gallstone (calculous) or due to dysfunction of gallbladder emptying in the absence of stones (acalculous). Acute cholecystitis is one possible complication of COVID-19 infection, particularly among critically ill patients.[2,4–8] When it occurs, acute cholecystitis is usually acalculous and the causal mechanism is unclear. Gallbladder wall hypomotility is common in critical illness; however, the identification of SARS-CoV2 RNA in gallbladder epithelial cells and bile could indicate a more specific causal role of the virus.[9–11] Few case reports have detailed the occurrence of gangrenous cholecystitis leading to perforation. In one case this was possibly due to the increased risk of thrombosis and organ ischemia associated with COVID-19.[12,13]

Antibiotics and percutaneous cholecystostomy should be attempted first in the management of acute cholecystitis among critically ill patients with COVID-19.[14,15] Cholecystectomy should be reserved for cases where percutaneous drainage has failed.[16] In a study conducted by the COVIDSurg Collaborative during the early phases of the pandemic, 145 patients with COVID-19 who underwent cholecystectomy had a 30-day mortality of 10.3%, despite most not being critically ill preoperatively. Mortality risk was particularly exacerbated among patients who had preoperative respiratory signs or symptoms of COVID-19 as compared with those who did not (19.2% vs 0.0%, $P < 0.001$).[17]

Acute Colonic Pseudoobstruction

Ogilvie syndrome or acute colonic pseudoobstruction refers to colonic distension in the absence of mechanical obstruction, and it is most commonly caused by infection, electrolyte imbalance, and opioids. Several cases of acute colonic pseudoobstruction have been reported among critically ill COVID-19 patients.[2,18–22]

The exact cause of acute colonic pseudoobstruction in critically ill patients with COVID-19 is unknown. Previously reported effects of SARS-CoV2 on the nervous system (eg, Guillain-Barré syndrome, transverse myelitis, encephalitis) suggest that a similar impact of the virus on mesenteric nerves could be the cause. Specifically, acute colonic pseudoobstruction might be caused by a loss of parasympathetic regulation of bowels if SARS-CoV2 invades the myenteric plexus.

In a stable patient without evident sepsis or shock, conservative management should be attempted first; this should include bowel rest, colonic decompression with a rectal tube or by colonoscopy, electrolyte replacement, administration of intravenous fluids, treatment of an underlying infection, and discontinuation of any drugs that could worsen the paralytic ileus (eg, opioids, sedatives). Although there have been some reports of clinical improvement with the use of acetylcholinesterase inhibitors such as neostigmine, the evidence supporting its use remains weak. Surgery is reserved for cases that failed conservative management, especially if there is progression to intestinal wall necrosis and perforation. Therefore, early diagnosis and appropriate management is essential for acute colonic pseudoobstruction, while maintaining a high index of suspicion for ischemia and perforation in case of clinical deterioration.

Acute Liver Injury and Transaminitis

Acute liver injury, defined as an elevated alanine aminotransferase (ALT) and aspartate aminotransferase (AST) levels, is a common complication of COVID-19 disease and can indicate a severe disease course.

In 2 large cohort studies from the United States, elevations in ALT and AST were detected in 29% to 63% of patients.[23,24] In a study of 2273 SARS-CoV-2-positive and 1108 SARS-CoV-2-negative hospitalized patients, SARS-CoV-2-positive patients had greater initial and peak ALT than those who had a similar clinical presentation but tested negative for SARS-CoV2.[25] Overall, 45% of SARS-CoV2-positive patients had mild liver injury (peak ALT <2 times the upper limit of normal [ULN]), 22% had moderate liver injury (peak ALT 2–5 times the ULN), and 6% had severe liver injury (peak ALT >5 times the ULN).

A systematic review including 9889 confirmed cases of COVID-19 from a single country reported an incidence of liver injury of 24.7%.[26] Patients with severe COVID-19 were twice as likely to suffer liver injury than those with nonsevere COVID-19.

The cause of acute liver injury in patients with COVID-19 is uncertain but likely involves direct, viral-mediated damage and an indirect, immune-mediated inflammatory response.[27] Direct viral-induced damage could be mediated through the angiotensin-converting enzyme 2 (ACE2) receptors found in biliary and hepatic endothelial cells.[28–30] Indirect immune-mediated damage results from cytokine storm with severe COVID-19, as evidenced by elevated C-reactive protein, serum ferritin, interleukin-6 (IL-6), and IL-2, which can lead to multisystem organ failure.[31,32] Additional liver damage could be the result of concomitant critical illness (eg, sepsis, shock). The degree of elevation of transaminases (notably peak ALT) was shown to be an independent predictor of mortality among patients with COVID-19.[25]

Some studies have supported regular testing of liver transaminases in patients with COVID-19.[33] The American Association for the Study of Liver Diseases (AASLD) recommends nonetheless keeping a broad differential when dealing with elevated transaminase levels in the setting of COVID-19 and exploring other causes (eg, hepatitis A, B, or C virus, myositis).[34]

Acute Pancreatitis

Acute pancreatitis is a complex disease resulting from inappropriate activation of digestive enzymes leading to autodigestion of the pancreas. Acute pancreatitis is an uncommon complication of COVID-19. According to a large cohort study of 11,883 hospitalized patients with COVID-19 from 12 hospitals, the incidence of acute pancreatitis was 0.27%.[35] In another retrospective study of more than 63,000 patients with COVID-19 seen in the emergency department, the incidence of acute pancreatitis was reported at 0.07%.[36]

It remains unclear whether acute pancreatitis that develops in the setting of COVID-19 disease is a direct result of SARS-CoV2 infection.[37] The presence of ACE2 receptors in pancreatic ductal, acinar, and islet cells as well as the isolation of SARS-CoV2 from a pancreatic pseudocyst point to a possible association.[38–40] Ex-vivo and in-vivo studies as well as human autopsies have demonstrated that SARS-CoV-2 infection can target β cells of the human pancreas and lead to metabolic dysregulation.[41,42] Similar studies are needed to ascertain the association between COVID-19 and pancreatitis.

COVID-19–related acute pancreatitis is treated similarly to non–COVID-19–related acute pancreatitis. Supportive therapy with fluid resuscitation, pain control, and nutritional support is the mainstay of treatment in uncomplicated cases. Percutaneous, endoscopic, or surgical debridement may be required if necrotizing pancreatitis supervenes.[43]

Ileus and Feeding Intolerance

Ileus refers to obstipation and feeding intolerance resulting from disruption of normal bowel peristalsis in the absence of mechanical obstruction. Significant ileus and feeding intolerance have been reported in 46% to 56% of critically ill patients with COVID-19 admitted to an intensive care unit.[2]

Critically ill patients with COVID-19 frequently require substantial doses of sedatives and opiates for ventilator synchrony, which can independently result in decreased intestinal function. It remains unclear whether SARS-CoV2 infection plays a direct role in causing this pathology.

Management of COVID-19–related ileus is no different from the management of ileus unassociated with COVID-19 infection. Supportive care is the mainstay of treatment and includes electrolyte replacement as necessary, maintenance of fluids, bowel rest, and intestinal decompression as needed.

Mesenteric Ischemia

Mesenteric ischemia can affect the small and/or large intestine and is caused either by a reduction in intestinal blood flow from systemic hypotension or by thromboembolic occlusion of the mesenteric vessels.[44] Its incidence was reported to be 3.8% to 4% in cohort studies of critically ill patients with COVID-19 admitted to one institution.[1,2]

Although the coagulopathy caused by COVID-19 is not fully understood, several studies show an association between SARS-CoV2 infection and mesenteric ischemia. Following matching based on baseline characteristics and clinical condition, critically ill patients with COVID-19 were significantly more likely to develop mesenteric ischemia than similarly ill patients without COVID-19.[45]

The diagnosis of mesenteric ischemia is typically confirmed by imaging. Contrast-enhanced computed tomography (CT) scan of the abdomen plays an important role in the detection of this disease and should be considered early on in the management of critically ill patients who exhibit GI symptoms.[46] Ischemic bowel should be suspected if pneumatosis intestinalis, thick edematous intestine, and/or portal venous gas are present.[47] When using intravenous contrast, arterial phase imaging may reveal filling defects in the thoracoabdominal aorta or mesenteric arteries, which could indicate acute thromboembolic events.[48–52] Alternatively, delayed venous phase imaging may reveal filling defects in the mesenteric and/or portal veins.[46,48,51] Finally, a considerable number of patients develop mesenteric ischemia despite having patent and well-perfusing mesenteric vessels on imaging.[1,2,53] Such findings suggest a microvascular cause of mesenteric ischemia in a significant number of patients. **Fig. 1** shows the CT scan findings of a patient with COVID-19 who developed mesenteric ischemia and small bowel perforation.

Laboratory findings can include increasing lactate, elevated D-dimers, leukocytosis, and unexplained metabolic acidosis; however, such laboratory tests might be normal early on before metabolic alterations occur. Those findings are also nonspecific and could be present in other conditions, such as severe viral sepsis in the absence of mesenteric ischemia.[54]

Surgical resection of any necrotic bowel is the mainstay treatment of mesenteric ischemia in the setting of COVID-19 disease. When there is evidence of proximal arterial thromboembolic disease, endovascular thrombectomy can be used to reopen blocked mesenteric arteries and restore blood flow to the intestines.[48,55] Anticoagulants may play a role in treating mesenteric ischemia; however, there is no compelling evidence to support their use prophylactically. The only available data come from case reports describing a reversal of bowel ischemia in hemodynamically stable patients who were treated conservatively with anticoagulation.[56,57]

On intraoperative gross examination of the bowel, many surgeons identified necrotic tissue, punctuate lesions, and/or frank perforation. Surgeons also reported peculiar findings of well-demarcated yellow discoloration with spotty or

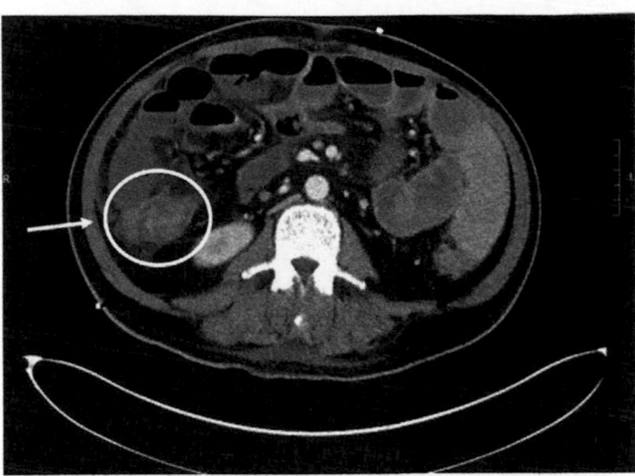

Fig. 1. Abdominal CT scan in a patient diagnosed with COVID-19 infection demonstrating small intestinal ischemia with perforation and loss of integrity of the small bowel wall in the right lower quadrant contiguous with a fluid and gas-containing collection.

circumferential distribution on the antimesenteric side.[53] Pathologic specimens may demonstrate sharp demarcation between areas of mucosal necrosis and viable mucosa, transmural infarction, and fibrin thrombi in small vessels underlying areas of necrosis.[58–60]

PATHOPHYSIOLOGY

The exact pathophysiology of COVID-related GI complications is unknown. The high rate of GI complications in patients with COVID-19 makes it more likely that they are not just a manifestation of critical illness but are at least in part caused by COVID-19. A propensity score–matched analysis of 184 critically ill patients with acute respiratory distress syndrome (ARDS) showed that more patients with COVID-19 ARDS developed mesenteric ischemia (4% vs 0%), elevated liver enzymes (55% vs 27%), and ileus (48% vs 22%).[61] In addition, certain GI complications might manifest differently in patients with versus without COVID-19. Although mesenteric ischemia in critical illness affects watershed areas, patients with COVID-19 often present with patchy areas of necrosis throughout the entire small bowel (**Fig. 2**).[1,2,53] As a result, illness severity alone is unlikely to explain the increased rates of GI complications, and other COVID disease-specific mechanisms may occur.

Identification of Severe Acute Respiratory Syndrome Coronavirus 2 in the Gastrointestinal Tract

SARS-CoV2 RNA or proteins have been isolated from several parts of the GI tract in patients known to have COVID-19 disease.

Several studies have reported elevated viral loads in fecal samples of patients with COVID-19 disease. In a systematic review and meta-analysis of 1636 patients with COVID-19, 43% of patients had evidence of fecal SARS-CoV-2 RNA. Patients with GI symptoms had a higher proportion of detectable fecal SARS-CoV-2 RNA as compared with those without GI symptoms (52.4% vs 25.9%; odds ratio [OR] = 2.4). The difference was most notable for patients who developed diarrhea (51.6% vs 24.0%; OR = 3.0) versus those without diarrhea. Fecal shedding also persisted longer than respiratory shedding (mean duration: 21.8 days vs 14.7 days; mean difference = 7.1 days).[62]

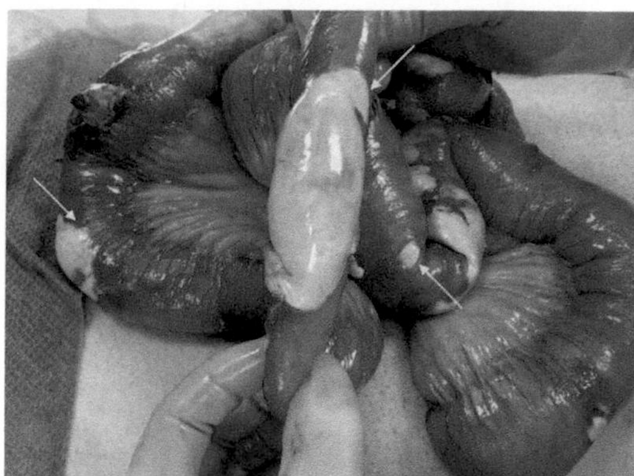

Fig. 2. Patchy antimesenteric bowel necrosis with bright yellow discoloration and clear demarcation in a patient diagnosed with COVID-19 infection. (*From* Kaafarani HMA, el Moheb M, Hwabejire JO, et al. Gastrointestinal Complications in Critically Ill Patients With COVID-19. Ann Surg. 2020;272(2):e61-e62. https://doi.org/10.1097/SLA.0000000000004004; with permission.)

High SARS-CoV2 viral loads have been documented by reverse transcription–polymerase chain reaction inside a pancreatic pseudocyst's fluid in the setting of COVID-19 disease.[40]

Viral proteins have been identified in the cytoplasm of gallbladder epithelial cells in several patients[9,10] and in the bile of one patient with COVID-19 disease.[11]

Angiotensin-Converting Enzyme 2 Receptor Interaction

Intestinal epithelium contains the second highest expression of ACE2 receptors in the body after the lungs.[49] Specifically, the ileum is the most commonly involved region of ischemia in COVID-related bowel disease and has a very high level of ACE2 expression.[1,2,48,53,63] Other sites of ACE2 expression include the epithelial cells of the gallbladder and ductal, acinar, and islet cells of the pancreas.[38,39] The virus could attach to the ACE2 receptors in the GI tract, translocate to the submucosal tissue, and damage the underlying tissue and vasculature, resulting in various pathologies.[64]

Microvascular Thrombosis

Thromboembolic events are a well-documented complication of SARS-CoV2 infection.[65] Presentation can include cerebrovascular accidents, strokes, deep vein thrombosis, renal failure, and mesenteric ischemia. In the latter, SARS-CoV2 has a higher propensity toward microvasculature and often spares large mesenteric arteries. Microscopic analysis of resected intestinal tissue revealed fibrin microthrombi in capillaries beneath necrotic zones.[66]

CLINICS CARE POINTS

- Although COVID-19 is primarily characterized as a respiratory infection, it has serious extrapulmonary manifestations including serious GI complications.
- Diarrhea, nausea, vomiting, and abdominal pain are the most common GI manifestations seen in patients with COVID-19, accounting for up to one-third of early symptoms.

- Critically ill patients with COVID-19 can experience a wide range of GI complications ranging from ileus to life-threatening mesenteric ischemia.
- The cause of GI manifestations in COVID-19 is multifactorial. The propensity of the virus for ACE2 receptors and their high expression in the GI tract, viral isolation in GI tissues, and microvascular coagulopathy support a role of SARS-CoV2 in the reported GI complications.

REFERENCES

1. El Moheb M, Christensen MA, Naar L, et al. Comment on "'gastrointestinal complications in critically ill patients with COVID-19'" an update. Ann Surg 2020; 274(6):e821–3. Published online.
2. Kaafarani HMA, el Moheb M, Hwabejire JO, et al. Gastrointestinal complications in critically ill patients with COVID-19. Ann Surg 2020;272(2):e61–2.
3. Tabesh E, Soheilipour M, Sami R, et al. Gastrointestinal manifestations in patients with coronavirus disease-2019 (COVID-19): Impact on clinical outcomes. J Res Med Sci 2022;27(1):32.
4. Sun JK, Liu Y, Zou L, et al. Acute gastrointestinal injury in critically ill patients with COVID-19 in Wuhan, China. World J Gastroenterol 2020;26(39):6087–97.
5. Hossein Hassani A, Beheshti A, Almasi F, et al. Unusual gastrointestinal manifestations of COVID-19: two case reports. Gastroenterol Hepatol Bed Bench 2020; 13(4):410–4.
6. Alhassan SM, Iqbal P, Fikrey L, et al. Post COVID 19 acute acalculous cholecystitis raising the possibility of underlying dysregulated immune response, a case report. Ann Med Surg 2020;60:434–7.
7. Puig G, Giménez-Milà M, Campistol E, et al. Development of concomitant diseases in COVID-19 critically ill patients. Rev Esp Anestesiol Reanim(Engl Ed) 2021;68(1):37–40.
8. Scutari R, Piermatteo L, Manuelli MC, et al. Long-term sars-cov-2 infection associated with viral dissemination in different body fluids including bile in two patients with acute cholecystitis. Life 2020;10(11):1–9.
9. Hong X, Ho J, Li P, et al. Evidence of SARS-CoV-2 infection in gallbladder and aggravating cholecystitis to septic shock: a case report. Ann Translational Med 2021;9(21):1631.
10. Balaphas A, Gkoufa K, Meyer J, et al. COVID-19 can mimic acute cholecystitis and is associated with the presence of viral RNA in the gallbladder wall. J Hepatol 2020;73(6):1566–8.
11. Liao Y, Wang B, Wang J, et al. SARS-CoV-2 in the bile of a patient with COVID-19-associated gallbladder disease. Endoscopy 2020;12(1148):52.
12. Bruni A, Garofalo E, Zuccalà V, et al. Histopathological findings in a COVID-19 patient affected by ischemic gangrenous cholecystitis. World J Emerg Surg 2020;15(1).
13. Alam W, Karam K. Gangrenous cholecystitis as a potential complication of COVID-19: a case report. Clin Med Insights: Case Rep 2021;14. https://doi.org/10.1177/11795476211042459.
14. Ying M, Lu B, Pan J, et al. COVID-19 with acute cholecystitis: a case report. BMC Infect Dis 2020;20(1). https://doi.org/10.1186/s12879-020-05164-7.
15. Çiyiltepe H, Yıldırım G, Fersahoğlu MM, et al. Clinical approach to patients admitted to the emergency room due to acute cholecystitis during the COVID-19 pandemic and percutaneous cholecystostomy experience. Ulus Travma Acil Cerrahi Derg 2021;27(1):34–42.

16. Mattone E, Sofia M, Schembari E, et al. Acute acalculous cholecystitis on a COVID-19 patient: a case report. Ann Med Surg 2020;58:73–5.
17. Gebran A, Gaitanidis A, Argandykov D, et al. Mortality & pulmonary complications in emergency general surgery patients with mortality COVID-19: a large international multicenter study. J Trauma Acute Care Surg 2022;93(1):59–65. Published online.
18. Sattar Y, Connerney M, Rauf H, et al. Three cases of COVID-19 disease with colonic manifestations. Am J Gastroenterol 2020;115(6):948–50.
19. Ibrahim YS, Karuppasamy G, Parambil Jv, et al. Case report: paralytic ileus: a potential extrapulmonary manifestation of severe COVID-19. Am J Trop Med Hyg 2020;103(4):1600–3.
20. Chong C, Airini IN, Abdul MN. Ogilvie's syndrome - a complication of severe COVID-19 infection. Mal J Med Health Sci 2022;18(1):375–7.
21. Zhang H, Li HB, Lyu JR, et al. Specific ACE2 expression in small intestinal enterocytes may cause gastrointestinal symptoms and injury after 2019-nCoV infection. Int J Infect Dis 2020;96:19–24.
22. Wang J, Marusca G, Tariq T, et al. Ogilvie Syndrome and COVID-19 infection. J Med Cases 2021;12(8):328–31.
23. Richardson S, Hirsch JS, Narasimhan M, et al. Presenting characteristics, comorbidities, and outcomes among 5700 patients hospitalized with COVID-19 in the New York City area. JAMA 2020;323(20):2052–9.
24. Goyal P, Choi JJ, Pinheiro LC, et al. Clinical characteristics of Covid-19 in New York City. N Engl J Med 2020;382(24):2372–4.
25. Phipps MM, Barraza LH, Lasota ED, et al. Acute liver injury in COVID-19: prevalence and association with clinical outcomes in a large. U.S Cohort 2020;72(3). https://doi.org/10.1002/hep.31404/suppinfo.
26. Zhao X, Lei Z, Gao F, et al. The impact of coronavirus disease 2019 (COVID-19) on liver injury in China A systematic review and meta-analysis. Medicine (United States) 2021;100(4). https://doi.org/10.1097/MD.0000000000024369.
27. Sun J, Aghemo A, Forner A, et al. COVID-19 and liver disease. Liver Int 2020; 40(6):1278–81.
28. Wang D, Hu B, Hu C, et al. Clinical characteristics of 138 hospitalized patients with 2019 novel coronavirus-infected pneumonia in Wuhan, China JAMA | original investigation | caring for the critically ill patient. JAMA 2020;323(11):1061–9.
29. Chai X, Hu L, Zhang Y, et al. Specific ACE2 expression in cholangiocytes may cause liver damage after 2019-nCoV infection. doi:10.1101/2020.02.03.931766
30. Hu S. Comment on "Organ-protective effect of angiotensin-converting enzyme 2 and its effect on the prognosis of COVID-19. J Med Virol 2020;92(9):1425–6.
31. Mehta P, McAuley DF, Brown M, et al. COVID-19: consider cytokine storm syndromes and immunosuppression. Lancet 2020;395(10229):1033–4.
32. Liu J, Li S, Liu J, et al. Longitudinal characteristics of lymphocyte responses and cytokine profiles in the peripheral blood of SARS-CoV-2 infected patients. EBioMedicine 2020;55. https://doi.org/10.1016/j.ebiom.2020.102763.
33. Yu D, Du Q, Yan S, et al. Liver injury in COVID-19: clinical features and treatment management. Virol J 2021;18(1). https://doi.org/10.1186/s12985-021-01593-1.
34. Fix OK, Hameed B, Fontana RJ, et al. Clinical best practice advice for hepatology and liver transplant providers during the COVID-19 pandemic: AASLD expert panel consensus statement. Hepatology 2020;72(1):287–304.
35. Inamdar S, Benias PC, Liu Y, et al. Prevalence, risk factors, and outcomes of hospitalized patients with coronavirus disease 2019 presenting as acute pancreatitis. Gastroenterology 2020;159(6):2226–8.e2.

36. Ò Miró, Llorens P, Jiménez S, et al. Frequency of five unusual presentations in patients with COVID-19: Results of the UMC-19-S1. Epidemiol Infect 2020;148: e189. Published online.
37. de-Madaria E, Capurso G. COVID-19 and acute pancreatitis: examining the causality. Nat Rev Gastroenterol Hepatol 2021;18(1):3–4.
38. Liu F, Long X, Zhang B, et al. ACE2 expression in pancreas may cause pancreatic damage after SARS-CoV-2 infection. Clin Gastroenterol Hepatol 2020;18(9): 2128–30.e2.
39. Hikmet F, Méar L, Å Edvinsson, et al. The protein expression profile of ACE2 in human tissues. Mol Syst Biol 2020;16(7). https://doi.org/10.15252/msb.20209610.
40. Schepis T, Larghi A, Papa A, et al. SARS-CoV2 RNA detection in a pancreatic pseudocyst sample. Pancreatology 2020;20(5):1011–2.
41. Müller JA, Groß R, Conzelmann C, et al. SARS-CoV-2 infects and replicates in cells of the human endocrine and exocrine pancreas. Nat Metab 2021;3(2): 149–65.
42. Steenblock C, Richter S, Berger I, et al. Viral infiltration of pancreatic islets in patients with COVID-19. Nat Commun 2021;12(1). https://doi.org/10.1038/s41467-021-23886-3.
43. Kumaran NK, Karmakar BK, Taylor OM. Coronavirus disease-19 (COVID-19) associated with acute necrotising pancreatitis (ANP). BMJ Case Rep 2020; 13(9). https://doi.org/10.1136/bcr-2020-237903.
44. Cerqueira NF, Hussni CA, Yoshida WB. Pathophysiology of mesenteric ischemia/reperfusion: a review. Acta Cir Bras 2005;20(4):336–43.
45. el Moheb M, Naar L, Christensen MA, et al. Gastrointestinal complications in critically Ill patients with and without COVID-19. JAMA - J Am Med Assoc 2020; 324(18):1899–901.
46. Keshavarz P, Rafiee F, Kavandi H, et al. Ischemic gastrointestinal complications of COVID-19: a systematic review on imaging presentation. Clin Imaging 2021; 73:86–95.
47. Bhayana R, Som A, Li MD, et al. Abdominal imaging findings in COVID-19: preliminary observations. Radiology 2020;297(1):E207–15.
48. de Barry O, Mekki A, Diffre C, et al. Arterial and venous abdominal thrombosis in a 79-year-old woman with COVID-19 pneumonia. Radiol Case Rep 2020;15(7): 1054–7.
49. Rodriguez-Nakamura RM, Gonzalez-Calatayud M, Martinez Martinez AR. Acute mesenteric thrombosis in two patients with COVID-19. two cases report and literature review. Int J Surg Case Rep 2020;76:409–14.
50. Beccara AL, Pacioni C, Ponton S, et al. Arterial mesenteric thrombosis as a complication of SARS-CoV-2 infection. Eur J Case Rep Intern Med 2020;7(5): 001690.
51. Norsa L, Valle C, Morotti D, et al. Intestinal ischemia in the COVID-19 era. Dig Liver Dis 2020;52(10):1090–1.
52. Osilli D, Pavlovica J, Mane R, et al. Case reports: mild COVID-19 infection and acute arterial thrombosis. J Surg Case Rep 2020;2020(9). https://doi.org/10.1093/jscr/rjaa343.
53. Gartland RM, Velmahos GC. Bowel necrosis in the setting of COVID-19. J Gastrointest Surg 2020;24(12):2888–9.
54. Klok FA, Kruip MJHA, van der Meer NJM, et al. Incidence of thrombotic complications in critically ill ICU patients with COVID-19. Thromb Res 2020;191:145–7.

55. Azouz E, Yang S, Monnier-Cholley L, et al. Systemic arterial thrombosis and acute mesenteric ischemia in a patient with COVID-19. Intensive Care Med 2020;46(7): 1464–5.
56. Thuluva SK, Zhu H, Tan MML, et al. A 29-year-old male construction worker from india who presented with left-sided abdominal pain due to isolated superior mesenteric vein thrombosis associated with SARS-CoV-2 infection. Am J Case Rep 2020;21:1–5.
57. Lakshmanan S, Toubia N. Pneumatosis intestinalis in COVID-19. Clin Gastroenterol Hepatol. Published online May 2020. 19(10):e99.doi:
58. Hwabejire JO, Kaafarani HM, Mashbari H, et al. Bowel ischemia in COVID-19 infection: one-year surgical experience. Am Surg 2021;87(12):1893–900.
59. Clark R, Waters B, Stanfill AG. Elevated liver function tests in COVID-19: causes, clinical evidence, and potential treatments. 2021. Available at: www.tnpj.com.
60. Naar L, Langeveld K, el Moheb M, et al. Acute kidney injury in critically-ill patients with COVID-19: a single-center experience of 206 consecutive patients. Ann Surg 2020;272(4):e280–1.
61. el Moheb M, Naar L, Christensen MA, et al. Gastrointestinal complications in critically ill patients with and without COVID-19. JAMA 2020;324(18):1899–901.
62. Zhang Y, Cen M, Hu M, et al. Prevalence and persistent shedding of fecal SARS-CoV-2 RNA in patients with COVID-19 infection: a systematic review and meta-analysis. Clin Translational Gastroenterol 2021;12(4):E00343.
63. Almafreji I, Ranganath S. Bowel ischemia in a patient with SARS CoV-2-like illness and negative real-time reverse transcription polymerase chain reaction test results during the peak of the pandemic. Cureus 2020. https://doi.org/10.7759/cureus.10442.
64. Chai X, Hu L, Zhang Y, et al. Specific ACE2 expression in cholangiocytes may cause liver damage after 2019-nCoV infection. bioRxiv 2020. https://doi.org/10.1101/2020.02.03.931766.
65. Llitjos JF, Leclerc M, Chochois C, et al. High incidence of venous thromboembolic events in anticoagulated severe COVID-19 patients. J Thromb Haemost 2020; 18(7):1743–6.
66. Cheung KS, Hung IFN, Chan PPY, et al. Gastrointestinal manifestations of SARS-CoV-2 infection and virus load in fecal samples from a hong kong cohort: systematic review and meta-analysis. Gastroenterology 2020;159(1):81–95.

Diarrhea and Coronavirus Disease 2019 Infection

David M. Friedel, MD[a], Mitchell S. Cappell, MD, PhD[b,*]

KEYWORDS

- COVID-19 • Pandemic
- SARS-CoV-2 (severe acute respiratory syndrome coronavirus-2) • Diarrhea
- Gastrointestinal symptoms • Colonoscopy • Stool studies • *C difficile* • Long COVID
- ACE-2 (angiotensin converting enzyme-2)

KEY POINTS

- Diarrhea occurs in approximately 10% to 20% of hospitalized patients with COVID-19 infection.
- The diarrhea is typically mild-to-moderate, watery, nonbloody, and generally lasts 2 to 6 days with some variability.
- The diarrhea is believed due to local infection of gastrointestinal mucosa mediated by the angiotensin converting enzyme-2 receptor.
- Approximtely 50% of patients with COVID-19 infection shed viral RNA particles in stool.
- Rarely the diarrhea can be severe and cause dehydration and electrolyte abnormalities. These abnormalities can require intravenous hydration, electrolyte repletion, and, rarely require hemodialysis for acute renal failure.
- Mild-to-moderate diarrhea from COVID-19 infection, without any specific identified cause, is often treated with antidiarrheals, such as Loperamide.
- Workup for severe diarrhoa in hospitalized adult patients with COVID-19 infection includes, aside from routine serum electrolytes, liver function tests, a basic metabolic panel, a hemogram, and a leukocyte differential; sometimes includes routine stool tests, a stool test for C. difficile, stool for calprotectin or lactoferrin, and occassionally abdominal computed tomography or colonoscopy.
- The diarrhea occasionally contributes to the morbidity and rarely contributes to the mortality of COVID-19 infection.

Both authors are equal first authors.
[a] Division of Therapeutic Endoscopy, Division of Gastroenterology, Department of Medicine, New York University Hospital, 259 First Street, Mineola 11501, NY, USA; [b] Department of Medicine, Gastroenterology Service, Aleda E. Lutz Veterans Administration Hospital at Saginaw, Building 1, Room 3212, 1500 Weiss Street, Saginaw, MI 48602, USA
* Corresponding author.
E-mail address: mitchell.cappell@va.gov

Gastroenterol Clin N Am 52 (2023) 59–75
https://doi.org/10.1016/j.gtc.2022.11.001
0889-8553/23/Published by Elsevier Inc.

INTRODUCTION

Coronavirus disease-2019 (COVID-19), caused by severe acute respiratory syndrome coronavirus-2 (SARS-CoV-2), is estimated to have infected more than 40% of the global population (>3 billion people) with more than 600 million documented infections and has claimed more than 6.5 million lives including more than one million Americans.[1] Pneumonia and respiratory complications account for most of the morbidity and mortality from COVID-19. However, angiotensin converting enzyme-2 (ACE-2), the entry receptor for the coronavirus SARS-CoV-2, is expressed in many extrapulmonary tissues and viral invasion and disruption occurs throughout the body. Extrapulmonary manifestations of COVID-19 infection include hemostatic abnormalities and thrombotic complications, cardiac dysfunction and arrhythmias, liver dysfunction and hepatitis, central nervous system/peripheral nervous system complications, acute kidney injury (AKI), and various skin rashes and eruptions.[2] Pyrexia, cough, dyspnea, pharyngitis, rhinorrhea, and malaise are the most common COVID-19 symptoms. ACE-2 receptors are more highly expressed in gastrointestinal (GI) mucosa than in respiratory mucosa, especially in the stomach and small intestine.[3] GI symptoms are relatively common, including prominently diarrhea, as well as nausea, emesis, anorexia, abdominal pain, and heartburn.[4]

The relationship between diarrhea and respiratory symptoms and between diarrhea and patient prognosis are variable. GI symptoms, including diarrhea, are sometimes the presenting symptoms with variable development of respiratory and hemostatic derangements. Diarrhea in the COVID-19-infected patient is typically mild-to-moderate but can occasionally be severe and life-threatening.[5,6]

METHODS

The relevant literature was reviewed using two independent computer search engines, PubMed and Ovid. The literature review was continuously updated until nearly submitting this review to the Journal on October 21, 2022. This work constitutes a semiquantitative review as defined in “The impact of COVID-19 infection on miscellaneous inflammatory disorders in the gastrointestinal tract” which is another article in this monograph. This semiquantitative review differs from a systematic review only by not listing articles identified by the computerized search which were excluded from this review and by not compiling the reason(s) for their exclusion.

This computerized literature review included the following search terms, key words, or phrases [with listing in brackets identifying the number of articles identified by PubMed per search term]: diarrhea and COVID [1805]; bloody diarrhea and COVID [19]; chronic diarrhea and COVID [181]; long COVID and diarrhea [34]; dehydration and diarrhea and COVID [12]; acute renal failure and diarrhea and COVID [79]; acute kidney injury and diarrhea and COVID [59]; fecal shedding of COVID [192]; fecal-oral transmission and COVID [267]; enterocytes and COVID [128]; colonocytes and COVID [3]; angiotensin converting enzyme-2 (ACE-2) receptor and intestines [214]; C difficile and COVID [63]; secretory diarrhea and COVID [3]; diarrhea therapy and COVID [711]; anti-diarrheals and COVID [9]; Loperamide and COVID [2]; kaolin pectin and COVID [0]; cholestyramine and COVID [1]; flavonoids and COVID [624]; intestinal ova and parasites and COVID [1]; amebiasis and COVID [14]; cytomegalovirus and COVID [297]; microscopic colitis and COVID [6]; bacterial infections and diarrhea and COVID [61]; colonoscopy and COVID [233], flexible sigmoidoscopy and COVID [11], enteroscopy and COVID [3], capsule colonoscopy and COVID [16], balloon enteroscopy (endoscopy) and COVID [0]; disposable endoscopes and COVID [39]; CT colonography and COVID [10]; fecal occult blood and COVID [88]; fecal immunological testing

(FIT) and COVID [13]; iron deficiency anemia and COVID [42]; colonoscopy screening and COVID [168]; colon and adenomas and COVID [13]; colon cancer screening and COVID [119]; colonoscopy surveillance and COVID [109]; colonic pseudo-obstruction and COVID [5]; long COVID and GI endoscopy [8]; GI endoscopy complications and COVID [36]; GI endoscopy guidelines and COVID [34]; gastrointestinal endoscopy and COVID transmission [195]; radiation proctitis and COVID [0]; rectal ulcer and COVID [12]; hemorrhoids and COVID [108]; rectal fissure and COVID [0]; SARS-CoV-2 viral RNA particles in stool [21]; diabetic diarrhea and COVID [156]; Diosmectite and COVID [2]; probiotics and COVID [353]; and microbiota and COVID [925].

Instructive case report: (moderately severe diarrhea from COVID-19 directly contributing to mortality (via acute renal failure from dehydration).

A 41-year-old woman with multiple, mild-to-moderate (asymptomatic) chronic health disorders and risk factors for COVID-19, all likely from the metabolic syndrome, including severe obesity (body mass index [BMI] = 37 kg/m^2), mild diabetes mellitus treated with metformin, hypertension treated with metoprolol, hypertriglyceridemia, and hypercholesterolemia, who worked as a nurse's aide, presented with moderately severe diarrhea with 7 to 10 moderately profuse watery bowel movements per day and minor upper respiratory symptoms of minimal cough, rhinorrhea, and low-grade pyrexia,[5] Physical examination revealed signs of dehydration and hypovolemia: decreased skin turgor, mild tachycardia at rest, orthostasis, and absent axillary sweat. There were no signs of respiratory distress: respiratory rate was 20 rpm, O_2 saturation was 97% on room air, lung fields were clear on auscultation and percussion, and lung fields were clear on chest roentgenogram.

Routine laboratory chemistries revealed multiple electrolyte derangements (hypokalemia, hyponatremia, and hypochloremia); mild prerenal azotemia, and an increased creatinine level; all of which were acutely abnormal from their previously normal baselines. The urine specific gravity was 1.029 (level highly consistent with severe dehydration). Stool workup revealed negative tests for *C difficile* toxins A and B, negative stool examinations for ova and parasites, negative stool cultures for enteric bacterial pathogens, and normal levels of fecal calprotectin and lactoferrin.

She received aggressive intravenous hydration, intravenous electrolyte repletion, and emergency dialysis while monitored in an intensive care unit (ICU) bed. She rapidly succumbed from acute renal failure associated with dehydration, electrolyte derangements, and prerenal azotemia, all attributed to the moderately severe COVID-19-associated diarrhea. The proximate cause of death was acute renal failure from the underlying cause of severe dehydration and electrolyte derangements attributed to the moderately severe diarrhea from acute COVID-19 infection (without her initially presenting with COVID-19 pneumonia): This patient presented in mid-March 2020 as one of the first 10 patients with COVID-19 infection diagnosed in Michigan and the case report was published in April 2020, as one of the first 40 publications in the world on the COVID-19 pandemic.[5]

DISCUSSION

Pathophysiology

SARS-CoV-2 viral RNA particles are detected in stool in approximately half of acutely infected subjects[7] (**Box 1**). Only a modest proportion of those with fecal shedding have GI symptoms, but viral RNA is still detectable in stool after pharyngeal clearance.[8,9] Fecal-oral transmission of COVID-19 is strongly implicated in infection but awaits further confirmation.[10–12] Fecal shedding often precedes COVID-19 symptoms and may continue after symptoms resolve.[13] The clinical utility of fecal testing for

Box 1
Diarrhea associated with COVID-19 infection

Pathophysiology

- Believed related to local infection of gastrointestinal mucosa mediated by local angiotensin converting enzyme-2 (ACE-2) receptor
- Approximately 50% of patients with COVID-19 infection have fecal shedding of SARS-CoV-2 (severe acute respiratory syndrome coronavirus-2)

Clinical characteristics

- Approximately 10% to 20% of patients with COVID-19 infection have diarrhea, with some variability reported among studies
- Diarrhea is typically moderate with $\leq$ 6 watery and non-bloody bowel movements per day
- Occasionally diarrhea is severe with >6 bowel movements per day. Such severe diarrhea is sometimes accompanied by patient dehydration and serum electrolyte abnormalities
- Duration of diarrhea is typically 2 to 6 days, with some variability among studies

COVID-19 is currently limited because it is costly and has limited availability, but it may be useful in patients with evident GI symptoms with delayed viral testing and in patients with unremitting diarrhea.[13]

The pathophysiology of acute diarrhea presenting during COVID-19 infection is multifactorial and variable. Putative mechanisms include viral entry through the abundant GI ACE-2 receptors with disruption of the absorptive surface of enterocytes and colonocytes; increased intracellular mucosal permeability; change of bowel flora; and gut ischemia, and possibly a calcium-dependent secretory diarrhea.[14–17] Endoscopic data are sparse, but GI mucosal inflammation appears mild to moderate, with bloody diarrhea decidedly unusual in COVID-19 infection.[3,14]

Antibiotic therapy for pulmonary and other local infections can induce diarrhea, especially from *C difficile* infection. Other medications or interventions, such as tube feeding, can also cause diarrhea. Diarrhea commonly occurs in post-COVID or 'long" COVID states. Diarrhea can begin after COVID-19 vaccination.

Epidemiology

GI symptoms, including anorexia, nausea/emesis, abdominal pain, and diarrhea, are common in patients with COVID-19 infection. Diarrhea is the most common or second most common GI complaint in most patient surveys, with a reported incidence ranging from 10% to 20%.[18] A meta-analysis of 60 studies noted approximately 18% had GI complaints, excluding the extremely common symptom of ageusia. In one survey of GI symptoms, 13% had diarrhea, 10% had nausea/emesis, and 9% had abdominal pain.[19] A systematic analysis of >18,000 patients reported diarrhea in 11.5%, nausea/emesis in 6.3%, and abdominal pain in 2.3%.[20] Various studies note a wide range of diarrhea prevalence, ranging from 2% to 49.5%,[21–24] and a meta-analysis of >132,000 COVID-19 subjects noted a diarrhea prevalence of 12%, and of anorexia of 22%.[25] An early meta-analysis noted the wide range of diarrhea prevalence among studies and reported a pooled prevalence of 10.4%.[26] Another meta-analysis of approximately 79,000 patients reported a 16.5% diarrhea prevalence.[27] A meta-analysis of >25000 COVID-19 subjects had a prevalence of anorexia in 20% and of diarrhea in 13%.[28]

Diarrhea is also common in the pediatric population. A meta-analysis of 2855 children or adolescents with COVID-19 reported a 4% diarrhea prevalence.[29] A systematic review of 2914 pediatric patients reported a 10.1% diarrhea prevalence.[30] A meta-analysis of 32 pediatric studies noted a 19% prevalence of diarrhea,[31] whereas another meta-analysis noted a pooled prevalence of 10%.[32] Children typically have a mild COVID-19 viral syndrome, with mild and self-limited diarrhea that is sometimes not even self-reported. However, 27% of pediatric COVID-19 patients with the dreaded Multisystem Inflammatory Syndrome in Children (MIS-C) had diarrhea in one meta-analysis.[33]

Diarrhea Characteristics

Diarrhea may be the first and occasionally the only COVID-19 symptom.[34,35] A systematic review noted 4.3% presented with diarrhea.[35] Diarrhea usually starts within 5 days of presentation and usually lasts for 2 to 6 days.[34,35] COVID-19 subjects with diarrhea as their only symptom are diagnosed later than those presenting with respiratory symptoms.[5] COVID-19 diarrhea is usually mild and self-limited, with less than six loose or watery bowel movements daily with each bowel movement typically consisting of modest volume[5,9,12,33,35](see **Box 1**). Stool is usually hemoccult negative, but occasionally hemorrhagic colitis is described.[23,36] One two-year-old child with COVID-19 had bloody dysentery as her only symptom of COVID-19 infection and recovered.[24,36] Severe diarrhea with up to 30 bowel movements per day rarely occurs.[8,37]

Clinical Correlations

Generally, GI symptoms of COVID-19, including diarrhea, are not correlated with demographic or clinical parameters.[18] One recent study suggested that age <80 years, immunosuppression, and a history of irritable bowel syndrome (IBS) may correlate with GI symptoms.[23] The presence of diarrhea is not clearly correlated with poor clinical outcomes, including death.[8,18,38] However, one American study correlated severe outcomes with diarrhea.[28] Another study correlated COVID-19 diarrhea with poor outcomes but noted that the correlation was stronger between abdominal pain and poor outcomes.[39] A meta-analysis suggested abdominal pain, but not diarrhea, was correlated with severe outcomes.[40] Contrariwise, three COVID-19 studies noted that diarrhea was correlated with improved clinical outcomes.[41–43] Overall, diarrhea in COVID-19 subjects does not clearly portend a bad prognosis. COVID-19 outcomes in children and adolescents are generally excellent in patients with or without diarrhea, except for patients with MIS-C.[30–32,34]

A comprehensive drug history must be obtained because medications that are used off-label as prophylaxis or treatment of COVID-19 infection may cause diarrhea.[19,44,45] The patient should be asked about non-prescription (over-the-counter) supplements because such drugs may cause diarrhea. This diagnosis should be strongly considered if the diarrhea correlates temporally with drug initiation. Drug discontinuation or substitution should be considered if clinically feasible.

Laboratory Tests

Blood tests for stable outpatient COVID-19 individuals are not required, except for those with abdominal pain or bloody diarrhea. In the hospital infected patients should undergo routine blood tests including a complete hemogram with leukocyte differential, serum electrolytes, and a basic metabolic panel (**Box 2**). A healthy outpatient with COVID-19 and diarrhea, but without recent antibiotic exposure, may be a candidate for expectant treatment without undergoing stool tests. However, patients who are elderly, present to the emergency department, are chronic residents in a health care facility, have fever, or have significant abdominal pain should have stool tests for *C difficile*. Stool testing for other bacterial pathogens has a modest yield, whereas stool tests for ova and parasites have a low yield except for patients with

Box 2
Laboratory workup of diarrhea associated with COVID-19 infection in hospitalized patients

Blood tests
- Hemogram with leukocyte differential
- Serum electrolytes, glucose, blood urea nitrogen and creatinine
- Basic metabolic panel, including routine liver function tests
- Blood cultures

Stool tests
- Stool for bacterial culture and sensitivity
- Stool for ova and parasites
- Stool for *C difficile* (confirm positive test by PCR)
- Fecal leukocytes (or more modern alternatives of stool for calprotectin or lactoferrin) to diagnose severe inflammatory diarrhea/colitis

Further tests
- KUB (kidneys ureter, bladder) or consider CT computerized tomography scan of abdomen for: notable abdominal pain, leukocytosis, or positive blood cultures
- Colonoscopy if patient relatively stable and concern for cytomegalovirus colitis

Unusual tests
- Spot stool with Sudan-4 stain (to evaluate qualitatively for steatorrhea)
- Stool electrolytes (to evaluate for secretory diarrhea)
- Neuroendocrine workup for diarrhea (plasma serotonin and chromogranin A)
- Stool elastase (to evaluate for chronic pancreatitis)

PCR–polymerase chain reaction

immunosuppression, with a prior history of such infections, or with a recent travel history. Hospitalized patients and patients with bloody diarrhea should undergo stool testing.

Stool determination for fecal leukocytes or for the more modern stool tests of calprotectin or lactoferrin should be performed to check for intestinal inflammation. Fecal COVID-19 patients with bloody, profuse, or unremitting diarrhea should be considered for colonoscopy. Cytomegalovirus colitis is an important consideration in immunocompromised subjects, including those receiving immunosuppressive therapy after organ transplantation. Conceivably, inflammatory bowel disease (IBD) may first present during COVID-19 infection. Scant data exist concerning endoscopy in COVID-19 subjects (see accompanying chapters on GI bleeding by Cappell and Friedel and on GI endoscopy by Sultan and coauthors). Physicians are now less reluctant to perform colonoscopy in patients with COVID-19 infection due to the advent of moderately effective vaccines, herd immunity, lower mortality with newer genetic variants, improved infection control in GI endoscopy units, and improved COVID-19 therapies. The sparse data on colonoscopy in COVID-19-infected patients usually relate to colonoscopy indications of GI hemorrhage or occasionally abdominal pain rather than diarrhea. A small COVID-19 cohort reported inflammatory and erosive abnormalities throughout the GI tract with COVID-19 infection,[46] a finding supported by other studies.[47–49]

Computerized tomography (CT) imaging is preferable to MRI to evaluate diarrhea in potentially unstable patients infected with COVID-19 because of its rapid turnaround time and lower cost. CT imaging should be considered for COVID-19 patients, once stabilized, if they present with diarrhea that is bloody, associated with abdominal pain, or significant laboratory abnormalities, including leukocytosis, acidosis, or prerenal azotemia (see **Box 2**). Colitis and other abdominal abnormalities may occur in patients without apparent respiratory symptoms, but thoracic CT windows should be obtained during abdominal CT because COVID-19 frequently causes pneumonia.[8,50]

CT findings in COVID-19 patients with diarrhea include colonic wall thickening and edema. CT Imaging can also diagnose GI perforation, pneumatosis coli, diverticulitis, or appendicitis.[51,52] The differential diagnosis for diffuse or segmental colitis in such patients includes COVID-19 itself, other pathogens such as *C difficile* or CMV, and bowel ischemia.

Chronic diarrhea including episodic diarrhea that becomes more manifest coincident with COVID-19 infection may arise from prior disorders exacerbated by COVID-19 infection, a new entity initiated by the infection, or incidental emergence of another disorder. Antecedent (possibly undiagnosed) disease may become more manifest during the pandemic, including IBS, small intestinal bacterial overgrowth, pancreatic insufficiency, microscopic colitis (MC), and ulcerative proctitis.[53] Chronic diarrhea has a broad differential including diseases classified as inflammatory, bloody, fatty, or dysenteric. Additional testing can include stool electrolytes (to differentiate secretory from non-secretory diarrhea), qualitative or quantitative fat (to detect steatorrhea), stool elastase (to diagnose chronic pancreatitis), stool for calprotectin or lactoferrin (to diagnose severe inflammatory diarrhea/colitis), and plasma serotonin and chromogranin A (to help diagnose neurosecretory diarrhea). Colonoscopy and CT imaging are often helpful to diagnose pancreatic diseases, IBD, or neuroendocrine tumors. The diagnosis of COVID-19 primary diarrhea is largely one of exclusion.[54]

Management

COVID-19 research is generally highly active and intense but is not focused on GI manifestations because these are usually not life-threatening. Specific novel treatments exist for COVID-19 infection, but none are designed to treat diarrhea per se.[26] Treatment for diarrhea is largely symptomatic and supportive. Judicious use of antidiarrheals, such as Loperamide (diphenoxylate-atropine), may be considered if the diarrhea is unremitting with negative stool tests for *C difficile* and no evidence of ileus, intestinal obstruction, or GI perforation (**Box 3**). Kaolin-pectin may be an effective and safe symptomatic therapy.[55] A bile acid sequestrant was used for COVID-19 diarrhea in a patient whose colonoscopy showed ileocolonic ulcers.[56] Antiparasitic drugs and flavonoids have been proposed as a treatment of COVID-19 diarrhea.[57–59] Diosmectite, an adsorbent clay with anti-inflammatory properties, may be effective therapy for COVID-19 diarrhea.[60] Traditional Chinese herbal medications may have

Box 3
Treatment of diarrhea associated with COVID-19 infection

Antidiarrheal therapy

- Antidiarrheals as symptomatic therapy after excluding specific causes (such as *C difficile* infection): Loperamide (diphenoxylate-atropine), Kaolin-pectin, and possibly flavonoids, Diosmectite, an adsorbent clay, or probiotics

Intravenous therapy

- Intravenous hydration and repletion of serum electrolytes for severe diarrhea accompanied by dehydration, serum electrolyte abnormalities, and possibly prerenal azotemia. Infants and young children may require special rehydration solutions.

Special treatments & monitoring in selected circumstances

- Monitor patient in an intensive care unit if patient exhibits hemodynamic compromise from hypovolemia
- Acute hemodialysis if necessary for severe electrolyte abnormalities and acute renal failure
- Special therapies for diarrhea from *C difficile* colitis, cytomegalovirus colitis, microcytic colitis, chronic pancreatitis, and neuroendocrine causes of diarrhea

a potential role in treating GI symptoms.[61] A Chinese group has examined massage therapy for COVID-19 diarrhea.[62]

Intravenous fluid is administered as necessary as guided by hypovolemia and prerenal azotemia, and serum electrolytes are supplemented as necessary as guided by the serum chemistries in hospitalized COVID-19 patients with diarrhea. Patients with hemodynamic compromise from severe dehydration from severe diarrhea may require aggressive intravenous hydration while monitored in an ICU and may require emergency dialysis. Intravenous fluids should be administered cautiously in patients with hypoxemia or cardiac failure associated with severe COVID-19 infection. Infants and young children may require specific rehydration solutions.

Probiotics have been considered for COVID-19 infection and specifically for associated diarrhea, with so far unsubstantiated benefits.[63–65] Moreover, probiotics are a heterogeneous group that should be administered cautiously in patients with multiorgan dysfunction and a potentially leaky gut.[65] China's National Health Commission supports probiotics for severe COVID-19 patients.[66] One Italian study noted a positive effect of "bacteriotherapy" on both diarrhea and respiratory status of COVID-19-infected patients.[67]

Diarrhea with Severe Coronavirus Disease-2019

Patients with severe COVID-19 infection are monitored in the ICU where they are exposed to hospital flora with risks of superinfection. Acute viral respiratory infections alter immune response and the ecology of respiratory and GI tract infections. Secondary, viral, bacterial, and fungal infections can occur, including Candida species, CMV, Aspergillus, Klebsiella, Mucormycosis, and Acinetobacter.[68] *Clostridioides difficile* is the most prevalent superinfection that causes diarrhea.[69] A patient with severe COVID-19 and CMV hemorrhagic enterocolitis survived with specific therapy.[70] Enteral feedings in COVID-19-infected patients (often via gastrostomy) are generally well tolerated, but the rate and feeding solution may have to be adjusted if diarrhea occurs.[71] MIS-C usually occurs in children and is often treated with parenteral immunoglobulin and corticosteroids.[34,72]

Clostridioides Difficile

Clostridioides (formerly Clostridium) *difficile* is the most common secondary GI infection in COVID-19 subjects (72.73). Stool tests for *C difficile* should be performed in all hospitalized patients with COVID-19 infection and diarrhea and in all COVID-19 infected outpatients with abdominal pain, fever, bloody diarrhea, or chronic diarrhea. This test should be repeated, even if negative, if the diarrhea persists. Treatment should be initiated expeditiously for a positive test. Some centers noted a decrease in *C difficile* stool testing during the early pandemic and the incidence of *C difficile* did not increase during the pandemic.[73–75] The unchanged rate may relate to judicious antibiotic stewardship and increased infectious precautions during the pandemic. In a small cohort of COVID-19 subjects, only 19% of co-infected patients had positive stool tests for *C difficile* on admission, and the rest developed *C difficile* infection after the COVID-19 diagnosis. Outcome data on co-infection is preliminary.[76] Theoretically, COVID-19 and *C difficile* may interact with each other to increase the virulence, transmissibility, and duration of each infection.[73] In one series, co-infection was associated with more severe and prolonged diarrhea and increased mortality as compared with those with COVID-19 without *C difficile* infection.[77] COVID-19 subjects generally initially had diarrhea attributable to the virus and some of these subjects developed diarrhea exacerbation from *C difficile* superinfection; the latter group had increased mortality.[78,79] Fecal microbiota transplantation (FMT) has continued during the pandemic and remains a viable therapeutic option for *C difficile* treatment though comprehensive donor testing is essential.[80]

Inflammatory Bowel Disease/Miscellaneous Inflammatory Disorders

Treatment of patients with ulcerative colitis and regional enteritis becomes more complex in patients with COVID-19 infection (see accompanying chapter on IBD by Summa and Hanauer). Two patients developed ulcerative colitis de novo simultaneous with COVID-19 infection, but the concurrence may have simply been coincidental.[81] COVID-19 enteritis may mimic regional enteritis, including one patient with multiple fistulae and a jejunal perforation.[82,83] COVID-19 symptoms are similar in IBD patients as compared with those in the general population, with 27% of IBD patients presenting with diarrhea in one meta-analysis.[84] Five out of twelve IBD patients noted diarrhea as their first COVID-19 symptom and two had diarrhea as their only symptom.[85] IBD patients do not seem to be more susceptible to COVID-19 infection, nor do they have more severe COVID-19 outcomes or higher mortality than patients without IBD.[84,86] Guidelines suggest using standard treatment of IBD during the pandemic while avoiding diarrhea exacerbation through recognition of immunosuppression inducing greater susceptibility to *C difficile* colitis.[87]

Analysis of a large Swedish cohort showed that MC subjects were more prone to contract COVID-19 infection and those with the subtype of collagenous colitis but not the subtype of lymphocytic colitis, had more severe COVID-19 disease and higher mortality.[88] Case reports documented new lymphocytic colitis or collagenous colitis with COVID-19 infection.[89,90] Colonoscopy with biopsies to exclude MC is a consideration in all patients who have apparently recovered from COVID-19 infection but have persistent diarrhea. The treatment of immune-checkpoint inhibitor colitis is challenging during the pandemic due to the need to maintain immunomodulatory therapy. Moderate-dose corticosteroids are a consideration in patients with less severe COVID-19 infection, but tocilizumab should be avoided because of the risk of intestinal perforation.[91]

Long Coronavirus Disease

Most COVID-infected subjects recover without sequelae, but a proportion have some symptoms that persist or reappear weeks to months after the original infection in a post-COVID-19 syndrome, also called long COVID (see accompanying chapter on long COVID by Trindade and colleagues). Approximately 40% of subjects in one Long COVID cohort manifested diarrhea[92] and approximately 13% of subjects in another long COVID cohort manifested diarrhea.[93] A systematic review noted that abdominal pain, nausea, and anorexia were more common than diarrhea in long COVID.[94] A Chinese group noted that at 90 days post-discharge from the hospital for COVID-19 infection, 15% had diarrhea with higher rates of anorexia or nausea.[95] In another long COVID-19 cohort approximately 18% had diarrhea five months after acute infection.[96] Diarrhea during the initial acute COVID-19 infection was correlated with the presence of diarrhea in long COVID-19.[97] Long COVID-19 can evolve into irritable bowel syndrome, as occurs in other postinfectious diarrheal states.[98] Antidiarrheals and antispasmodics may be used after negative stool studies, including studies for *C difficile*. However, other causes of chronic diarrhea should be considered with performance of colonoscopy, if not already performed. Chronic symptoms after acute COVID-19 infection are uncommon in children.[99]

Vaccine

Approximately 3% of subjects in a large COVID-19 vaccine database reported diarrhea but prolonged diarrhea is unusual.[100] The Pfizer vaccine informational site reported 11% of adults had diarrhea, with almost 90% of these cases being mild.[101] Diarrhea is more common after the adenovirus vector vaccine than mRNA vaccines, and the frequency of the incidence of diarrhea increased with increased adjuvant concentration in the vaccine preparation.[102] Multisystem inflammatory syndrome was reported in one adult after COVID-19 vaccination.[103]

Clinical Implications and Emerging Trends

The COVID pandemic is a rapidly evolving pandemic due to rapidly emerging new viral strains with greater contagiousness but apparently lower mortality; vaccines that prevent and protect against infection; the development of herd immunity; development of moderately effective antibiotic therapy; and implementation of infection controls to reduce population exposure. Diarrhea is a minor symptom in the overwhelming majority of COVID-19 patients that typically requires only symptomatic therapy and exclusion of more specific causes of diarrhea exacerbation, such as *C difficile* superinfection. However, given the huge magnitude of the pandemic with pandemic mortality numbering in the many millions, even the mostly minor symptom and disorder of diarrhea can contribute to pandemic mortality due to the huge number of infected patients. It is critical to recognize life-threatening dehydration and electrolyte depletion early to expeditiously initiate intravenous hydration and electrolyte repletion, and even perform emergency dialysis as necessary in an ICU setting.

This review is best considered as a snapshot of the current state of diarrhea with COVID, with likely future advancements and improvements in clinical therapy, management, and prognosis over time.

SUMMARY

COVID-19 morbidity and mortality largely results from respiratory disease and sometimes from the development of a hypercoagulable state. However, extrapulmonary disorders are common including GI complaints of anorexia, nausea/emesis, abdominal pain, or diarrhea. The GI pathophysiology is largely due to the abundant ACE-2 receptors within GI mucosa promoting SARS-CoV-2 viral entry. Diarrhea is the most common or second most common GI symptom in most COVID-19 patient surveys. COVID-19 diarrhea is usually non-bloody and moderate. It can be the presenting symptom of COVID-19 infection, but most commonly occurs within several days after the onset of other COVID-19 symptoms. It usually lasts for only several days but can be prolonged. Fecal–oral transmission of the virus is likely but requires further substantiation. Stool analysis for COVID-19 currently has limited clinical utility. Mortality is increased in some studies of COVID-19 cohorts with diarrhea, but this is not reported in most studies. Diarrhea presenting later in the hospitalization for COVID-19 infection is often related to *C difficile* infection. Late–presenting diarrhea is usually associated with a worse prognosis. Mild diarrhea from COVID-19 infection is usually treated symptomatically with anti-diarrheal medications, whereas severe diarrhea may require intravenous fluid infusion and electrolyte replacement therapy as necessary. The differential diagnosis for diarrhea includes potential medicine side-effects, such as from antibiotics, and *C difficile* infection. Diarrhea is an increasingly common complaint in subjects who have long COVID.

CLINICS CARE POINTS

- The coronavirus disease-2019 (COVID-19) pandemic has infected more than 600,000,000 patients worldwide and has killed more than 6,000,000 patients. Most of the mortality from COVID-19 arises from COVID-19 pneumonia and pulmonary complications.

- Diarrhea is common with COVID-19 infection. It is reported in approximately 10% to 20% of cases. It is recognized as one of the presenting symptoms of this infection.
- The diarrhea is typically mild-to-moderate, watery, and non-bloody; it typically lasts 2 to 6 days, with somewhat variable duration.
- The diarrhea is believed to be due to local invasion of the virus via the angiotensin-converting enzyme-2 receptor, which is highly expressed in gastrointestinal mucosa, especially in the stomach and small intestine. The virus is often shed in stool.
- Rarely the diarrhea can be severe and cause dehydration and electrolyte abnormalities that require intravenous hydration and electrolyte repletion. In extreme instances, the diarrhea can contribute to acute renal failure from hypovolemia associated with COVID-19 infection.
- The diarrhea when mild is typically treated symptomatically with antidiarrheals such as Loperamide.
- Workup for severe diarrhea in hospitalized adults with COVID-19 infection includes routine serum electrolytes, liver function tests, and a basic metabolic panel; a hemogram and leukocyte differential; sometimes routine stool tests including a test for *C difficile*; and very occasionally abdominal computerized tomography or colonoscopy.
- The differential diagnosis of persistent diarrhea with COVID-19 infection includes, in addition to primary COVID-19 diarrhea, medication-associated diarrhea, especially from antibiotics; hyperalimentation via percutaneous endoscopic gastrostomy or other tube feedings; *C difficile* infection; and, occasionally, irritable bowel syndrome; lymphocytic colitis; or other diarrheal disorders.
- The diarrhea typically has a favorable prognosis in the absence of COVID-19 pneumonia. However, it is variably reported that diarrhea associated with COVID-19 infection may have a worse prognosis.
- Diarrhea is increasingly reported persisting for more than four weeks after acute COVID-19 infection, as part of long COVID-19. Although inadequately characterized, long COVID diarrhea appears to have a good prognosis.

ACKNOWLEDGMENTS

Dr Cappell is a full-time employed gastroenterologist at the Aleda E. Lutz Veterans Administration Hospital in Saginaw, of the United States Government. All opinions expressed in this article are not necessarily those of the Aleda E. Lutz Veterans Administration Hospital in Saginaw or of the United States Government.

REFERENCES

1. COVID-19 Cumulative Infection Collaborators. Estimating global, regional, and national daily and cumulative infections with SARS-CoV-2 through Nov 14, 2021: a statistical analysis. Lancet 2022;399(10344):2351.
2. Gupta A, Madhavan MV, Sehgal K, et al. Extrapulmonary manifestations of COVID-19. Nat Med 2020;26(7):1017–32.
3. Zhang J, Garrett S, Sun J. Gastrointestinal symptoms, pathophysiology and treatment in Covid-19. Genes Dis 2021;8(4):385–400.
4. Cha MH, Regueiro M, Sandhu DS. Gastrointestinal and hepatic manifestations of Covid-19: a comprehensive review. World J Gastroenterol 2020;26(19): 2323–32.
5. Cappell MS. Moderately severe diarrhea and impaired renal function with COVID-19 infection. Am J Gastroenterol 2020;115(6):947–8.

6. Pan L, Mu M, Yang P, et al. Clinical characteristics of Covid–19 patients with digestive symptoms in Hubei, China: a descriptive cross–sectional, multicenter study. Am J Gastroenterol 2020;115(5):766–73.
7. Chen Y, Chen L, Deng Q, et al. The presence of SARS-Cov-2 RNA in the feces of Covid–19 patients. J Med Virol 2020;90(7):833–70.
8. Ramachandran P, Onukogu I, Ghanta S, et al. Gastrointestinal symptoms and outcomes in hospitalized coronavirus disease 2019 patients. Dig Dis 2020;38: 373–9.
9. Carvalho A, Alqusairi R, Adams A, et al. SARS-CoV-2 gastrointestinal infection causing hemorrhagic colitis: Implications for detection and transmission of COVID-19 disease. Am J Gastroenterol 2020;115:942–6.
10. Park SK, Lee CW, Park DI, et al. Detection of SARS-CoV-2 in fecal samples from patients with asymptomatic and mild COVID–19 in Korea. Clin Gastroenterol Hepatol 2021;19(7):1387–94.
11. Jones DL, Baluja MQ, Greaham DW, et al. Shedding of SARS-CoV-2 in feces and urine and its potential role in person–to–person transmission and the environment of COVID 19. Sci Tot Environ 2020;749:141364.
12. Han C, Duan C, Zhang S, et al. Digestive symptoms in COVID-19 patients with mild disease severity: Clinical presentation, stool viral RNA testing, and outcomes. Am J Gastroenterol 2020;115:916–23.
13. Tian Y, Rong L, Nian W, et al. Review article: Gastrointestinal features and COVID-19 and the possibility of faecal transmission. Aliment Pharmacol 2020; 51(9):843–51.
14. Khoury NC, Russo TJ. A case of gastrointestinal-predominant Covid–19 demonstrates value of stool PCR test. J Med Virol 2021;93(2):662–3.
15. Galanopoulos M, Gkeros F, Doukatas A, et al. COVID–19 pandemic: Pathophysiology and manifestations from the gastrointestinal tract. World J Gastroenterol 2020;26(31):4579–88.
16. Yeoh YK, Zuo T, Lui GC, et al. Gut microbiota composition reflects disease severity and dysfunctional immune responses in patients with COVID–19. Gut 2021;70(4):698–706.
17. Parel S, Parikh C, Verma D, et al. Bowel ischemia in COVID–19: a systematic review. Int J Clin Pract 2021;75(12):e14930.
18. Silva FAFD, Brito BB, Santos MLC, et al. COVID-19 gastrointestinal manifestations: a systematic review. Rev Soc Bras Trop Rev 2020;25(53):e20200714.
19. Singh S, Samanta J, Suri V, et al. Presence of diarrhea associated with better outcomes in patients with COVID-19 - A prospective evaluation. Indian J Med Microbiol 2022;40(3):404–8.
20. Cheung KS, Hung IFN, Chan PPY, et al. Gastrointestinal manifestations of SARS-CoV-2 infection and virus load in fecal samples from a Hong Kong cohort: Systematic review and meta-analysis. Gastroenterology 2020;159(1):81–95.
21. Megyeri K, Dernovics Á, Al-Luhaibi ZII, et al. COVID-19-associated diarrhea. World J Gastroenterol 2021;27(23):3208–22.
22. Guan WJ, Ni ZY, Hu Y, et al. China Medical Treatment Expert Group for Covid-19. Clinical characteristics of coronavirus disease 2019 in China. NEJM 2020; 382:1708–20.
23. Xiao F, Tang M, Zheng X, et al. Evidence for gastrointestinal infection of SARS-CoV-2. Gastroenterology 2020;158(6):1831–3.e3.
24. Leung WK, To KF, Chan PK, et al. Enteric involvement of severe acute respiratory syndrome-associated coronavirus infection. Gastroenterology 2003;125: 1011–7.

25. Chen N, Zhou M, Dong X, et al. Epidemiological and clinical characteristics of 99 cases of 2019 novel coronavirus pneumonia in Wuhan, China: a descriptive study. Lancet 2020;395:507–13.
26. Al Maqbali M, Al Badi K, Sinani M Al, et al. Clinical features of COVID-19 patients in the first year of pandemic: A systematic review and meta-analysis. Biol Res Nurs 2022;24(2):172–85.
27. D'Amico F, Baumgart DC, Danese S, et al. Diarrhea during COVID-19 infection: Pathogenesis, epidemiology, prevention, and management. Clin Gastroenterol Hepatol 2020;18(8):1663–72.
28. Shehab M, Alrashed F, Shuaibi S, et al. Gastroenterological and hepatic manifestations of patients with COVID-19, prevalence, mortality by country, and intensive care admission rate: systematic review and meta-analysis. BMJ Open Gastroenterol 2021;8(1):e000571.
29. Elshazli RM, Kline A, Elgaml A, et al. Gastroenterology manifestations and COVID-19 outcomes: a meta-analysis of 25,252 cohorts among the first and second waves. J Med Virol 2021;93(5):2740–68.
30. Mantovani A, Rinaldi E, Zusi C, et al. Coronavirus disease 2019 (COVID-19) in children and/or adolescents: a meta-analysis. Pediatr Res 2021;89(4):733–7.
31. Patel NA. Pediatric COVID-19: Systematic review of the literature. Am J Otolaryngol 2020;41(5):102573.
32. Mansourian M, Ghandi Y, Habibi D, et al. COVID-19 infection in children: a systematic review and meta-analysis of clinical features and laboratory findings. Arch Pediatr 2021;28(3):242–8.
33. Radia T, Williams N, Agrawal P, et al. Multi-system inflammatory syndrome in children & adolescents (MIS-C): A systematic review of clinical features and presentation. Paediatr Respir Rev 2021;38:51–7.
34. Wang J, Yuan X. Digestive system symptoms and function in children with COVID-19: A meta-analysis. Medicine (Baltimore) 2021;19;100(11):e24897.
35. Jin X, Lian JS, Hu JH, et al. Epidemiological, clinical and virological characteristics of 74 cases of coronavirus-infected disease 2019 (COVID-19) with gastrointestinal symptoms. Gut 2020;69:1002–9.
36. Tariverdi M, Farahbakhsh N, Gouklani H, et al. Dysentery as the only presentation of COVID-19 in a child: a case report. J Med Case Rep 2021;15(1):65
37. Maslennikov R, Pouluektova E, Ivashkin V, et al. Diarrhoea in adults with coronavirus-beyond incidence and mortality: a systematic review and meta-analysis. Infect Dis (Lond) 2021;53(5):348–60.
38. Aroniadis OC, Wang X, Gong T, et al. Factors associated with the development of gastrointestinal symptoms in patients hospitalized with Covid-19. Dig Dis Sci 2022;67(8):3860–71.
39. Rogers HK, Choi WW, Gowda N, et al. Frequency and outcomes of gastrointestinal symptoms in patients with Corona Virus Disease-19. Indian J Gastroenterol 2021;40(5):502–11.
40. Zeng W, Qi K, Ye M, et al. Gastrointestinal symptoms are associated with severity of coronavirus disease 2019: A systematic review and meta-analysis. Eur J Gastroenterol Hepatol 2022;34(2):168–76.
41. Hayashi Y, Wagatsuma K, Nojima M, et al. The characteristics of gastrointestinal symptoms in patients with severe COVID-19: A systematic review and meta-analysis. J Gastroenterol 2021;56(5):409–20.
42. Schettino M, Pellegrini L, Picascia D, et al. Clinical characteristics of COVID-19 patients with gastrointestinal symptoms in Northern Italy: a single-center cohort study. Am J Gastroenterol 2021;116(2):306–10.

43. Fallouh NA, Naik KH, Udochi CO, et al. Better clinical outcomes in hospitalized COVID-19 minority patients with accompanying gastrointestinal symptoms. J Natl Med Assoc 2022;113(6):626–35.
44. Singh B, Ryan H, Kredo T, et al. Chloroquine or hydroxychloroquine for prevention and treatment of COVID-19. Cochrane Database Syst Rev 2021;2(2): CD013587.
45. Wen W, Chen C, Tang J, et al. Efficacy and safety of three new oral antiviral treatment (molnupiravir, fluvoxamine and Paxlovid) for COVID-19: A meta-analysis. Ann Med 2022;54(1):516–23.
46. Chiu MN, Bhardwaj M, Sah SP, et al. Safety profile of COVID-19 drugs in a real clinical setting. Eur J Clin Pharmacol 2022;78(5):733–53.
47. Kuftinec G, Elmunzer BJ, Amin S, et al. The role of endoscopy and findings in COVID-19 patients: An early North American Cohort. BMC Gastroenterol 2021;21(1):205.
48. Massironi S, Viganò C, Dioscoridi L, et al. Endoscopic findings in patients infected with 2019 novel coronavirus in Lombardy, Italy. Clin Gastroenterol Hepatol 2020;18(10):2375–7.
49. Vanella G, Capurso G, Burti C, et al. Gastrointestinal mucosal damage in patients with COVID-19 undergoing endoscopy: an international multicentre study. BMJ Open Gastroenterol 2021;8(1):e000578.
50. Xie XP, Sheng LP, Han CQ, et al. Features of capsule endoscopy in COVID-19 patients with a six-month follow-up: A prospective observational study. J Med Virol 2022;94(1):246–52.
51. Boraschi P, Giugliano L, Mercogliano G, et al. Abdominal and gastrointestinal manifestations in COVID-19 patients: Is imaging useful? World J Gastroenterol 2021;14(27):4143–59.
52. Caruso D, Zerunian M, Pucciarelli F, et al. Imaging of abdominal complications of COVID-19 infection. BJR Open 2021;2(1):20200052.
53. Gubatan J, Zikos T, Spear Bishop E, et al. Gastrointestinal symptoms and health care utilization have increased among patients with functional gastrointestinal and motility disorders during the COVID-19 pandemic. Neurogastroenterol Motil 2022;34(4):e14243.
54. Aguila E, Cua I. Dumagpi J When do you say it's SARS-CoV-2-associated diarrhea? J Gastroenterol Hepatol 2020;35(9):1652–3.
55. Kow CS, Hasan SS. The use of antimotility drugs in COVID-19 associated diarrhea. J Infect 2021;82(2):e19.
56. Shirohata A, Ariyoshi R, Fujigaki S, et al. A case of COVID-19 diarrhea relieved by bile acid sequestrant administration. Clin J Gastroenterol 2022;15(2): 393–400.
57. Shimizu K, Hirata H, Kabata D, et al. Ivermectin administration is associated with lower gastrointestinal complications and greater ventilator-free days in ventilated patients with COVID-19: A propensity score analysis. J Infect Chemother 2022;28(4):548–53.
58. Uyaroğlu OA, Güven GS, Güllü İ. Can Levamisole be used in the treatment of COVID-19 patients presenting with diarrhea? J Infect Dev Ctries 2020;14(8): 844–6.
59. Paul AK, Jahan R, Bondhon TA, et al. Potential role of flavonoids against SARS-CoV-2-induced diarrhea. Trop Biomed 2021;38(3):360–5.
60. Poeta M, Cioffi V, Buccigrossi V, et al. Diosmectite inhibits the interaction between SARS-CoV-2 and human enterocytes by trapping viral particles, thereby

preventing NF-kappaB activation and CXCL10 secretion. Sci Rep 2021;11(1): 21725.
61. Shi S, Wang F, Li J, et al. The effect of Chinese herbal medicine on digestive system and liver functions should not be neglected in COVID-19: An updated systematic review and meta-analysis. IUBMB Life 2021;73(5):739–60.
62. Zhou KL, Dong S, Fu GB, et al. Tuina (massage) therapy for diarrhea in COVID-19: a protocol for systematic review and meta-analysis. Medicine (Baltimore) 2020;99(28):e21293.
63. Wang H, Wang Y, Lu C, et al. The efficacy of probiotics in patients with severe COVID-19. Ann Palliat Med 2021;10(12):12374–80.
64. Mak JWY, Chan FKL, Ng SC. Probiotics and COVID-19: One size does not fit all. Lancet Gastroenterol Hepatol 2020;5(7):644–5.
65. Mikucka A, Deptuła A, Bogiel T, et al. Bacteraemia caused by probiotic strains of Lacticaseibacillus rhamnosus: Case studies highlighting the need for careful thought before using microbes for health benefits. Pathogens 2022;11(9):977.
66. Gao QY, Chen YX, Fang JY. 2019 Novel coronavirus infection and gastrointestinal tract. J Dig Dis 2020;21(3):125–6.
67. Ceccarelli G, Borrazzo C, Pinacchio C, et al. Oral bacteriotherapy in patients with COVID-19: A retrospective cohort study. Front Nutr 2021;7:613928.
68. Garcia-Vidal C, Sanjuan G, Moreno-García E, et al. Incidence of co-infections and superinfections in hospitalized patients with Covid-19: A retrospective cohort study. Clin Microbiol Infect 2021;27(1):83–8.
69. Laszkowska M, Kim J, Faye AS, et al. Prevalence of Clostridioides difficile and other gastrointestinal pathogens in patients with COVID-19. Dig Dis Sci 2021; 66(12):4398–405.
70. Carll WC, Rady MY, Salomao MA, et al. Cytomegalovirus haemorrhagic enterocolitis associated with severe infection with COVID-19. BMJ Open Gastroenterol 2021;8(1):e000556.
71. Osuna-Padilla I, Rodríguez-Moguel NC, Aguilar-Vargas A, et al. Safety and tolerance of enteral nutrition in COVID-19 critically ill patients, a retrospective study. Clin Nutr ESPEN 2021;43:495–500.
72. Mahmoud S, El-Kalliny M, Kotby A, et al. Treatment of MIS-C in children and adolescents. Curr Pediatr Rep 2022;10(1):1–10.
73. Azimirad M, Noori M, Raeisi H, et al. How does COVID-19 pandemic impact on Incidence of Clostridioides difficile infection and exacerbation of Its gastrointestinal symptoms? Front Med (Lausanne) 2021;8:775063.
74. Hawes AM, Desai A, Patel PK. Did Clostridioides difficile testing and infection rates change during the COVID-19 pandemic? Anaerobe 2021;70:102384.
75. Yadlapati S, Jarrett SA, Lo KB, et al. Examining the rate of Clostridioides (formerly Clostridium) difficile infection pre- and post-COVID-19 pandemic: An institutional review. Cerus 2021;13(12):e20397.
76. Granata G, Petrosillo N, Al Moghazi S, et al. The burden of Clostridioides difficile infection in COVID-19 patients: A systematic review and meta-analysis. Anaerobe 2022;74:102484.
77. Sehgal K, Fadel HJ, Tande AJ, et al. Outcomes in patients with SARS-CoV-2 and Clostridioides difficile coinfection. Infect Drug Resist 2021;14:1645–8.
78. Maslennikov R, Ivashkin V, Ufimtseva A, et al. Clostridioides difficile co-infection in patients with COVID-19. Future Microbiol 2022;17:653–63.
79. Maslennikov R, Svistunov A, Ivashkin V, et al. Early viral versus late antibiotic-associated diarrhea in novel coronavirus infection. Medicine (Baltimore) 2021; 100(41):e27528.

80. Khanna S, Tande A, Rubin DT, et al. Fecal microbiota transplantation for recurrent C difficile infection during the COVID-19 pandemic: Experience and recommendations. Mayo Clin Proc 2021;96(6):1418–25.
81. Elbadry M, Medhat MA, Zaky S, et al. Ulcerative colitis as a possible sequela of COVID-19 infection: The endless story. Arab J Gastroenterol 2022;23(2):134–7.
82. Abbassi B, Deb A, Costilla V, et al. Subacute enteritis two months after COVID-19 pneumonia with mucosal bleeding, perforation, and internal fistulas. Am Surg 2021;1. 31348211023461.
83. Parigi TL, Bonifacio C, Danese S. Is it Crohn's disease? Gastroenterology 2020; 159(4):1244–6.
84. Singh AK, Jena A, Kumar -MP, et al. Clinical presentation of COVID-19 in patients with inflammatory bowel disease: A systematic review and meta-analysis. Intest Res 2022;20(1):134–43.
85. Taxonera C, Sagastagoitia I, Alba C, et al. 2019 novel coronavirus disease (COVID-19) in patients with inflammatory bowel diseases. Aliment Pharmacol Ther 2020;52(2):276–83.
86. Al-Ani AH, Prentice RE, Rentsch CA, et al. Review article: Prevention, diagnosis and management of COVID-19 in the IBD patient. Aliment Pharmacol Ther 2020; 52(1):54–72.
87. Magro F, Rahier JF, Abreu C, et al. Inflammatory bowel disease management during the COVID-19 outbreak: The ten do's and don'ts from the ECCO-COVID Taskforce. J Crohn Colitis 2020;14(14 Suppl 3):S798–806.
88. Khalili H, Zheng T, Söderling J, et al. Association between collagenous and lymphocytic colitis and risk of severe coronavirus disease 2019. Gastroenterology 2021;160(7):2585–7.e3.
89. Nassar IO, Langman G, Quraishi MN, et al. SARS-CoV-2-triggered lymphocytic colitis. BMJ Case Rep 2021;14(8):e243003.
90. Brennan GT. COVID-19-induced collagenous colitis. Gastro Hep Adv 2022; 1(6):976.
91. Amin R, Thomas AS, Khurana S, et al. Management of immune-related colitis during the COVID-19 pandemic. Inflamm Bowel Dis 2020;26(10):e110–1.
92. Zapata E, Monsalve DM, Acosta-Ampudia Y, et al, Post-COVID study group. Post-COVID syndrome. A case series and comprehensive review. Autoimmun Rev 2021;20(11):102947.
93. Wu Q, Ailshire JA, Crimmins EM. Long COVID and symptom trajectory in a representative sample of Americans in the first year of the pandemic. Sci Rep 2022;12(1):11647.
94. Choudhury A, Tariq R, Jena A, et al. Gastrointestinal manifestations of long COVID: a systematic review and meta-analysis. Therap Adv Gastroenterol 2022;15. 17562848221118403.
95. Weng J, Li Y, Li J, et al. Gastrointestinal sequelae 90 days after discharge for COVID-19. Lancet Gastroenterol Hepatol 2021;6(5):344–6.
96. Noviello D, Costantino A, Muscatello A, et al. Functional gastrointestinal and somatoform symptoms five months after SARS-CoV-2 infection: A controlled cohort study. Neurogastroenterol Motil 2022;34(2):e14187.
97. Augustin M, Schommers P, Stecher M, et al. Post-COVID syndrome in non-hospitalised patients with COVID-19: a longitudinal prospective cohort study. Lancet Reg Health Eur 2021;6:100122.
98. Settanni CR, Ianiro G, Ponziani FR, et al. COVID-19 as a trigger of irritable bowel syndrome: a review of potential mechanism. World J Gastroenterol 2021;27(43): 7433–45.

99. Borch L, Holm M, Knudsen M, et al. Long COVID symptoms and duration in SARS-CoV-2 positive children - a nationwide cohort study. Eur J Pediatr 2022; 181(4):1597–607.
100. Akaishi T, Takahashi T, Sato S. Prolonged diarrhea following COVID-19 vaccination: A case report and literature review. Tohoku J Exp Med 2022;257(3):251–9.
101. https://www.cdc.gov/vaccines/covid-19/info-by-product/pfizer/reactogenicity.html. (Accessed 4 October 2022).
102. Pormohammad A, Zarei M, Ghorbani S, et al. Efficacy and safety of COVID-19 vaccines: A systematic review and meta-analysis of randomized clinical trials. Vaccines (Basel) 2021;9(5):467.
103. Nune A, Iyengar KP, Goddard C, et al. Multisystem inflammatory syndrome in an adult following the SARS-CoV-2 vaccine (MIS-V). BMJ Case Rep 2021;14(7): e243888.

Gastrointestinal Bleeding in COVID-19-Infected Patients

Mitchell S. Cappell, MD, PhD[a,*], David M. Friedel, MD[b]

KEYWORDS

- COVID-19 • Pandemic • SARS • Gastrointestinal bleeding
- Esophagogastroduodenoscopy • Colonoscopy • Therapeutic endoscopy
- Endoscopy safety

KEY POINTS

- Gastrointestinal bleeding occurs in about 1.5% to 3.0% of patients hospitalized with COVID-19 infection.
- GI bleeding is generally mild-to-moderate with findings of mild-to-moderate mucosal inflammation, but the bleeding is occasionally severe and life-threatening, especially when from peptic ulcer disease or stress gastritis associated with severe COVID-19 pneumonia.
- Lower GI bleeding associated with COVID-19 infection is frequently due to ischemic colitis, associated with thromboembolism and a hypercoagulable state, that is in turn associated with COVID-19 infection.
- GI bleeding can occasionally contribute to morbidity in COVID-19 infected patients, but rarely contribute to mortality in patients hospitalized with COVID-19 infection.
- Although at the pandemic onset, GI bleeding was rarely evaluated by GI endoscopy in COVID-19-infected patients, patients with moderate GI bleeding from COVID-19 infection are increasingly undergoing semi-elective GI endoscopy.
- Patients with COVID-19 infection were initally intubated before undergoing EGD, but now patients undergoing EGD are generally intubated only for pneumonia and respiratory decompensation from COVID-19 infection.

INTRODUCTION

COVID-19 (coronavirus disease of 2019) infection caused by the highly contagious severe acute respiratory virus coronavirus 2 (SARS-CoV-2 virus) is responsible for the current global pandemic that has caused about 600 million proven acute infections

The two authors are equal first authors.
[a] Division of Gastroenterology, Department of Medicine, Aleda E. Lutz Veterans Hospital at Saginaw, Main Building, Room 3212, 1500 Weiss Street, Saginaw, MI 48602, USA; [b] Division of Therapeutic Endoscopy, Division of Gastroenterology, Department of Medicine, New York University Langone Hospital, 259 1st Street, Mineola, NY 11501, USA
* Corresponding author.
E-mail address: mitchell.cappell@va.gov

Gastroenterol Clin N Am 52 (2023) 77–102
https://doi.org/10.1016/j.gtc.2022.10.004
0889-8553/23/Published by Elsevier Inc.

and about 6 million deaths worldwide as of September 2022, including about 1 million deaths in the United States.[1] It predominantly causes respiratory disease, most prominently pneumonia that can cause respiratory failure. The initial phase of the pandemic in the United States (March-May 2020) caused considerable mortality, especially in those with risk factors of obesity, diabetes mellitus, immunosuppression, other significant comorbidities, and old age. Subsequent phases were characterized by decreased mortality, but increased contagiousness associated with newly emerging viral strains from genetic mutations. Vaccines are now available in much of the developed world that are moderately effective in preventing infection as are specific medications, such as nirmatrelvir (Paxlovid) and ritonavir, that can decrease infection severity and shorten disease duration. Public health measures, such as facemasks and patient isolation techniques, that vary regionally, likely blunted the pandemic spread. Nonetheless, COVID-19 infection remains an ongoing global crisis with notable morbidity and mortality.

Respiratory and systemic manifestations of COVID-19 infection, including dyspnea, cough, rhinorrhea, pyrexia, and malaise, predominate, but extrapulmonary manifestations occur frequently, including gastrointestinal (GI) and hepatic manifestations, such as anorexia, nausea, emesis, diarrhea, abdominal pain, and elevated transaminase levels. GI manifestations can produce morbidity and occasionally contribute to mortality.[2]

GI bleeding in COVID-19 subjects is uncommon. A meta-analysis of symptoms among greater than 25,000 COVID-19 subjects noted anorexia in 20%, diarrhea in 13%, and hematemesis in 9%.[3] However, the incidence of GI bleeding in this study is much higher than that reported in most clinical studies at 1.5% to 3.0%. GI bleeding is rarely the initial manifestation of COVID-19 infection[4] and most commonly manifests after hospitalization for COVID-19 infection.[5–7] GI bleeding usually arises from the upper GI tract, and manifests as anemia, melena, or hematemesis and less commonly arises from the lower GI tract and manifests as hematochezia, or occasionally melena. GI bleeding occurs more frequently in older patients, especially men, and especially in those with comorbidities.[8]

In a large meta-analysis, about 27% of infected subjects shed COVID-19 RNA in their stool.[3] The SARS-CoV-2 angiotensin-converting enzyme-2 receptor is highly expressed in the gut and this receptor provides a portal of entry for the virus, especially in the stomach and small intestine, which can cause local GI infection and clinical manifestations, including GI inflammation and GI bleeding.[9] The host immune response, including potential cytokine storm, multiorgan viral involvement, and side reactions of administered medications, such as corticosteroids or anticoagulants, may contribute to gut inflammation and exacerbate the GI bleeding.[10] GI bleeding from COVID-19 is usually self-limited even when caused by a "double-hit" of an initial viral cytopathic effect and secondary immune-mediated or medication-induced side effects.[11] Patients with severe COVID-19 infection may occasionally develop massive GI bleeding from physiologic stress, caused by sepsis, severe pneumonia, and respiratory or multiorgan failure, akin to the historically important phenomena of Cushing ulcer, related to increased intracranial pressure, and Curling ulcer, related to severe and extensive burns.[12] Stress gastritis and peptic ulcer disease (PUD) are common in patients with pneumonia and respiratory failure from COVID-19 infection, which constituted a common outcome in the early pandemic.[13] The propensity of the GI tract to bleed is somewhat related to the disparate effects of hypercoagulopathy in COVID-19-infected patients (perhaps reducing their bleeding tendency), administration of prophylactic anticoagulation to counteract this hypercoagulopathy that potentially promotes GI bleeding, and occurrence of thromboses potentially causing mucosal ischemia or necrosis with GI bleeding from sloughing of

GI mucosa or necrotic mucosal ulcers.[14] In one case report a patient with COVID-19 infection and sickle cell disease had GI bleeding with nonerosive gastroduodenitis secondary to microthrombi.[15]

METHODS

The literature was reviewed using two independent computer search engines, PubMed and Ovid. The literature review was continuously updated until nearly submitting this review to the Journal in September 2022. This work constitutes a semiquantitative review as defined in the article "The Impact of COVID-19 Infection on Miscellaneous Inflammatory Disorders in the Gastrointestinal Tract," elsewhere in this issue. This semiquantitative review differs from a systematic review only by not listing articles identified by the computerized search, which were excluded from this review, and by not compiling their reasons for exclusion. This computerized literature review included the following search terms, key words, or phrases (with listing in parentheses identifying the number of articles found by PubMed per search term): esophagogastroduodenoscopy (EGD) and COVID (465), colonoscopy and COVID (220), flexible sigmoidoscopy and COVID (11), therapeutic GI endoscopy and COVID (139), enteroscopy and COVID (2), capsule endoscopy and COVID (29), balloon enteroscopy (endoscopy) and COVID (5), nasal endoscopy and COVID (135), endoscopic retrograde cholangiopancreatography and COVID (64), disposable endoscopes and COVID (39), computed tomography colonography and COVID (10), GI bleeding scan and COVID (3), mesenteric angiography and GI bleeding and COVID (5), therapeutic angiography and GI bleeding and COVID (3), hematemesis and COVID (25), GI bleeding and COVID (182), melena and COVID (35), hematochezia and COVID (148), fecal occult blood and COVID (84), fecal immunologic testing and COVID (610), iron deficiency anemia and COVID (40), colonoscopy screening and COVID (156), colonoscopy surveillance and COVID (104), colonic pseudo-obstruction and COVID (5), colonoscopy and decompression and COVID (2), peroral endoscopic myotomy and COVID (9), long COVID and GI endoscopy (8), GI endoscopy complications and COVID (33), GI endoscopy guidelines and COVID (33), and GI endoscopy and COVID transmission (193).

Specific GI disorders/diseases in the literature review included (with number of cited articles per search term listed in parentheses) included: Mallory-Weiss tear and COVID (2), esophageal toxicity and medications and COVID (2), nasogastric tube erosions and COVID (2), Kaposi sarcoma and COVID (24), peptic ulcer and COVID (41), gastric ulcers and COVID (21), duodenal ulcers and COVID (16), hemorrhagic esophagitis and COVID (34), Barrett esophagus and COVID (13), gastroesophageal reflux disease and COVID (38), gastrointestinal stromal tumor and COVID (10), gastric antral vascular ectasia and COVID (1), gastric leiomyoma and COVID (1), colon and adenomas and COVID (12), colon cancer screening and colonoscopy and COVID (32), mucosal associated lymphoid tissue-OMA and COVID (9), Cameron lesion and COVID (1), Dieulafoy lesion and COVID (0), gastric lymphoma and COVID (0), esophageal adenocarcinoma and COVID (12), esophagus squamous cell cancer and COVID (4), gastric adenocarcinoma and COVID (22), linitis plastica and COVID (0), paraesophageal hernia and COVID (7), hemobilia and COVID (1), hemosuccus pancreaticus and COVID (0), marginal or anastomotic ulcer and COVID (35), Billroth II and COVID (6), radiation proctitis and COVID (0), radiation-associated vascular ectasia and COVID (0), gastric varices and COVID (10), bleeding esophageal varices and COVID (7), portal hypertensive gastropathy and COVID (1), rectal ulcer and COVID (11), bleeding hemorrhoids and COVID (10), and rectal fissure and COVID (0).

DISCUSSION

Prevalence

The current literature review reveals a low rate of GI bleeding in COVID-19 subjects, with most studies reporting a rate of 1.5% to 3%, with notable statistical outliers and considerable study variability. Moreover, much GI bleeding in COVID-19-infected patients is subclinical and decidedly less significant than the typical pulmonary manifestations of COVID-19. A global compilation of COVID-19 endoscopies noted up to nearly half of subjects had GI mucosal abnormalities, such as mucosal erosions.[16] A large, COVID-19 cohort, mostly from Egypt, reported a high rate of GI bleeding from hematemesis in 9%, melena in 5.3%, hematochezia in 0.6%, and fecal-occult positive stools in 5%.[3] Contrariwise, systematic review of 12 studies reported a prevalence of GI bleeding of only 0.06%.[17] After excluding two outlier studies, another meta-analysis of 91,887 COVID-19 subjects noted a 2.0% pooled prevalence of GI bleeding of whom 77% had upper GI bleeding.[18] A European cohort of 4,128 COVID-19 subjects noted a 1.8% prevalence of GI bleeding.[19] An Italian cohort of 4,871 COVID-19-infected patients noted a 0.5% prevalence of upper GI bleeding.[20] A New York cohort of 11,158 COVID-19 subjects reported a prevalence of 3% of GI bleeding,[21] whereas another New York cohort of 1,206 COVID-19-infected patients reported a 3.1% prevalence of GI bleeding.[22] A Spanish cohort of 74,814 COVID-19-infected patients had a prevalence of GI bleeding of 1.1%,[23] whereas a Chinese cohort of 36,358 COVID-19 subjects reported a 2% prevalence of GI bleeding.[24] These disparate results reflect differences in criteria for GI bleeding, different patient demographics, different countries, different rates of COVID-19 infection, and different study designs (letters to the editor,[11] case reports, case series,[4,12] case-controlled studies, retrospective studies, prospective studies, systematic reviews,[17] and meta-analyses[3,18]). The literature on GI bleeding associated with COVID-19 infection has been sparse until recently relative to the overall number of COVID-19-related publications and much less than that reported for several other GI manifestations. In particular, few studies have reported on GI endoscopic findings because of the scarcity of performing EGD for GI bleeding in patients with COVID-19 infection.

Evaluation of Gastrointestinal Bleeders Before Endoscopy

Gastroenterologists should promptly obtain a complete but directed medical history with a focus on GI disease in any patient with acute, overt GI bleeding, but particularly when associated with severe COVID-19 infection. The GI history should focus on prior GI bleeding and its cause, prior GI endoscopies and their findings, and endoscopic therapies because patients often bleed from the same GI lesions that they had previously bled from.[25] Patients should be asked about prior GI surgery and prior GI radiologic findings. The patient should be specifically asked about medicines administered for GI diseases, including histamine-2 receptor antagonists; proton pump inhibitors (PPIs); medications for inflammatory bowel disease; chemotherapy for GI cancers; gastrotoxic medications that increase the risk of GI bleeding, such as aspirin; cyclooxygenase-II inhibitors; nonsteroidal anti-inflammatory drugs; esophagotoxic medications (bisphosphonates, doxycycline); and anticoagulants (including coumadin, unfractionated heparin, low molecular heparin, clopidogrel, and rivaroxaban).

The medical history provides clues to the cause of the GI bleed. A history of alcoholism, jaundice, or liver disease increases the likelihood of cirrhosis, portal hypertension, and bleeding from esophageal varices or portal hypertensive gastropathy.[25] A history of smoking cigarettes increases the risk of duodenal ulcers. The patient should be asked about prior *Helicobacter pylori* infection and its therapy.

The patient with acute and overt GI bleeding should undergo a focused physical examination that includes vital signs to help assess the need for fluid resuscitation or blood transfusions; careful abdominal examination including the presence, location, intensity, and pitch of bowel sounds; abdominal tenderness; presence of rebound tenderness; and presence of splenomegaly. Stigmata of chronic liver disease should be searched for, including hepatomegaly, spider angiomas, palmar erythema, caput medusa, Dupuytren contracture, jaundice, asterixis, and ascites because such signs suggest GI bleeding from portal hypertension or cirrhosis. Abdominal tenderness is uncommon with upper GI bleeding, except occasionally from PUD. Severe abdominal pain suggests bowel ischemia, GI obstruction, or GI perforation. Severe direct abdominal tenderness, rebound tenderness, or involuntary guarding suggests a possible acute (surgical) abdomen, which must be excluded before performing EGD for GI bleeding. Air under the diaphragm (free intraperitoneal air) on abdominal roentgenogram or on abdominal computed tomography strongly suggests an acute abdomen. Rectal examination should be carefully performed to assess the patient for the presence, type, and quantity of rectal bleeding and check for anal masses, hemorrhoids, anal fissures, and anal stenoses. Nasogastric tube aspiration can help check for gross blood in the upper GI tract and clear the stomach of residual blood for unobstructed gastric visualization at EGD.

The presentation and appearance of the blood offers clues to the site of GI bleeding, its acuity, and its severity. Melena, recognized as black and tarry stools, mostly (90%) arises from an upper GI lesion because of degradation of blood with GI transit, but occasionally (10%) arises from small intestinal or right colonic lesions in the presence of slowed intestinal transit. Hematemesis indicates bleeding proximal to the ligament of Treitz.[25] Hemorrhoidal bleeding classically presents with a clinical triad of bright red blood per rectum caused by arterialized blood from the hemorrhoidal plexus, blood coating rather than admixed with stools, and postdefecatory bleeding caused by traumatic stool evacuation. Hypotension, orthostatic hypotension, tachycardia at rest, mental confusion, orthostatic dizziness, cold and clammy extremities, angina, and severe palpitations may suggest hemodynamic compromise from severe GI bleeding.[25] Cutaneous ecchymoses or petechia are signs of a coagulopathy.

Laboratory Evaluation for the Gastrointestinal Bleeder

Patients should have blood samples determined for routine electrolytes, chemistries, blood sugar, blood urea nitrogen (BUN), creatinine, liver function tests, lipase, and other standard biochemical parameters. Patients should have a complete blood count, including hematocrit, hemoglobin, mean corpuscular volume, mean corpuscular hemoglobin concentration, platelet count, leukocyte count, and leukocyte differential. The international normalized ratio of the prothrombin time should be determined. Patients with upper GI bleeding typically have an elevated BUN level with a BUN/creatinine ratio greater than 20:1 because of the combined effects of prerenal azotemia from hypovolemia and BUN elevation from GI resorption of degraded blood during intestinal transit.[25] Iron level, ferritin level, and percent iron saturation are useful to demonstrate iron deficiency from chronic GI blood loss. The medical history, physical examination, and initial laboratory values are important to assess resuscitation requirements for intravenous fluids or blood transfusions, triage to regular hospital beds versus monitored beds versus an intensive care unit (ICU), and timing of endoscopy including emergency or urgent endoscopy versus delayed or deferred endoscopy. Other consultative services may be urgently required for the GI bleeder, including surgery, radiology, and the intensivist.

Patient Stabilization Before Gastrointestinal Endoscopy

All patients with acute GI bleeding require hemodynamic evaluation and stabilization of vital signs before evaluation for potential GI endoscopy. Evaluation and stabilization is particularly important in patients with significant COVID-19 infection who may suffer from multiorgan failure including respiratory compromise from severe pneumonia, acute kidney injury or chronic kidney disease with chronically depressed glomerular filtration rate, and coagulation disorders. Respiratory compromise from COVID-19 pneumonia may not necessarily present with overt hypoxia but may be subtly suggested by other abnormal vital signs, unexplained acidosis, restlessness, or unexplained severe pyrexia or sepsis. Prerenal azotemia contributed by GI bleeding may exacerbate acute kidney injury. Hematocrit levels should be followed serially with time. A serial hematocrit decline may signify significant GI blood loss because of hemodilution to compensate for acute blood loss, but a hematocrit decline is a lagging indicator of blood loss.

Patients with overt GI bleeding should have two secure, large-bore, intravenous lines placed to ensure adequate fluid infusion for volume resuscitation. Patients with overt bleeding should be typed and crossed for potential transfusions of packed erythrocytes. All patients with acute upper GI bleeding should initially receive PPI therapy continuously and intravenously. This is most important for PUD or hemorrhagic esophagitis because these disorders are related to gastric acidity, but PPI therapy is also recommended for upper GI bleeding of any cause before performing EGD because the cause of the GI bleeding is usually uncertain before EGD and maintaining the intraluminal gastric pH greater than five stabilizes a gastric clot and prevents rebleeding of GI lesions.

Patients with potential hemodynamic instability manifested by systemic hypotension, orthostatic hypotension, or significant orthostatic changes (orthostasis) with evident active GI bleeding should be evaluated for an ICU bed. Admission to an ICU bed for blood transfusions is even more important in patients with concomitant COVID-19 pneumonia because of potential respiratory decompensation from fluid overload. In patients with active GI bleeding the preferred therapy for hypovolemia is transfusion of packed erythrocytes rather than intravenous colloid infusion or normal saline. Despite a current shortage of blood products attributed to the effects of the omicron surge during the pandemic,[26] blood transfusions for acute GI bleeders are generally considered a medical emergency.

Conservative Management with Deferral of Gastrointestinal Endoscopy

COVID-19 is usually transmitted from infected individuals via fine respiratory droplets. Aerosolization promotes spread with some potential for viral transmission when droplets land on surfaces. GI endoscopy, especially EGD, is a moderately high-risk procedure for COVID-19 transmission to the endoscopist and endoscopy staff because of aerosolization of droplets expired by COVID-19-infected patients. This transmission risk and the diversion of medical resources to counter the COVID-19 pandemic underlies the reluctance or deferral of performing GI endoscopy for hospitalized patients for nonurgent indications. This approach was historically reflected in publications noting the “dilemma” of performing endoscopy and the “less is more” attitude regarding performing GI endoscopy for GI bleeding in patients with COVID-19 infection.[27–29] A higher threshold for performing endoscopy for GI bleeding was proposed in COVID-19-infected patients, reflected semiquantitatively by higher Glasgow-Blatchford scores of GI bleeding severity.[30,31] Guidelines promulgated by different national professional gastroenterology societies throughout the world reflect a conservative approach to GI endoscopy in COVID-19-infected patients, including deferral of GI endoscopy if possible.[32–34] In the early pandemic (Spring 2020) rates of GI endoscopy plummeted by 10-fold from the prepandemic baseline rate.[35] Most GI bleeding is subclinical and therefore does not require GI endoscopy, but even overt GI bleeding was sometimes approached conservatively without GI endoscopy in COVID-19-infected patients. The pandemic generally diminished endoscopic volume for COVID-19 and non-COVID-19 patients, but this diminished volume did not adversely affect patient outcomes in a Canadian cohort study.[36] Nonetheless, COVID-19-infected patients with hemodynamically significant bleeding should be strongly considered for EGD after patient stabilization including volume resuscitation or packed erythrocyte transfusions and stabilization of the respiratory status.[37]

COVID-19-infected patients with GI bleeding are more likely to have a longer hospital stay, and less frequently undergo GI endoscopy than GI bleeders without COVID-19 infection.[38] Furthermore, upper GI hemorrhage in COVID-19 patients is positively associated with ICU admission and mechanical ventilation.[39] Longer time to GI endoscopy in COVID-19 subjects does not negatively impact their clinical outcomes.[20,40] GI bleeding in COVID-19 subjects is often subclinical or at least self-

Box 1
General principles of GI bleeding in COVID-19-infected patients

1. Literature on GI bleeding in COVID-19-infected patients is sparse relative to respiratory manifestations or many other GI disorders. This may relate to relative infrequency of performing GI endoscopy because of perceived risks to patients and endoscopy staff from the infection.
2. Higher threshold and less urgency for performing GI endoscopy on COVID-19-infected patients. May relate to perceived risks to patients and to endoscopy staff during the pandemic.
3. Often GI bleeding in COVID-19-infected patients is clinically mild and does not require GI endoscopy.
4. GI endoscopy may be deferred in acutely ill patients with mild-to-moderate GI bleeding because such patients often have multiple acute medical problems, especially respiratory failure.
5. Concern about transmission of COVID-19 to endoscopic staff during GI endoscopy. However, the risk to GI endoscopic staff of contracting COVID-19 infection during GI endoscopy is apparently not high if strict universal precautions are applied to all GI endoscopies performed during the pandemic.
6. Concern about prophylactic endotracheal intubation for EGD. In the initial stages of the pandemic (March-April 2020), endotracheal intubation was nearly universally performed for EGD, but subsequently endotracheal intubation is rarely and selectively performed for EGD.
7. Most critically ill COVID-19-infected patients receive anticoagulation, which must usually be withheld periprocedurally.
8. Modest need for endoscopic hemostasis during GI endoscopy in COVID-19-infected patients because the bleeding is often not severe. Endoscopic therapy may not be feasible in patients receiving anticoagulation (see point 7).
9. Need for percutaneous endoscopic gastrostomy in intubated and ventilated patients with COVID-19 infection but fortunately rarely causes bleeding complications.
10. Therapies often used in patients with COVID-19 infection, including corticosteroids, anticoagulation, and tocilizumab, negatively impact the GI tract and enhance GI bleeding.

limited.[41] A conservative approach may be justified. A small cohort of COVID-19 subjects with GI hemorrhage did well with conservative management and the author suggested a 24-hour waiting period before evaluating GI bleeders for GI endoscopy, a position endorsed by a journal editorial.[42,43] The general principles of managing bleeders with COVID-19 infection are summarized in **Box 1**, with an emphasis on differences between COVID-19-infected versus noninfected patients.

In a retrospective study, 24 (1.8%) of 1342 patients with COVID-19 presented with GI bleeding of whom 23 patients had upper GI bleeding, including 22 (91.6%) with evident cirrhosis and 21 presented with upper GI bleeding from esophageal varices. Two patients without cirrhosis were presumed to have nonvariceal bleeding. Medical therapy for esophageal variceal bleeding included vasoconstrictors, either somatostatin in 17 (73.9%) or terlipressin in four (17.4%). All patients with upper GI bleeding received PPIs and antibiotics. Fourteen patients (60.9%) were transfused packed erythrocytes, with a median transfusion of one unit. Initial control of upper GI bleeding was achieved in all 23 patients and none required emergency GI endoscopy. At 5-day follow-up, none rebled or died. Two patients later rebled; one from intermittently bleeding gastric antral vascular ectasia, and another rebled 19 days after hospital discharge. Three (12.5%) patients with cirrhosis succumbed to acute hypoxemic respiratory failure during the hospitalization. This study suggests that conservative management strategies including pharmacotherapy, and restrictive transfusions with close hemodynamic monitoring can successfully manage GI bleeding in COVID-19 patients and reduce their need for urgent GI endoscopy. The decision to proceed to GI endoscopy should be performed by a multidisciplinary team emphasizing limited use of GI endoscopy.[44]

Concerns regarding endoscopists contracting COVID-19 infection while performing conventional (tube) GI endoscopy have promoted alternative tests for diagnosis and treatment of GI bleeding, such as disposable endoscopes,[45] experimental robotic endoscopes,[46] telemetric sensor capsules,[47] small intestinal capsules for screening before GI enteroscopy,[48] and colonic capsules for screening before colonoscopy[49] to reduce the endoscopist's risks. A novel barrier device may minimize viral transmission from infected patients to endoscopists.[50] For example, positioning the endoscopist's head away from the patient's mouth during EGD decreased the endoscopist's facial exposure to visible droplets from 87% at 70 cm distance to 0% at 100 cm distance ($P < 0.001$) and thereby theoretically reduced transmission of COVID-19 infection to the endoscopist during EGD. Moreover, a physical barrier device reduced endoscopist's exposure to droplets to 0% at all distances.[50] A European study suggested an interventional radiologic approach to GI bleeding among 11 COVID-19 subjects to reduce transmission of COVID-19 to examining physicians.[51] The current supply of intravenous contrast medium is insufficient because of the pandemic.[52]

Suggested Approach to Gastrointestinal Bleeding in COVID-19 Subjects

The advent of COVID-19 vaccination and personalized protective equipment (PPE) for endoscopic staff minimizes potential COVID-19 transmission during GI endoscopy resulting in greater safety to endoscopic staff. PPE should optimally include an N95 mask or equivalent, a disposable, waterproof (impervious) surgical gown, safety goggles, face shield, hair cap, and protective footwear.[53] The endoscopist and the endoscopy staff should be offered such PPE. Endoscopists should be fitted for appropriately sized N95 masks and briefly trained on how to wear them. It is important to use new N95 masks at least daily. The endoscopist should be offered the option of thicker surgical gloves (eg, Microflex NeoPro NPG888 synthetic chloroprene disposable gloves) insead of the standard thin disposable gloves.

The endoscopy suite should be thoroughly cleaned between endoscopic cases with viricidal antiseptic, sterilizing solutions that are highly effective against COVID-19, concentrating on endoscopic equipment, endoscopic accessories, and the endoscopy cart to prevent COVID-19 transmission during GI endoscopy. At the endoscopy center where I worked antiseptic solutions were changed to use antiseptic solutions with proven high efficacy against COVID-19 soon after the pandemic onset throughout all clinical areas, including the sinks of bathrooms.[35] With all the aforementioned precautions, COVID-19 transmission to endoscopy staff during endoscopy is reported but highly uncommon.[54] GI endoscopy should be performed judiciously and conservatively in COVID-19 subjects, with less urgency and lower priority than that recommended for noninfected patients. Elective or semielective endoscopy in COVID-19-infected patients may be reasonably deferred until after the patient becomes noninfected, as proven by nasal swabs testing for the viral RNA of COVID-19. It may be helpful to perform GI endoscopy on COVID-19-infected patients as the last case on the normal daily endoscopy schedule to permit extra time to disinfect the room after this last case. Endoscopy staff should minimize their time exposed to a COVID-19-infected patient. For example, they should generally avoid being present in the endoscopy suite during intubation and extubation in infected patients.

In the early pandemic (March-May 2020), GI fellows were excused from performing GI endoscopy on their patients and attending GI endoscopists were required to perform GI endoscopy by themselves. This concept was irrational and unsubstantiated by data. GI fellows tend to be young, healthy, and at low risk of serious complications from COVID-19 infection, whereas GI attendings are often old (with about half of them older than 65 years old),[55,56] less healthy, with a higher incidence of comorbidities, and at high risk of severe COVID-19 complications. This recommendation negatively impacted endoscopic training of GI fellows who performed few GI endoscopies in March-May 2020 and this recommendation was withdrawn by May 2020.[35,56] Even currently, in 2022, GI fellows report less training in GI endoscopy

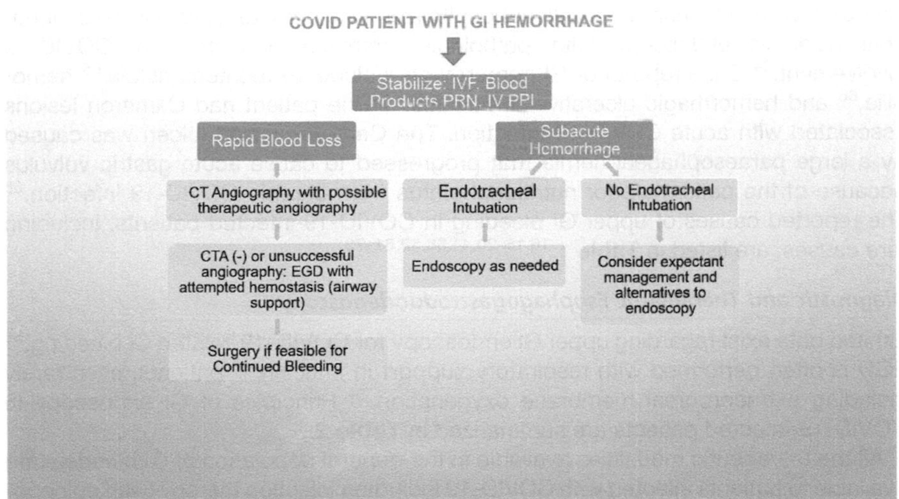

Fig. 1. Approach to GI bleed in COVID patient. Expectant management: monitor, transfuse PRN, reversal anticoagulation, and antiplatelet drugs if feasible. Alternative methods: nuclear bleeding scan, CTA, capsule endoscopy. CT, computed tomography; CTA, computed tomography angiography; IV, intravenous; IVF, intravenous fluids.

than fellows trained before the pandemic began because of not performing GI endoscopy during the pandemic onset and the lingering effects of the ongoing pandemic on somewhat restricting GI endoscopy.

In the beginning of the pandemic, all patients with proven COVID-19 infection were intubated prophylactically before EGD.[25] However, universal endotracheal intubation for EGD in COVID-19 patients entails potential difficulty of patient extubation postprocedure, especially for patients with COVID-19 pneumonia and respiratory compromise with consequent deleterious effects on patient prognosis.[57] Thus, endotracheal intubation for GI endoscopies should generally be avoided, if possible, when advocated solely for the indication of COVID-19 infection without additional reasons. However, this practice varies according to local endoscopy practice patterns, local prevalence of COVID-19 infection, and institutional policies. Ancillary services, such as interventional radiology, nuclear medicine, or GI surgery, may decrease the need for GI endoscopic intervention (**Fig. 1**).

Cause of Upper Gastrointestinal Tract Bleeding Proximal to Ligament of Treitz

PUD, including erosive gastritis and duodenitis, is the most common cause of upper GI bleeding in COVID-19-infected patients.[16,18–20,58] A small series of COVID-19 subjects noted a poor prognosis from gastric ulcers.[59,60] However, generalized mucosal inflammation and friability is a common leitmotif of GI infection with COVID-19 that causes minor GI blood loss.[16] A multicenter study of 87 upper GI endoscopies reported upper GI ulcers in one-quarter of patients, with gastroduodenitis in 16%, and petechial/hemorrhagic gastropathy in 9%.[16] In a New York cohort of 41 endoscopies in COVID-19-infected patients, EGD commonly revealed gastric/duodenal ulcers.[60] An Italian cohort of 38 COVID-19 subjects undergoing EGD reported 37% had esophagitis, erosive gastritis, or peptic ulcers.[61] Gastric erosions/ulcers in COVID-19 subjects may preferentially occur in the proximal stomach.[62] Reflux esophagitis was a common cause of GI bleeding but was significantly less common than PUD.[16,61] Esophageal variceal hemorrhage was also common in patients with COVID-19 infection,[16,44,62,63] likely reflecting that liver disease is a risk factor for severe COVID-19 infection. One patient hospitalized with hematemesis had an esophageal ulcer at endoscopy with pathologic demonstration of local COVID-19 involvement.[64] Case reports of GI hemorrhage include aortoenteric fistula,[65] hemobilia,[66] and hemorrhagic ulcerative duodenitis.[67] One patient had Cameron lesions associated with acute COVID-19 infection. The Cameron lesion (ulcer) was caused by a large paraesophageal hernia that progressed to cause acute gastric volvulus because of the patient's poor nutritional status from chronic COVID-19 infection.[68] The reported causes of upper GI bleeding in COVID-19-infected patients, including rare causes, are listed in **Table 1**.[16,18–20,44,58,59,61–73]

Diagnostic and Therapeutic Esophagogastroduodenoscopy

Limited data exist regarding upper GI endoscopy for COVID-19-related GI bleeding.[58] EGD is often performed with respiratory support in critically ill patients, even rarely including extracorporeal membrane oxygenation.[74] Principles of GI endoscopy in COVID-19-infected patients are summarized in **Table 2**.

All the therapeutic modalities available in the general population of GI bleeders are available to patients infected with COVID-19 including injection therapy (with epinephrine or sclerosants), ablative therapy (electrocoagulation with bipolar electrocoagulation probe or Gold Probe [Boston Scientific, Marlborough, MA), noncontact methods (argon plasma coagulation), mechanical therapy (band ligation, hemoclips, or detachable snares), or Hemospray (Cook Medical, Bloomington, IN).[75,76] However, COVID-

Table 1
Reported causes of upper GI bleeding proximal to the ligament of Treitz in patients with COVID-19 infection

Lesion	Putative Mechanisms	Selected References
Angiodysplasia	1 case reported in a large series of 87 EGDs performed mostly for overt GI bleeding	Vanella et al,[16] 2021
Aortoenteric fistula	Case report	González-Sagredo et al,[65] 2021
Dieulafoy lesion	1 case reported in a large series of 87 EGDs mostly performed for overt GI bleeding	Vanella et al,[16] 2021
Cameron lesion associated with acute COVID-19 infection	Case report Cameron lesion/ulcer was caused by a large paraesophageal hernia that progressed to cause acute gastric volvulus because of patient's poor nutritional status from COVID-19 infection	Deliwala et al,[68] 2021
Esophageal candidiasis (without bleeding)	2 cases among 87 patients undergoing EGD	Vanella et al,[16] 2021
Esophageal ulcer	1 case caused by primary COVID-19 infection 5 cases reported in a large endoscopic series of 87 EGDs performed mostly for overt GI bleeding	Vanella et al,[16] 2021, Bisseling et al,[64] 2021
Esophageal variceal hemorrhage	Increased reporting of esophageal variceal hemorrhage in COVID-19 infection may result from increased susceptibility of patients with cirrhosis, chronic liver disease, or advanced alcoholic liver disease to contracting COVID-19 infection	[16,44,62,63]
Esophagitis moderately frequent	Hemorrhagic esophagitis from gastroesophageal reflux disease is moderately common but less frequently reported in COVID-19 patients than peptic ulcer disease	Vanella et al,[16] 2021, Kuftinec et al,[61] 2021
Gastric leiomyoma/inflammatory fibroid polyp	1 case report of a patient with COVID-19-associated severe pneumonia requiring extracorporeal membrane oxygenation who had upper GI	Mur-Murota et al,[70] 2021

(continued on next page)

Table 1
(continued)

Lesion	Putative Mechanisms	Selected References
	bleeding from a gastric inflammatory polyp successfully treated with endoscopic hemostasis	
Gastrointestinal stromal tumor	Case report	Aguayo et al,[71] 2020
Gastropathy- petechial/hemorrhagic	Common reported finding (occurring in 9.2%) in a large study of COVID-19 patients undergoing EGD	Vanella et al,[16] 2021
Hemobilia	2 case reports of hemobilia	Koc and Çiçek,[66] 2021
Marginal (anastomotic) ulcer	Case report	Galvez et al,[72] 2020
Portal hypertensive duodenopathy	1 case reported in a large endoscopic series of 87 endoscopies mostly performed for overt GI bleeding	Vanella et al,[16] 2021
Portal hypertensive gastropathy	Case report	Philips et al,[73] 2020

Table 2
Gastrointestinal endoscopy for GI bleeding in patients with COVID-19 infection

General Principles/Topic	Clinical Applications	Reasons
PCR testing for COVID-19 infection.	Many institutions with high institutional prevalence of COVID-19 infection standardly screen all patients scheduled for GI endoscopy by PCR testing for COVID-19 infection. Alternatively, institutions screen all patients with planned GI endoscopy for history of exposure to someone with known COVID-19 within <14 d, and for symptoms suspicious of COVID-19 (eg, cough, dyspnea, or diarrhea). Patients who have at least 1 such exposure or symptom should undergo PCR testing for SARS-CoV-2.	Reduce COVID-19 exposure of endoscopy staff.
EGD is theoretically a high-risk procedure for transmitting COVID-19 infection from a patient with COVID-19 to endoscopy staff because of the presence of aerosolized infective droplets. However, the actual risk of transmission seems to be manageable. Risk to endoscopy staff may be higher in an infected patient with active overt hematemesis.	Endoscopy staff should strongly consider using PPE, including wearing an N95 face mask during endoscopy performed on COVID-19-infected patients.	Reduce personnel exposure to COVID-19 infection from infected patients.
Much less performance of EGD for elective indications in patients with active COVID-19 infection as compared with noninfected patients.	Generally, defer EGD for elective indications until patient recovers from acute COVID-19 infection.	Some risks to endoscopy staff from exposure to patient with COVID-19 infection during GI endoscopy. Patient with complicated acute COVID-19 infection may not tolerate EGD. Some patients with COVID-19 infection (eg, patients with severe pneumonia) may require prophylactic endotracheal intubation for EGD.
Similar frequency of performing EGD for emergency/urgent indications in patients with	Perform EGD for overt life-threatening GI bleeding, when therapeutic EGD is likely	Cannot wait for patient to recover from acute COVID-19 infection when EGD is required

(*continued on next page*)

Table 2
(continued)

General Principles/Topic	Clinical Applications	Reasons
acute COVID-19 infection versus noninfected patients.	needed, and when EGD is needed before contemplated GI surgery.	emergently or urgently. Maximize patient hemodynamic stability and respiratory status before performing EGD.
Deferral of elective GI endoscopy in a COVID-19-infected patient.	Wait a few weeks after the acute infection until the patient tests negative by PCR on a new COVID-19 test.	Reduce risk to endoscopy staff and reduce risks of endoscopy in a patient with active COVID-19 infection.
Prophylactic intubation for EGD in COVID-19-infected patients.	In the initial pandemic surge (March-May 2020) patients were generally intubated before EGD. From June 2020 onward only selected patients underwent prophylactic intubation for specific reasons.	Reason for current selective policy for endotracheal intubation before EGD is difficulty in extubating patients with respiratory compromise (especially from COVID-19 pneumonia).
Precautions during EGD in COVID-19-infected patients.	Endoscopy staff should exercise universal precautions when performing EGD on all patients during the pandemic, but especially in performing EGD on COVID-19-infected patients.	EGD properly performed with precautions seems to result in a low risk of COVID-19 transmission to endoscopy staff.
Routine screening and surveillance colonoscopy often deferred in patients with active COVID-19 infection until after the patient clears the virus as proven by nasal swab.		No reason to subject patient to increased risks of elective colonoscopy when the patient has active COVID-19 infection. No reason to subject the endoscopy staff to the risks of contracting the virus from infected patients.
Patients with GI bleeding associated with COVID-19 infection may have higher risks of morbidity and mortality than patients with GI bleeding without COVID-19 infection.	Patients with GI bleeding associated with severe COVID-19 pneumonia, respiratory compromise, and other serious complications of COVID-19 should generally be followed by an intensivist in an ICU.	Patients with severe pneumonia, respiratory compromise, and other serious complications of COVID-19 are at higher risk of mortality.
Protecting endoscopy personnel during EGD performed on a COVID-19-infected patient.	Endoscopy personnel in the endoscopy suite should be minimized during intubation and	Reduce exposure of endoscopy staff to COVID-19 infection.

	extubation of patients with COVID-19 infection.	
Management of anticoagulation in COVID-19 patients with GI bleeding: these patients seem to have higher rates of thrombotic complications. Anticoagulation can complicate the management of GI bleeding. This may be particularly important in planning endoscopic therapy for overt, active GI bleed, which may require withholding anticoagulation just before and after therapeutic endoscopy.	Contemplated endoscopic therapy for overt, active GI bleed may require withholding anticoagulation just before and just after therapeutic endoscopy.	COVID-19 patients likely have higher rates of thrombotic complications. Anticoagulation can complicate the management of GI bleeding. This may be particularly important in planning endoscopic therapy for overt, active GI bleed, which may require withholding anticoagulation just before and after therapeutic endoscopy.
Telemedicine.	May be considered as an alternative to ambulatory physical patient visits for follow-up after GI endoscopy.	Reduce hospital staff exposure to COVID-19-infected patients.

Abbreviation: PCR, polymerase chain reaction.

Table 3
Reported causes of jejunal and ileal bleeding in patients with COVID-19 infection

Lesion	Putative Mechanisms	Selected References
Jejunal ulcers and multiple proximal jejunojejunal fistulae	Scattered reported cases (1 with only jejunal ulcers)	16,84,86
Hemorrhagic enteritis	2 independent case reports Lesions attributed to COVID-19 infection	Amarapurkar et al,[85] 2020, Francese et al,[88] 2022
Small and large intestinal mucosal sloughing	1 case report	Yamakawa et al,[83] 2022
Gastrointestinal stromal tumor in jejunum	Case report	Jablońska et al,[89] 2022
Ileal angiodysplasia		Francese et al,[88] 2022

19-infected patients have special considerations in selecting endoscopic therapy. First, performing therapeutic EGD in patients with active upper GI bleeding may place the endoscopist and the endoscopy staff at higher risk of contracting COVID-19 infection. Exposure should therefore be minimized by performing therapeutic endoscopy by a senior "master" endoscopist with considerable experience in therapeutic endoscopy in patients at high risk to perform the therapy expeditiously.[77] Second, patients with active upper GI bleeding should be intubated endotracheally before performing EGD to protect the endoscopy staff from contracting the infection and to protect the patient's airway from aspiration of blood during EGD. Third, patients undergoing therapeutic EGD who have recently received prophylactic anticoagulation to reduce their risk of thromboembolism associated with COVID-19 infection may be best served by receiving endoscopic therapy providing the most secure and stable hemostasis (even in the face of anticoagulation in the recent past or contemplated in the future), such as endoscopic clips or band ligation.[78] Endoscopic band ligation may be performed in COVID-19-infected patients for esophageal variceal hemorrhage.[63] Fourth, endoscopic therapeutic modalities can be selected according to ease of performance and speed of therapy, such as favoring argon plasma coagulation, to minimize exposure of the endoscopist and the endoscopy staff to potentially infectious aerosolized blood from patients with active upper GI bleeding. This may be a highly personal professional decision in that endoscopists may feel more comfortable with therapeutic modalities because of personal experience. Fifth, endoscopists may elect not to apply therapeutic endoscopy altogether in patients with borderline indications for endoscopic therapy, such as a peptic ulcer that is slowly oozing blood (Forrest IB lesion).[79] Similarly, an endoscopist may elect not to decapitate a nonbleeding adherent clot (by guillotine by snare) and expose an underlying lesion to determine whether an ulcer with stigmata of recent hemorrhage lies underneath the clot[80] to prevent active bleeding after clot decapitation to reduce endoscopist exposure to actively bleeding infected patients. Patients with upper GI bleeding with flat spots or clean-based ulcers do not require endoscopic therapy regardless of the presence or absence of COVID-19 infection.[80] Sixth, COVID-19-infected patients who fail endoscopic therapy but are good surgical candidates may reasonably be sent for GI surgery or angiographic embolization, rather than persist at an unsuccessful endoscopic therapy or perform repeat endoscopic therapy.

In a highly selective multicenter North American cohort, only about 1% of subjects underwent GI endoscopy for GI bleeding and only two patients (about 0.1%) of the entire group underwent therapeutic endoscopy.[61] Ten of 18 subjects who underwent EGD for GI hemorrhage had reported esophagitis, gastritis, or ulcer, but did not receive endoscopic therapy. The authors noted low utilization of GI endoscopy despite prevalent COVID-19 GI symptoms, that inflammatory and erosive mucosal abnormalities were common in COVID-19 patients, and that most of these abnormalities were related to the underlying critical illness and not a local viral cytopathic effect.[61] In another New York cohort, 10 patients deemed to have significant bleeding underwent EGD with eight having gastric or duodenal ulcers and four requiring single or combined endoscopic hemostatic therapy to control the bleeding; four patients had recurrent bleeding, but no fatalities occurred because of the GI bleeding.[81] Three of four COVID-19 pneumonia patients hospitalized in ICUs required endoscopic hemostasis for bleeding ulcers in one series.[37] Three patients with COVID-19 duodenal hemorrhage were successfully treated with endoscopic vacuum therapy.[82]

Small Intestine Beyond Ligament of Treitz

The vast small intestinal surface area with its high density of angiotensin-converting enzyme-2 receptors renders this organ particularly susceptible to direct COVID-19 infection and injury. Infections usually manifest subclinically as only inflammation and erosions.[16,17] One patient had documented small and large intestinal mucosal sloughing with infection.[83] Another had a Crohn-like presentation with GI bleeding and fistulas.[84] Another patient underwent segmental resection for hemorrhagic enteritis, without Crohn disease, attributed directly to COVID-19 infection.[85] He required surgery and survived the surgery.

Jejunal and ileal causes of GI bleeding in COVID-19-infected patients are summarized in **Table 3**.[16,48,83–89]

Capsule Endoscopy and Enteroscopy to Evaluate Small Intestinal Bleeding

Mucosal abnormalities were commonplace in COVID-19 subjects undergoing capsule endoscopy.[48,86] Capsule endoscopy was touted as a primary diagnostic modality because of hesitancy about performing traditional tube endoscopy in COVID-19-infected patients.[87] For example, in one study,[48] 146 patients with COVID-19 infection first underwent capsule endoscopy as a triage tool to investigate GI bleeding as compared with 72 historical control subjects undergoing standard of care (SOC) evaluation for GI bleeding initially using EGD in the prepandemic era of January 1 to January 31, 2020. Active bleeding or stigmata of recent hemorrhage were observed in 44 (59.5%) patients in the COVID-19-infected group versus 18 (25.0%) in the SOC group (adjusted odds ratio, 5.23; 95% confidence interval, 2.23–12.27). Only 36 patients (48.7%) in the COVID-19-infected group required any invasive procedure during the hospitalization, compared with 70 (97.2%) in the SOC group (adjusted odds ratio, 0.01; 95% confidence interval, 0.001–0.08). The mean (standard deviation) number of invasive procedures was statistically significantly lower in the capsule endoscopy group: 0.59 (0.77) per patient in the COVID-19 group versus 1.18 (0.48) per patient in the SOC group (adjusted difference, −0.54; 95% confidence interval, −0.77 to −0.31). The authors concluded that the number of invasive GI endoscopies could be significantly decreased in COVID-19 patients when capsule endoscopy was performed as the initial test without increasing the rate of rebleeding or other complications.

Only one case report of push enteroscopy has been reported in COVID-19-infected patients: a 34-year-old man suffered sequelae of subacute GI obstruction and failure to thrive 2 months after a prolonged admission for COVID-19 infection.[84] He subsequently underwent push enteroscopy, which was performed safely and was diagnostic: it revealed residual jejunal ulcers and multiple proximal jejunojejunal fistulae.

The push enteroscopy directly led to laparotomy, which revealed strictures with dense intra-abdominal adhesions, a large jejunojejunal fistula, and evident prior jejunal perforation from severe COVID-19 infection. The patient recovered after small bowel resection with anastomoses and was discharged home, but represented with dyspnea, acute chest pain, and cardiac arrest 6 weeks postoperatively and subsequently died. The death was believed unrelated to the push enteroscopy 6 weeks earlier. A literature review revealed no data on single or double balloon enteroscopy performed in COVID-19-infected patients. Small intestinal bleeding from Crohn disease is reviewed in the accompanying article by Summa and Hanauer elsewhere in this issue.

Cause of Colonic Bleeding

Sparse colonoscopic data report ischemic colitis is a common cause of lower GI bleeding.[90] Ischemic or hemorrhagic colitis was noted in 13% to 33% of patients in several colonoscopy series.[16,61,90,91] Ischemic colitis has also been reported after tocilizumab therapy,[92] and after COVID-19 vaccination.[93] Hemorrhagic colitis can occur with COVID-19 infection, with concomitant cytomegalovirus reported in one case.[94,95] Other colonoscopic studies revealed rectal ulcers,[60,82] often caused by indwelling rectal tubes.[81] For GI bleeding in COVID-19 patients with inflammatory bowel disease, either ulcerative colitis or Crohn disease, see the accompanying article by Summa and Hanauer elsewhere in this issue. Five COVID-19 patients with GI bleeding underwent colonoscopy in one study with nonspecific findings, including presumptive bleeding from colonic diverticulosis or internal hemorrhoids.[16] Clinically manifest lower GI bleeding including hematochezia is uncommon with colonoscopy often showing minor mucosal lesions consistent with the same pattern for upper GI bleeding. Some bleeding may be incidental to COVID-19 infection.[16–19,61] Colonoscopy is generally deferred in COVID-19-infected patients, with colon capsule examination proposed as an initial diagnostic alternative to colonoscopy.[49] Interventional radiology should be considered for colonic bleeding if resources are available.[29,51,96] **Table 4** lists causes of colonic bleeding in COVID-19-infected patients.[16,61,81,90,92–95]

Outcomes of Gastrointestinal Bleeding

The spectrum of upper GI bleeding in COVID-19 patients commonly includes presentation with subclinical bleeding related to mucosal friability, anemia and hemoccult positive stools possibly requiring transfusions, but also includes clinically apparent bleeding in critically ill patients with COVID-19 pneumonia. COVID-19 infection may be incidental to the presentation with GI hemorrhage, especially in areas where COVID-19 infection is omnipresent.[4] Rarely, GI bleeding in a COVID-19 patient may be massive and fatal.[12,97,98] The literature has somewhat conflicting results concerning predisposing factors and the relationship of GI bleeding to outcome, including mortality. This variability may reflect differences in study design, demographics, and statistical analysis. A consistent finding was decreased use of GI endoscopy for GI bleeding and greater length of stay for patients with GI bleeding during the pandemic than for patients before the pandemic.[30,99]

In an Italian cohort, 78% had GI bleeding associated with thromboprophylaxis with anticoagulants.[20] A European study also noted this strong association.[19] Other studies have not reported anticoagulation as a significant risk factor.[21,81,100]

Mortality secondary to GI bleeding was often not stratified and outcome seemed most related to pulmonary or multisystem failure, including sepsis and thrombosis. GI hemorrhage in COVID-19 subjects in some analyses was not clearly associated with increased overall mortality, although COVID-19-infected patients had greater

Table 4
Reported causes of lower GI bleeding associated with COVID-19 infection

Lesion	Putative Mechanisms	References
Ischemic colitis	Reported in 13%–33% of patients with COVID-19 infection undergoing colonoscopy Association believed caused by COVID-19 infections promoting thrombosis	[16,61,90]
Ischemic colitis	Associated with tocilizumab therapy	Forneiro Pérez et al,[92] 2021
Ischemic colitis	After COVID-19 vaccination	Cui et al,[93] 2022
Rectal ulcers	Often related to placement of rectal tubes	Martin et al,[81] 2020
Hemorrhagic colitis	Acute hemorrhagic diarrhea without evident ulcerative colitis or ischemic colitis on colonoscopy including pathologic examination of colonoscopic biopsies. Attributed to "traveler's diarrhea" due to recent visit to Egypt from the United States with negative work-up for bacterial cultures of stool and negative examinations for ova and parasites of stool.	Carvalho et al,[94] 2020
Hemorrhagic colitis can occur with COVID-19 infection	1 case associated with concomitant cytomegalovirus infection	Leemans et al,[95] 2020
Colonic angiodysplasia	2 cases reported in a review of 27 colonoscopies mostly performed for overt GI bleeding	Vanella et al,[16] 2021
Bleeding hemorrhoids	1 case reported in a review of 27 colonoscopies mostly performed for overt GI bleeding	Vanella et al,[16] 2021
Colonic diverticulosis with bleeding	4 cases reported in a review of 27 colonoscopies mostly performed for overt GI bleeding	Vanella et al,[16] 2021

mortality than non-COVID-19 subjects, at least for all patients presenting with upper GI bleeding.[23,40] Other studies found GI bleeding was associated with increased COVID-19 mortality.[3,101]

Emerging Trends

COVID-19 infection is a moving and evolving target because of emergent new viral mutations that are likely more infections and less lethal, changes in the biology of the infection caused by improved host defenses from vaccinations and improved antiviral treatments including improved critical care, better management of respiratory compromise, and the introduction of moderately effective antiviral therapy. These changes are reflected in decreasing mortality and likely decreasing morbidity from the virus, which may reduce the burden of GI disease including GI bleeding. Long COVID is being increasingly appreciated, but it does not seem so far to frequently cause significant GI bleeding (See the article by Tindade and colleagues on long COVID elsewhere in this issue.). Although there is a theoretical risk of transmission of COVID-19 infection to uninfected patients, endoscopy staff, and the GI endoscopist from aerosolization of viral particles, particularly in patients with active upper GI bleeding, the risk of spread to these groups seems to be less than initially feared, partly caused by use of PPE, isolation techniques, viricidal cleaning solutions, and universally recommended vaccinations. This change has allowed a gradual increase in the use of GI endoscopy from less than 10% of baseline rate during the pandemic onset to substantial but still incomplete recovery in the use of GI endoscopy toward the prepandemic baseline. Although the data on GI endoscopy were particularly sparse early in the pandemic, these data have been accumulating recently with the recovery of GI endoscopy toward prepandemic levels. This review is best considered a snapshot of the current state of GI bleeding with COVID, with likely future advancements and improvements in clinical therapy, management, and prognosis over time.

SUMMARY

GI symptoms and GI pathology are common in COVID-19 infection, but overt GI bleeding is uncommon. Mucosal abnormalities are frequently noted at GI endoscopy and capsule endoscopy. However, GI hemorrhage associated with COVID-19 is often subclinical. The presentation of GI bleeding in COVID-19 ranges from the bleeding patient incidentally found to have COVID-19 infection to the critically ill COVID-19 subject with pneumonia and multisystem disorders. Use of anticoagulant and antiplatelet drugs and the known association of physiologic "stress" GI bleeding in critically ill patients with respiratory illness may be predisposing factors in this population. Modest endoscopic data suggest that PUD, including erosive gastroduodenitis, are common causes of GI bleeding. Ischemic colitis has a known association with COVID-19, but uncommonly manifests as overt bleeding. The approach to COVID-19 subjects with GI bleeding resembles that of the general population with the cogent exception of often deferring endoscopy for patients with mild GI bleeding and reserving endoscopy for patients with more severe GI bleeding likely requiring therapeutic endoscopy. International and national guidelines reflect this philosophy and practice. Better understanding of COVID-19 pathogenesis and the advent of preventive measures, such as vaccination and improved medications, such as Paxlovid, may ultimately render a conservative approach to GI endoscopy no longer tenable.

The editor of this monograph on GI manifestations and therapy for COVID hopes to contribute to this general advancement on COVID-19 therapy and prognosis by hereby offering the first volume or monograph devoted exclusively to the GI, liver, and pancreatic manifestations of COVID infection. Although COVID-19 is primarily a respiratory disease with prominent respiratory symptoms and frequent respiratory compromise, GI manifestations play an important secondary role in the morbidity and even rarely in the mortality of this infection.

CLINICS CARE POINTS

- COVID-19 has produced >6,000,000 deaths worldwide since March 2020 primarily from pneumonia and respiratory failure.

- GI manifestations of COVID-19 infection, especially diarrhea and GI bleeding, have sometimes produced morbidity and rarely contributed to mortality from this viral infection.
- GI bleeding occurs in 1.5% to 3.0% of patients hospitalized with acute COVID-19 infection.
- GI bleeding is typically mild-to-moderate and associated with mild mucosal erosions/abnormalities but can occassionally cause severe bleeding, especially from peptic ulcer disease or stress gastritis associated with pneumonia or respiratory failure from COVID-19 infection.
- In the pandemic onset, GI bleeding was rarely evaluated by GI endoscopy due to the risks of endoscopy staff contracting the infection from infected patients and the feared risks of infected patients suffering complications from undergoing GI endoscopy.

ACKNOWLEDGEMENTS

Dr Cappell is employed as a gastroenterologist at the Aleda E. Lutz VA Medical Center at Saginaw Michigan. The Saginaw VA Hospital and the federal government take no position on the opinions expressed in this article. This article is a review article that does not require Internal Review Board approval because there is no original patient data contained in this article.

REFERENCES

1. Cascella M, Rajnik M, Aleem A, et al. Features, evaluation, and treatment of coronavirus (COVID-19). StatPearls [Internet]. Treasure Island (FL): StatPearls Publishing; 2022. https://www.ncbi.nlm.nih.gov/books/NBK554776/. Accessed May 23, 2022.
2. Cappell MS. Moderately severe diarrhea and impaired renal function with COVID-19 infection. Am J Gastroenterol 2020;115(6):947–8.
3. Elshazli RM, Kline A, Elgaml A, et al. Gastroenterology manifestations and COVID-19 outcomes: a meta-analysis of 25,252 cohorts among the first and second waves. J Med Virol 2021;93(5):2740–68.
4. Gulen M, Satar S. Uncommon presentation of COVID-19: gastrointestinal bleeding. Clin Res Gastroenterol Hepatol 2020;44(4):e72–6.
5. Wang P, Tan X, Li Q, et al. Extra-pulmonary complications of 45 critically ill patients with COVID-19 in Yichang, Hubei province, China: a single centered, retrospective, observation study. Medicine (Baltimore) 2021;100(9):e24604.
6. Lin L, Jiang X, Zhang Z, et al. Gastrointestinal symptoms of 95 cases with SARS-CoV-2 infection. Gut 2020;69(6):997–1001.
7. Perisetti A, Gajendran M, Mann R, et al. COVID-19 extrapulmonary illness: special gastrointestinal and hepatic considerations. Dis Mon 2020;66(9):101064.
8. Ion D, Panduraru D, Bolocan A, et al. Gastro-intestinal bleeding in COVID-19 patients: is there any causal relation? Chirurgia 2021;116(6 Suppl):S69–76.
9. Zhang J, Garrett S, Sun J. Gastrointestinal symptoms, pathophysiology, and treatment in COVID-19. Genes Dis 2021;8(4):385–400.
10. Ye Q, Wang B, Zhang T, et al. The mechanism and treatment of gastrointestinal symptoms in patients with COVID-19. Am J Physiolog Gastrointest Liver Physiol 2020;319(2):G245–52.
11. Dioscoridi L, Giannetti A, Massad MT, et al. A "double-hit" damage mechanism can explain self-limited GI bleeding in COVID-19 pneumonia. Gastrointest Endosc 2021;93(5):1192–3.

12. Mohamed M, Nassar M, Nso N, et al. Massive gastrointestinal bleeding in a patient with COVID-19. Arab J Gastroenterol 2021;22(2):177–9.
13. Cook D, Guyatt G. Prophylaxis against upper gastrointestinal bleeding in hospitalized patients. N Engl J Med 2018;378(26):2506–16.
14. Sarkar M, Madabhavi IV, Quy PN, et al. COVID-19 and coagulopathy. Clin Resp J 2021;15(12):1259–74.
15. Buckholz A, Kaplan A, Jessurun J, et al. Microthrombosis associated with GI bleeding in COVID-19. Gastrointest Endosc 2021;93(1):263–4.
16. Vanella G, Capurso G, Burti C, et al. Gastrointestinal mucosal damage in patients with COVID-19 undergoing endoscopy: an international multicentre study. BMJ Open Gastroenterol 2021;8(1):e000578.
17. Ashktorab H, Russo T, Oskrochi G, et al. Clinical and endoscopic outcomes in coronavirus disease-2019 patients with gastrointestinal bleeding. Gastro Hep Adv 2022;1(4):487–99.
18. Marasco G, Maida M, Morreale GC, et al. Gastrointestinal bleeding in COVID-19 patients: a systematic review with meta-analysis. Can J Gastroenterol Hepatol 2021;2021:2534975.
19. Zellmer S, Hanses F, Muzalyova A, et al. Gastrointestinal bleeding and endoscopic findings in critically and non-critically ill patients with corona virus disease 2019 (COVID-19): results from Lean European Open Survey on SARS-CoV-2 (LEOSS) and COKA registries. United Eur Gastroenterol J 2021;9(9):1081–90.
20. Mauro A, De Grazia F, Lenti MV, et al. Upper gastrointestinal bleeding in COVID-19 inpatients: incidence and management in a multicenter experience from Northern Italy. Clin Res Gastroenterol Hepatol 2021;45(3):101521.
21. Trindade AJ, Izard S, Coppa K, et al. Gastrointestinal bleeding in hospitalized COVID-19 patients: a propensity score matched cohort study. J Intern Med 2021;289(6):887–94.
22. Makker J, Mantri N, Patel HK, et al. The incidence and mortality impact of gastrointestinal bleeding in hospitalized COVID-19 patients. Clin Exp Gastroenterol 2021;14:405–11.
23. González Maker R, Jacob J, Miro O, et al. Incidence, clinical characteristics, risk factors, and outcomes of upper gastrointestinal bleeding in patients with COVID-19: results of the UMC-19-S12. J Clin Gastroenterol 2022;56(1):e38–46.
24. Zhang H, Wu Y, He Y, et al. Age-related risk factors and complications of patients with COVID-19: a population-based retrospective study. Front Med (Lausanne) 2021;8:757459.
25. Cappell MS, Friedel D. Initial management of acute upper gastrointestinal bleeding: from initial evaluation up to gastrointestinal endoscopy. Med Clin North Am 2008;92(3):491–509, xi.
26. American Red Cross. Red Cross declares first-ever blood crisis amid omicron surge. Available at: https://www.redcross.org/about-us/news-andevents/press-release/2022/blood-donors-needed-now-as-omicron-intensifies.html. Accessed September 28, 2022.
27. Duan Z, Liu K, Zhou S. The dilemma in the management of suspected upper GI bleeding in patients with COVID-19 pneumonia. Gastrointest Endosc 2020;92(6):1273–4.
28. Edwards C, Penman ID, Coleman M. Gastrointestinal endoscopy during COVID-19: when less is more. Frontline Gastroenterol 2020;11(4):256–7.

29. Holzwanger EA, Bilal M, Stallwood CG, et al. Acute lower gastrointestinal bleeding during the COVID-19 pandemic: less is more. Endoscopy 2020; 52(9):816–7.
30. Laursen SB, Gralnek IM, Stanley AJ. Raising the threshold for hospital admission and endoscopy in upper gastrointestinal bleeding during the COVID-19 pandemic. Endoscopy 2020;52(10):930–1.
31. Duan Z, Zhou S, Niu Z. Use of the Glasgow-Blatchford score during the COVID-19 pandemic needs more rigorous research. Endoscopy 2021;53(2):209.
32. Soetikno R, Teoh AY, Kaltenbach T, et al. Considerations in performing endoscopy during the COVID-19 pandemic. Gastrointest Endosc 2020;92:176–83.
33. Gralnek IM, Hassan C, Beilenhoff U, et al. ESGE and ESGENA Position Statement on gastrointestinal endoscopy and the COVID-19 pandemic. Endoscopy 2020;52(6):483–90.
34. Iqbal U, Patel PD, Pluskota CA, et al. Outcomes of acute gastrointestinal bleeding in patients with COVID-19: a case-control study. Gastroenterol Res 2022;15(1):13–8.
35. Cappell MS. Local COVID-19 epicenter in Detroit metropolitan area causing profound and pervasive reorganization of clinical, educational, research, and financial programs of a large academic gastroenterology division with a GI fellowship and primary medical school affiliation. Dig Dis Sci 2021;66(11):3635–58.
36. Khan R, Saha S, Gimpaya N, et al. Outcomes for upper gastrointestinal bleeding during the first wave of the COVID-19 pandemic in the Toronto area. J Gastroenterol Hepatol 2022;37(5):878–82.
37. Pradhan F, Alishahi Y. Gastrointestinal bleeding and endoscopic outcomes in patients with SARS-CoV-2. Clin Endosc 2021;54(3):428–31.
38. Chiu PWY, Ng SC, Inoue H, et al. Practice of endoscopy during COVID-19 pandemic: position statements of the Asian Pacific Society for Digestive Endoscopy (APSDE-COVID statements). Gut 2020;6:991–6.
39. Rosevics L, Fossati BS, Teixeiba S, et al. COVID-19 and digestive endoscopy: emergency endoscopic procedures and risk factors for upper gastrointestinal bleeding. Arq Gastroenterol 2021;58(3):337–43.
40. Benites-Goñi H, Pascacio-Fiori M, Monge-Del Valle F, et al. Impact of the COVID-19 pandemic in the time to endoscopy in patients with upper gastrointestinal bleeding. Rev Gastroenterol Peru 2020;40(3):219–23.
41. Barrett LF, Lo KB, Stanek SR, et al. Self-limited gastrointestinal bleeding in COVID-19. Clin Res Gastroenterol Hepatol 2020;44(4):e77–80.
42. Cavaliere K, Levine C, Wander P, et al. Management of upper GI bleeding in patients with COVID-19 pneumonia. Gastrointest Endosc 2020;92(2):454–5.
43. Sbeit W, Mari A, Pellicano R, et al. When and whom to scope in case of gastrointestinal bleeding in the COVID-19 era? Minerva Gastroenterol (Torino) 2021; 67(4):307–9.
44. Shalimar Vaishnav M, Elhence A, Kumar R, et al. Outcome of conservative therapy in coronavirus disease-2019: patients presenting with gastrointestinal bleeding. J Clin Exp Hepatol 2021;11(3):327–33.
45. Xu F, Yang Y, Ding Z. Esophagogastroduodenoscopy procedure using disposable endoscope to detect the cause of melena in a patient with COVID-19. Dig Endosc 2021;33(1):e1–2.
46. Onaizah O, Koszowska Z, Winters C, et al. Guidelines for robotic flexible endoscopy at the time of COVID-19. Front Robot A 2021;8:612852.

47. Elsayed I, Meier B, Caca K, et al. Potential use of a novel telemetric sensor capsule in patients with suspected gastrointestinal bleeding during the COVID-19 pandemic. Endoscopy 2021;53(3):337–8.
48. Hakimian S, Raines D, Reed G, et al. Assessment of video capsule endoscopy in the management of acute gastrointestinal bleeding during the COVID-19 pandemic. JAMA Netw Open 2021;4(7):e2118796.
49. MacLeod C, Wilson P, Watson AJM. Colon capsule endoscopy: an innovative method for detecting colorectal pathology during the COVID-19 pandemic? Colorectal Dis 2020;22(6):621–4.
50. Suzuki S, Kusano C, Ikehara H. Simple barrier device to minimize facial exposure of endoscopists during COVID-19 pandemic. Dig Endosc 2020;32(5):e118–9.
51. Ierardi AM, Del Giudice C, Coppola A, et al. Gastrointestinal hemorrhages in patients with COVID-19 managed with transarterial embolization. Am J Gastroenterol 2021;116(4):838–40.
52. American Hospital Association. Shortage of contrast media for CT imaging affecting hospitals and health systems | AHA. Available at: https://www.aha.org/advisory/2022-05-12-shortage-contrast-media-ct-imaging-affecting-hospitals-and-health-systems. Accessed June 23, 2022.
53. Jayasena H, Abeynayake D, De Silva A, et al. The use of personal protective equipment in endoscopy: what should the endoscopist wear during a pandemic? Exp Rev Gastroenterol Hepatol 2021;15(12):1349–59.
54. Agarwal A, Chowdhury SD, Sachdeva S, et al. Low risk of transmission of SARS-CoV2 and effective endotherapy for gastrointestinal bleeding despite challenges supports resuming optimum endoscopic services. Dig Liver Dis 2021;53(1):4–7.
55. www.aamc.org/data-reports/workforce/interactive-data/active-physicians-age-and-specialty-2019. Accessed October 10, 2022.
56. Vignesh S, Butt AS, Alboraie M, et al. Impact of COVID-19 on endoscopy training: perspectives from a global survey of program directors and endoscopy trainers. Clin Endosc 2021;54(5):678–87.
57. Yang X, Yu Y, Xu J. Clinical course and outcomes of critically ill patients with SARS-CoV-2 pneumonia in Wuhan, China: a single-centered, retrospective, observational study. Lancet Respir Med 2020;8(5):475–81.
58. Melazzini F, Lenti MV, Mauro A, et al. Peptic ulcer disease as a common cause of bleeding in patients with coronavirus disease 2019. Am J Gastroenterol 2020; 115(7):1139–40.
59. Deb A, Thongtan T, Costilla V. Gastric ulceration in Covid-19: an ominous sign? BMJ Case Rep 2021;14(7):e244059.
60. Blackett JW, Kumta NA, Dixon RE, et al. Characteristics and outcomes of patients undergoing endoscopy during the COVID-19 pandemic: a multicenter study from New York City. Dig Dis Sci 2020;60:1–10.
61. Kuftinec G, Elmunzer BJ, Amin S, et al. The role of endoscopy and findings in COVID-19 patients, an early North American Cohort. BMC Gastroenterol 2021;21(1):205.
62. Papanikolaou IS, Lazaridis LD, Rizos E, et al. Untying the knot: acute variceal bleeding in a COVID-19 patient. What should the gastroenterologist keep in mind? Eur J Gastroenterol Hepatol 2021;33(3):450–1.
63. El Kassas M, Al Shafie A, Abdel Hameed AS, et al. Emergency endoscopic variceal band ligation in a COVID-19 patient presented with hematemesis while on mechanical ventilation. Dig Endosc 2021;32(5):812–5.
64. Bisseling TM, van Laarhoven A, Huijbers A, et al. Coronavirus disease-19 presenting as esophageal ulceration. Am J Gastroenterol 2021;1;116(2):421–4.

65. González-Sagredo A, Iborra Ortega E, Herranz Pinilla C, et al. Covid-19 and aorto-enteric fistula. Rev Esp Enferm Dig 2021;113(12):852–3.
66. Koç ES, Çiçek B. COVID-19 induced haemobilia: a novel entity. J Gastrointest Liver Dis 2021;30(4):528–30.
67. Awwad I, Greuel S, Tacke F, et al. Haemorrhagic ulcerative duodenitis in a patient with COVID-19 infection: clinical improvement following treatment with budesonide. BMJ Open Gastroenterol 2021;8(1):e000757.
68. Deliwala SS, Hussain MS, Ponnapalli A, et al. Black oesophagus, upside-down stomach and Cameron lesions: cascade effects of a large hiatal hernia. BMJ Case Rep 2021;14(11):e246496.
69. Pérez Roldán F, Malik Javed Z, Yagüe Compadre JL, et al. Gastric ulcers with upper gastrointestinal bleeding in patients with severe SARS-CoV-2. Rev Esp Enferm Dig 2021;113(2):122–4.
70. Mur-Murota A, Yoshi S, Okuda R, et al. Successful hemostasis of bleeding gastric inflammatory fibroid polyp by endoscopic treatment in a patient with severe COVID-19. Clin J Gastroenterol 2021;14(4):1008–13.
71. Aguayo WG, Moyon FX, Molina GA, et al. A bleeding GIST in pandemic times, a cooperative approach to a delayed complication, a case report. Int J Surg Case Rep 2020;77:880–4.
72. Galvez A, King K, El Chaar M, et al. Perforated marginal ulcer in a COVID-19 patient. Laparoscopy in these trying times? Obes Surg 2020;30(11):4605–8.
73. Philips CA, Kumbar S, Ahamed R, et al. Managing acute portal hypertensive gastropathy bleed during the time of COVID-19 pandemic: novelty or necessity? Cureus 2020;12(5):e8333.
74. Casper M, Lepper P, Danziger G, et al. Gastrointestinal endoscopy during extracorporeal membrane oxygenation (ECMO) for COVID-19. J Gastrointestin Liver Dis 2020;29(3):471–3.
75. Cappell MS. Therapeutic endoscopy for acute upper gastrointestinal bleeding. Nat Rev Gastroenterol Hepatol 2010;7(4):214–29.
76. Hagel AF, Albrecht H, Nägel A, et al. The application of Hemospray in gastrointestinal bleeding during emergency endoscopy. Gastroenterol Res Pract 2017; 2017:3083481.
77. Cappell MS. Gastrointestinal endoscopy in high-risk patients. Dig Dis 1996; 14(4):228–44.
78. Lanas Á. Hemorragia gastrointestinal [gastrointestinal bleeding]. Gastroenterol Hepatol 2015 Sep;38(Suppl 1):56–63. Spanish.
79. Jensen DM, Eklund S, Persson T, et al. Reassessment of rebleeding risk of Forrest IB (Oozing) peptic ulcer bleeding in a large international randomized trial. Am J Gastroenterol 2017;112(3):441–6.
80. Laine L, Jensen DM. Management of patients with ulcer bleeding. Am J Gastroenterol 2012;107(3):345–60 [quiz: 361].
81. Martin TA, Wan DW, Hajifathalian K, et al. Gastrointestinal bleeding in patients with coronavirus disease 2019: a matched case-control study. Am J Gastroenterol 2020;115(10):1609–16.
82. de Moura DTH, de Moura EGH, Hirsch BS, et al. Modified endoscopic vacuum therapy for duodenal hemorrhage in patients with severe acute respiratory syndrome coronavirus 2. Endoscopy 2022;54(S 02):E837–9.
83. Yamakawa T, Ishigami K, Takizawa A, et al. Extensive mucosal sloughing of the small intestine and colon in a patient with severe COVID-19. DEN Open 2022; 2(1):e42. Epub 2021.

84. Abbassi B, Deb A, Costilla V, et al. A subacute enteritis two months after COVID-19 pneumonia with mucosal bleeding, perforation, and internal fistulas. Surg 2021. https://doi.org/10.1177/00031348211023461. Online ahead of print.
85. Amarapurkar AD, Vichare P, Pandya N, et al. Haemorrhagic enteritis and COVID-19: causality or coincidence. J Clin Pathol 2020;73(10):686.
86. Li L, Yang L, Li J, et al. Diagnosis of suspected small bowel bleeding by capsule endoscopy in patients with COVID-19. Inter Med 2021;60(15):2425–30.
87. McAlindon M. COVID-19: impetus to the adoption of capsule endoscopy as a primary diagnostic tool? Frontline Gastroenterol 2021;12(4):263–4.
88. Francese M, Ferrari C, Lotti M, et al. The thin red line: ileal angiodysplasia versus SARS-CoV-2-related haemorrhagic enteritis. J Clin Pathol 2022. https://doi.org/10.1136/jclinpath-2021-207754. jclinpath-2021-207754.
89. Jablońska B, Szmigiel P, Wosiewicz P, et al. A jejunal gastrointestinal stromal tumor with massive gastrointestinal hemorrhage treated by emergency surgery: a case report. Medicine (Baltimore) 2022;101(35):e30098.
90. Paul T, Joy AR, Alsoub HARS, et al. Case report: ischemic colitis in severe COVID-19 pneumonia: an unforeseen gastrointestinal complication. Am J Trop Med Hyg 2021;104(1):63–5.
91. Massironi S, Vigano C, Dioscoridi L, et al. Endoscopic findings in patients infected with 2019 novel coronavirus in Lombardy. Clin Gastroenterol Hepatol 2020;18:2375–7.
92.. Forneiro Pérez R, Dabán López P, Zurita Saavedra MS, et al. Tocilizumab as a possible cause of ischemic colitis. Gastroenterol Hepatol 2021;44(5):373–4.
93. Cui MH, Hou XL, Liu JY. Ischemic colitis after receiving the second dose of a COVID-19 inactivated vaccine: a case report. World J Clin Cases 2022;26;10(12):3866–71.
94. Carvalho A, Alqusairi R, Adams A, et al. SARS-CoV-2 gastrointestinal Infection causing hemorrhagic colitis: implications for detection and transmission of COVID-19 disease. Am J Gastroenterol 2020;115(6):942–6.
95. Leemans S, Maillart E, Van Noten H, et al. Cytomegalovirus haemorrhagic colitis complicating COVID-19 in an immunocompetent critically ill patient: a case report. Clin Case Rep 2020;9(5):e03600.
96. Kumar MA, Krishnaswamy M, Arul JN. Post COVID-19 sequelae: venous thromboembolism complicated by lower GI bleed. BMJ Case Rep 2021;14(1):e241059.
97. Chen T, Yang Q, Duan H. A severe coronavirus disease 2019 patient with high-risk predisposing factors died from massive gastrointestinal bleeding: a case report. BMC Gastroenterol 2020;20(1):318.
98. Mitrovic M, Tadic B, Jankovic A, et al. Fatal gastrointestinal bleeding associated with acute pancreatitis as a complication of Covid-19: a case report. Int Med 2022;50(5). 3000605221098179.
99. Kim J, Doyle JB, Blackett JW, et al. Effect of the coronavirus 2019 pandemic on outcomes for patients admitted with gastrointestinal bleeding in New York City. Gastroenterology 2020;159(3):1155–7.
100. Rustgi SD, Yang JY, Luther S, et al. Anticoagulation does not increase risk of mortality or ICU admission in hospitalized COVID-19 patients with gastrointestinal bleeding: results from a New York health system. Clin Res Gastroenterol Hepatol 2021;45(3):101602.
101. Zuin M, Rigatelli G, Fogato L, et al. Higher risk of death in COVID-19 patients complicated by gastrointestinal bleeding events: a meta-analysis. Minerva Gastroenterol (Torino) 2021;67(4):408–10.

COVID-19 and Inflammatory Bowel Disease

Keith C. Summa, MD, PhD, Stephen B. Hanauer, MD*

KEYWORDS

- Inflammatory bowel disease • Ulcerative colitis • Crohn disease
- Immunosuppression • COVID-19 • SARS-CoV-2 • COVID vaccination
- Long COVID

KEY POINTS

- Patients with inflammatory bowel disease (IBD) are not at significantly increased risk of infection, severe disease, or death from the SARS-CoV-2 virus.
- Among IBD treatments, only systemic corticosteroids have been associated with increased risk for severe COVID-19 disease and death.
- COVID-19 vaccination is safe, well-tolerated, and effective in most IBD patients.
- IBD patients should undergo COVID-19 vaccination, including booster doses after the initial vaccine series, to reduce the morbidity and mortality from COVID-19.
- Gastroenterologists have a role in promoting uptake of vaccination recommendations among IBD patients.

INTRODUCTION

In late 2019, the novel coronavirus, now known as severe acute respiratory syndrome coronavirus-2 (SARS-CoV-2), began circulating in Wuhan, China, and subsequently spread worldwide causing a global pandemic, with SARS-CoV-2 now likely transitioning to become a widely circulating endemic virus. SARS-CoV-2 is an RNA virus that causes infection by binding of the receptor-binding domain from the viral spike protein to the host receptor angiotensin-converting enzyme-2, which triggers viral entry.[1,2] Angiotensin-converting enzyme-2 receptors are widely expressed throughout the body, including on gastrointestinal epithelial cells.[3,4] SARS-CoV-2 infection causes the clinical syndrome of coronavirus disease-2019 (COVID-19), which is heterogeneous, ranging from asymptomatic infection, to mild and self-limited symptoms, to severe disease requiring hospitalization, and to excessive immune activation and cytokine storm leading to multiple organ failure, shock, and death.[1] Gastrointestinal

Division of Gastroenterology and Hepatology, Department of Medicine, Northwestern University Feinberg School of Medicine, 676 North Saint Clair Street, Suite 1400, Chicago, IL 60611, USA
* Corresponding author.
E-mail address: shanauer@northwestern.edu

Gastroenterol Clin N Am 52 (2023) 103–113
https://doi.org/10.1016/j.gtc.2022.10.005
gastro.theclinics.com

symptoms, such as anorexia, diarrhea, nausea, and abdominal pain, are common in COVID-19, and were widely reported in the early descriptions of COVID-19.[5] Gastrointestinal symptoms of SARS-CoV-2 infection are presumably related to local effects of viral infection and host immune responses because SARS-CoV-2 viral RNA is isolated from the stool of infected individuals.[6,7]

The emergence of the COVID-19 pandemic generated widespread uncertainty and concern for patients with inflammatory bowel diseases (IBD), because the risks of SARS-CoV-2 infection for IBD patients, many of whom are treated with immunosuppressive therapies associated with increased risk of infection,[8,9] were initially unknown. In addition, the dramatic societal responses to the pandemic presented challenges to IBD patients, who had to quickly adapt to a new environment characterized by changing public health recommendations, reduced opportunity for in-person clinical visits with providers, and shifts to use of telemedicine technologies. Furthermore, the rapid development and deployment of COVID-19 vaccines, including the use of novel messenger RNA (mRNA)-based vaccine technology, led to new questions and uncertainties for IBD patients who were excluded from initial clinical trials leading to the emergency use authorization and subsequent approval by the Food and Drug Administration in the United States. It was not initially known whether these vaccines would be safe and/or effective, nor whether vaccination would adversely impact their IBD. Finally, the development of persistent symptoms after SARS-CoV-2 infection, known as "long COVID" or postacute COVID-19 syndrome (PACS), represented another unknown for IBD patients who struggled to discern the potential long-term consequences of infection.

This article addresses the incidence of COVID-19 and the risk for severe disease from COVID-19 in patients with IBD, gleaned mainly from large-scale IBD patient databases. The impact of IBD treatments on COVID-19 risk is reviewed. The sequelae and aftereffects of SARS-CoV-2 infection are discussed, including the concept of long COVID, also known as PACS. COVID-19 vaccination in IBD patients is then discussed, including humoral and cell-mediated immune responses to vaccination in patients, and the effects of various IBD medications on vaccine responses. This review concludes with clinical recommendations regarding COVID-19 vaccination in IBD patients.

DISCUSSION

COVID-19 Incidence in Patients with Inflammatory Bowel Disease

An immediate concern present at the onset of the pandemic was whether IBD patients were at increased risk of COVID-19 given the underlying immune dysregulation driving their IBD and their IBD treatments, most of which are immunosuppressive or immunomodulatory in nature. A total of eight initial studies were summarized and combined in a rapid review and meta-analysis published in the fall of 2020, which described an overall incidence of COVID-19 in IBD patients of 0.3%.[10] Six of these studies included patient numbers sufficient to combine in a meta-analysis of 9177 primarily European IBD patients (two studies from Italy, two studies from Spain, one study from France and Italy, and one study from China). From this pooled patient cohort, a total of 32 confirmed cases of COVID-19 were identified during the study period (ranging from January 2020 in the Chinese study to early April 2020 in the Spanish studies). This rate of 0.3% was comparable with the rate in the general population, with similar demographics at that time (0.2%–0.4%).[10]

Shortly thereafter, the results of an analysis of COVID-19 infection rates in a large multinational cohort of IBD patients (n = 23,879) from 12 centers in Europe and Israel was published.[11] This study, which evaluated the time period from February 21 to

June 30, 2020, identified a cumulative incidence of 0.406% (97 IBD patients with confirmed SARS-CoV-2 infection), which nearly matched the incidence observed in a matched general population without IBD (0.402%).[11]

An important caveat of this and much of the early research on COVID-19 is the substantial heterogeneity in the early phases of the pandemic, because different parts of the world were affected by waves of COVID-19 infections at different times, and different parts of the world had substantially variable COVID test availability and patterns of public health and societal responses to the pandemic that shifted over time and in relation to one another. It is thus difficult to interpret, understand, and compare reported rates of incidence given these temporal dynamics of the pandemic and responses to it. For example, individual IBD patients, given their concerns about potential increased disease susceptibility and/or severity, may have more carefully adhered to recommendations for social distancing, isolation, and masking than the general population. If such behavioral patterns were adopted by large numbers of IBD patients, these behaviors may have reduced the reported incidence of COVID-19 in IBD patients compared with what would have been observed in a hypothetical environment characterized by similar behaviors for IBD patients and control subjects.

Despite these potential limitations and theoretical concerns related to initial studies, the conclusion that patients with IBD are not at significantly increased risk for SARS-CoV-2 infection has been borne out and confirmed over time. As SARS-CoV-2 transitions from a global pandemic to an endemic virus, ongoing research and monitoring should continue to evaluate whether IBD patients are at increased risk over time.

COVID-19 Severity in Patients with Inflammatory Bowel Disease

A related early concern among IBD patients and providers was whether SARS-CoV-2 infection was more severe in IBD patients compared with matched individuals without IBD. Similar limitations impacted early research into risks for severe COVID-19 in IBD patients. In addition, the initial phases of the pandemic likely exhibited significant selection bias because severe cases were scrutinized closely, whereas the high rate of asymptomatic infection was not initially appreciated. An early case-control study involving COVID-19-positive patients (confirmed or highly suspected) at two New York City hospitals compared disease severity in 80 IBD patients versus 160 matched non-IBD control patients, finding similar overall rates of a composite end point of severe disease, consisting of intensive care unit admission, endotracheal intubation, or death (24% for IBD patients vs 35% for non-IBD patients; $P = 0.352$).[12] This study demonstrated that the most significant risk factor for severe COVID-19 in IBD patients was increased age, the same risk factor for those without IBD.[12] Older age was associated with increased risk for severe disease in the IBD and non-IBD cohorts, highlighting the theme that the risk factors for severe COVID-19-related disease, such as age and comorbidities, are not unique to IBD and are instead similar between IBD patients and those without IBD. An intriguing additional finding from this study was that rates of several gastrointestinal symptoms in the setting of SARS-CoV-2 infection were significantly higher in IBD patients compared with those without IBD: diarrhea (45% vs 19%; $P < 0.001$) and abdominal pain (20% vs 5%; $P < 0.001$).[12]

A longitudinal component of this early study described an association between moderate-to-severe IBD disease and SARS-CoV-2 infection rate, because IBD patients with COVID-19 were significantly more likely to have clinically active disease, endoscopic disease activity, and baseline elevation of the inflammatory biomarkers C-reactive protein and fecal calprotectin.[12] In addition, an increased risk for COVID-19 was seen in IBD patients receiving corticosteroids.[12] A subsequent retrospective observational study of an Italian cohort of IBD patients (n = 122; the Sicilian Network for IBD [SN-IBD] cohort) infected with SARS-CoV-2 during the second pandemic wave in the fall of 2020 found, on multivariate analysis, that severe IBD activity was the only independent predictor of severe COVID-19, as defined by a composite end point consisting of the need for respiratory support or death.[13]

One of the best resources for comprehensive, longitudinal research on COVID-19 in IBD patients has been the SECURE-IBD database (Surveillance Epidemiology of Coronavirus [COVID-19] Under Research Exclusion for Inflammatory Bowel Disease; covidibd.org). The initial report of data from the SECURE-IBD database consisting of 525 cases of COVID-19 in IBD patients from 33 countries during the early phases of the pandemic indicated that increasing age, increasing number of comorbidities (two or more), and use of corticosteroids were associated with an increased risk of severe disease.[14] Interestingly, the use of 5-aminosalicylate or sulfasalazine was associated with increased risk of severe disease, whereas the use of tumor necrosis factor (TNF)-α antagonist therapy was not associated with an increased risk of severe disease. Among these cases of COVID-19, 161 patients were hospitalized (31%), 37 patients had severe COVID-19 (7%), and 16 patients died (case fatality rate of 3%).

The overall mortality in this IBD patient database did not differ significantly from mortality reported in the United States, Europe, and China, strengthening the conclusion that there was not an increased risk of death from COVID-19 in IBD patients compared with the general population. Overall, these findings reinforce the notion that the most significant risk factors for severe COVID-19 in IBD patients are shared with those individuals without IBD, namely increased age and medical comorbidities. Indeed, a subsequent, updated analysis of the SECURE-IBD database reported that most of the severe COVID-19 and COVID-19-related deaths occurred in older IBD patients.[15]

Inflammatory Bowel Disease Treatments and COVID-19

A particular benefit of the SECURE-IBD database has been to evaluate the impact of different IBD treatments on COVID-19 disease risk; an important challenge given the number of medications and the different mechanisms of action currently used by IBD patients. This comprehensive registry was used in a recently published evaluation of different IBD medication classes on COVID-19 risk using 6144 individual reports of SARS-CoV-2 infection in IBD patients since the inception of the SECURE-IBD database on March 13, 2020, until May 21, 2021.[16] Confirming prior reports, including a previous publication from the SECURE-IBD registry,[15] systemic corticosteroids were associated with an increased risk of hospitalization or death (from any cause) or both (adjusted odds ratio [aOR], 2.45; 95% confidence interval [CI], 1.81–3.31), an increased risk of severe COVID-19 (aOR, 3.49; 95% CI, 2.62–4.65), and an increased risk of death because of COVID-19 (aOR, 4.77; 95% CI, 3.36–6.77). Methotrexate was marginally associated with an increased risk of hospitalization or death or both (aOR, 1.26; 95% CI, 1.00–1.57), which did not persist in models evaluating associations between methotrexate and severe COVID-19 (aOR, 1.04; 95% CI, 0.39–2.81) or between methotrexate and death because of COVID-19 (aOR, 0.79; 95% CI, 0.20–3.08).

Biologic therapy with monoclonal antibodies targeting TNF, IL12/23, or α4β7 integrins was associated with decreased risk of hospitalization, death, or both (aOR, 0.58 [95% CI, 0.50–0.69]; 0.44 [95% CI, 0.36–0.54]; and 0.66 [95% CI, 0.56–0.78], respectively). Combination therapy using a TNF antagonist plus thiopurine was associated with significantly increased risk for hospitalization or death, but not with severe COVID-19. In contrast, combination therapy using a TNF antagonist plus methotrexate was not associated with significantly elevated risk for adverse COVID-19-related outcomes (hospitalization, death, or severe disease). No statistically significant differences in risk of adverse COVID-19 outcomes were observed when comparing patients on different classes of biologic medications (TNF antagonist, IL12/23 antagonist, or integrin antagonist).[16]

In contrast to prior reporting from the SECURE-IBD database,[14] in this analysis, no significant increase in risk of adverse COVID-19 outcomes was observed in patients on aminosalicylates or sulfasalazine therapy.[16] The larger body of evidence used in this most recent publication, and evidence from an independent cohort of IBD patients,[17] supports the conclusion that neither aminosalicylate nor sulfasalazine therapy is associated with increased risk of severe COVID-19 or COVID-19-related complications. It may be that the unexpected association between 5-aminosalicylate or sulfasalazine therapy and adverse COVID-19 outcomes that was initially reported was actually driven by delays in reporting and/or reporting bias because of early pandemic-associated factors discussed previously.

A potentially protective effect was seen with the Janus kinase (JAK) inhibitor, tofacitinib (aOR, 0.48; 95% CI, 0.30–0.76), although the sample size was small, consisting of only nine infections.[16] A dedicated analysis of SECURE-IBD database patients treated with tofacitinib did not identify significantly increased risks for COVID-19-related adverse events or venous thromboembolism in patients receiving tofacitinib.[18] Furthermore, a recent meta-analysis of six studies including 11,145 patients receiving systemic JAK inhibitor therapy (for any indication) with moderate-to-severe COVID-19 infection found a probable decrease in all-cause mortality at 28 and at 60 days post-infection (relative risk [RR], 0.72 [95% CI, 0.57–0.91] and RR, 0.69 [95% CI, 0.56–0.82], respectively), without an increase in adverse effects.[19] Patients on newer agents from medication classes including sphinogosine 1 phosphate receptor modulators, IL23 antagonists, and selective JAK inhibitors were not part of the SECURE-IBD database at the time of the data collection period and thus were not included in this analysis.

Taken together, the totality of evidence at present indicates that systemic corticosteroid use is unequivocally associated with increased risk for adverse outcomes from SARS-CoV-2 infection, and that advanced therapies for IBD, with the possible exception of combination therapy using a TNF antagonist and thiopurine, are not associated with an increased risk of COVID-19-related adverse events. Thus, in concordance with international guidelines for treating IBD, corticosteroid-sparing therapies should be used to wean patients off corticosteroids as soon as possible to reduce the risk of corticosteroid-related (including adverse COVID-19-related) risks. Likewise, patients should be informed of the safety of other IBD medications in the setting of COVID-19 infections to provide reassurance and enhance adherence to therapy. The SECURE-IBD database has been an invaluable resource for the field to facilitate practical research to inform clinical care in the setting of a rapidly evolving global pandemic. Ongoing use and maintenance of SECURE, and similar disease-related Internet databases, offer unique and powerful opportunities to advance clinical research for global IBD, immune-related inflammatory diseases, transplant, and cancer communities.

Postacute COVID-19 Syndrome or Long COVID

An important development from the COVID-19 pandemic has been the recognition of persistent symptoms lasting at least 4 weeks or longer after SARS-CoV-2 infection. This phenomenon has been labeled as PACS, commonly referred to as long COVID. For this review, these two terms (PACS and long COVID) are considered synonymous, and PACS is used for consistency. PACS involves many different and often nonspecific symptoms, such as chronic fatigue, headache, brain fog, cognitive dysfunction, chronic pain, shortness of breath, and chest pain.[20] Manifestations of PACS may range from mild and self-limited to severe and debilitating symptoms.[20]

Gastrointestinal symptoms are present in about half of patients with acute COVID-19 infection and persist at 6 months in approximately 10% to 25% COVID-19 patients.[21,22] A recently published systematic review and meta-analysis estimated the prevalence of persistent gastrointestinal symptoms in the setting of PACS to be 22%, although the underlying studies included in this meta-analysis were limited by small size and heterogeneity.[23] Gastrointestinal symptoms of PACS include diarrhea, constipation, nausea/vomiting, dyspepsia, anorexia, abdominal pain, and heartburn, among others.[21–23] They are often associated with symptoms of anxiety and depression, which usually precede SARS-CoV-2 infection, and they tend to gradually wane over time. The underlying cause of long-term and persistent gastrointestinal symptoms of PACS is unknown. Potential mechanisms may include persistent viral antigen presence in mucosal tissues triggering ongoing host responses, changes in the microbiome induced by SARS-CoV-2 infection, aftereffects or sequelae of host immune responses to the SARS-CoV-2 virus, persistent activation or alteration of immune cells and inflammatory signaling pathways, or postinfectious irritable bowel syndrome. These are not mutually exclusive processes and may interact in different ways in different patients to contribute to the reported symptoms.

A study of 46 European patients with IBD that underwent upper endoscopy and colonoscopy at a median of 7 months after SARS-CoV-2 infection (range, ~3–8.5 months) demonstrated that SARS-CoV-2 RNA expression was present in mucosal tissue of most patients (69.5%), and that SARS-CoV-2 viral antigen was present in intestinal epithelial tissue and $CD8^+$ T cells in more than half of patients (52.1%).[24] Despite these viral (or remnant) markers persisting in many patients, infectious virions of SARS-CoV-2 were unable to be retrieved from mucosal tissues and live virus was not able to be cultured from any of the patients; suggesting that patients were experiencing inadequate or incomplete viral clearance as opposed to active subclinical, latent, or recurrent viral infection. Importantly, only those patients with persistence of viral antigens experienced post-COVID symptoms, whereas no symptoms were reported in patients without detectable viral antigens. Viral antigen persistence was not related to the severity of COVID-19 infection, underlying endoscopic inflammatory activity at the time of endoscopy, or IBD-related immunosuppressive treatment.[24]

This finding of SARS-CoV-2 viral antigen persistence has been explored in individuals without IBD. In a small study of 14 individuals evaluated at an average of 4 months (range, 2.8–5.7 months) after acute SARS-CoV-2 infection, five patients (35.7%) had detectable viral antigen (SARS-CoV-2 N protein) in intestinal enterocytes.[25] Although these individuals did not have PACS, this establishes that viral antigen persistence occurs in the intestine in a subset of patients after acute SARS-CoV-2 infection. Taken together, these findings demonstrate that SARS-CoV-2 viral antigens can persist within the gastrointestinal tract after acute infection with SARS-CoV-2, raising the intriguing possibility that viral antigen persistence may induce a chronic inflammatory response or host immune perturbation that contributes to ongoing symptoms of PACS. Further research with validation and replication of these findings in independent cohorts in conjunction with longer-term monitoring of patients with PACS, including those with IBD, may help clarify the natural history of this entity and its underlying mechanisms.

COVID Vaccination in Patients with Inflammatory Bowel Disease

A defining feature of the COVID-19 pandemic has been the rapid development, testing, and deployment of vaccinations against the SARS-CoV-2 virus, including the use of novel mRNA-based technologies. Despite the political and cultural challenges related to vaccine uptake and use among the population at large, the creation of highly effective and safe vaccines targeting this novel virus is a resounding success of the biomedical establishment that has resulted in significant reductions in hospitalizations, severe illness, and death from COVID-19. Although the initial mRNA vaccines granted approval for use (Pfizer-BioNTech BNT162b2 and Moderna mRNA1273) were shown to be safe and effective in trials leading to emergency use authorization, patients with IBD were excluded from these initial clinical trials. This led to initial concerns about the safety and efficacy of these vaccines in IBD patients, given their underlying disease and their potential use of immunosuppressive and/or immunomodulatory medications.

In a similar manner to the SECURE-IBD database to study COVID-related adverse outcomes in IBD patients, the PREVENT-COVID and CLARITY-IBD initiatives were launched to examine the safety and efficacy of COVID-19 vaccination for IBD patients. Initial results from the PREVENT-COVID study demonstrated that vaccination is safe, well-tolerated, and effective in IBD patients.[26] This has been confirmed in additional studies and meta-analyses.[27–29] A meta-analysis published in July 2022 including 46 studies evaluating responses to COVID-19 vaccination in IBD patients found that most IBD patients receiving COVID-19 vaccination achieve adequate immunogenic responses, as determined by seropositivity for anti-SARS-CoV-2 spike and/or anti-SARS-CoV-2 receptor binding domain antibodies.[27] For studies with complete immunization data ($n = 31$ studies; 9447 patients), the pooled seroconversion rate for vaccinated IBD patients was 0.96 (95% CI, 0.94–0.97), which was slightly less than the rate for vaccinated control patients of 0.98 (95% CI, 0.98–0.99). Among vaccinated IBD patients, the pooled positivity of neutralization assays (testing the ability of patient antibodies to neutralize the virus) was 0.80 (95% CI, 0.70–0.87). Furthermore, there were no statistically significant differences in vaccine responses among IBD patients taking different medication classes. In addition, pooled rates of breakthrough infection risk after vaccination were similar in IBD patients and the vaccinated general population (RR, 0.60; 95% CI, 0.25–1.42).[27] Taken together, these findings indicate that COVID-19 is highly effective, safe, and well-tolerated in IBD patients. Furthermore, there has been no evidence that undergoing vaccination can trigger activation of underlying IBD activity or inflammation.

In addition to these large-scale studies confirming the safety and efficacy of COVID-19 vaccination in IBD patients, detailed studies have explored the immunogenic responses to vaccination in patients receiving different medication classes. Several studies have shown that antibody responses are attenuated in patients on TNF antagonist therapy,[30–32] but the clinical significance of these findings is unclear, and these results should not be construed as indicating that patients on these therapies should not undergo vaccination.

As the COVID-19 pandemic transitions to an endemic virus that will likely circulate widely in a seasonal pattern common to many infections spread via respiratory droplets and aerosols, it will be important to determine how frequently IBD patients, according to IBD subtypes or therapies, should undergo vaccination with booster doses. Studies examining the durability of antibody responses in vaccinated IBD patients have shown that antibody titers begin to decline approximately 4 weeks after vaccination, and this reduction is accelerated in patients receiving a TNF antagonist therapy or combination therapy with a TNF antagonist and immunomodulator.[27] Although such reductions in titers have been described, the clinical significance of these reductions is unknown, because the underlying antibody titer has not been shown to be directly related to susceptibility to infection, and patients may generate protective cell-mediated immune responses that are independent of antibody titers.

For now, it seems prudent to recommend that IBD patients, especially those at increased risk because of older age and those receiving immunosuppressive therapies, receive booster COVID-19 doses approximately every 4 to 6 months pending further evidence-based guidance. The continued use of registries and databases, such as PREVENT-COVID and SECURE-IBD, can be leveraged for ongoing research on the durability and efficacy of vaccination in IBD patients, which may inform recommendations on frequency of booster doses.

SUMMARY

The initial global pandemic caused by the SARS-CoV-2 virus confronted patients with IBD with uncertainties, anxieties, questions, and challenges. These centered on individual personal risks for severe COVID-19-related disease and death, the impact of COVID-19 on their underlying IBD, the safety of their IBD medications in the setting of the global pandemic, the efficacy and safety of COVID-19 vaccination, and the long-term consequences of SARS-CoV-2 infection on their health and quality of life. In addition, societal changes induced by the COVID-19 pandemic exerted a significant burden related to uncertainties associated with often changing public health guidance and changes to health care access and delivery. Fortunately, a currently large and growing body of evidence from prospectively monitored cohorts of IBD patients has consistently demonstrated that patients are not at significantly increased risk of severe disease or death from COVID-19. Furthermore, COVID-19 vaccination is now known to be safe, effective, and durable for most individuals with IBD. Although some studies have shown decreased antibody concentrations in response to vaccination in IBD patients, in particular in older patients and patients treated with anti-TNF monotherapy, combination therapy with anti-TNF and a conventional immunomodulator, tofacitinib, and systemic corticosteroids; the cumulative body of evidence indicates that COVID-19 vaccination is a powerful and proven tool to reduce morbidity and mortality from SARS-CoV-2 infection.

Gastroenterologists have an important role in promoting COVID-19 vaccination adherence and should provide reassurance for all gastroenterologic patients, including those with IBD, regarding the safety and efficacy of COVID-19 vaccination. This guidance should be delivered clearly and consistently for IBD patients to receive vaccinations in accordance with updated professional guidelines. IBD patients should receive COVID-19 vaccination, preferably with an mRNA vaccine. Patients receiving immunosuppressive therapies should have an additional mRNA vaccine dose 4 weeks after completion of the two-dose primary vaccine series and a booster dose about 3 months thereafter. Individuals not on immunosuppressive therapy should have a booster dose about 5 months after completion of the initial two-dose vaccine series. These recommendations are in accordance with guidelines and consensus opinion from the International Organization for the Study of Inflammatory Bowel Disease,[33] the British Society of Gastroenterology,[34] the Crohn's & Colitis Foundation, and the Centers for Disease Control and Prevention Advisory Committee on Immunization Practices. Although the Advisory Committee on Immunization Practices position included individuals treated with systemic corticosteroids (at a dose of $\geq$20 mg/day), anti-TNF therapy, and immunomodulators, it did not provide specific recommendations for patients taking vedolizumab, ustekinumab, risankizumab, ozanimod, tofacitinib, or upadacitinib. Despite this limitation, it seems reasonable and prudent to also apply these recommendations to patients receiving these particular therapies.

As vaccine-induced immunity wanes over time and as new SARS-CoV-2 variants emerge, it will be incumbent on gastroenterologists to maintain clear communication with IBD patients regarding updated COVID-19 vaccination recommendations and guidance. Ongoing prospective monitoring of clinical studies in IBD patients are expected to inform clinical practice with respect to the optimal timing of booster vaccination doses to maintain adequate immunity to prevent and minimize COVID-related morbidity and mortality. In addition, future studies offer the potential to describe and clarify longer-term effects of SARS-CoV-2 infection in IBD patients, because an initial study has reported long-term persistence of SARS-CoV-2 viral antigens in intestinal tissue of IBD patients, a finding of unknown clinical significance. Given the growing number of IBD (and non-IBD) patients suffering from persistent gastrointestinal symptoms after COVID-19 infection, such information is critical to understand the prevalence, natural history, and progression of post-COVID-19 sequelae, and the impact of COVID-19 vaccination on long-term SARS-CoV-2 infection-related outcomes.

CLINICS CARE POINTS

- Patients with IBD are not at significantly increased risk for severe disease or death from COVID-19.
- Systemic corticosteroid use is associated with increased risk of COVID-19-related severe disease and death, rendering weaning off and reducing use of systemic corticosteroids key priorities for gastroenterologists taking care of IBD patients.
- COVID-19 vaccination is safe and effective in IBD patients, including those on immunosuppressive therapies.
- Individuals with IBD should undergo COVID-19 vaccination, preferably with an mRNA vaccine, including a booster dose for those that are not immunosuppressed and an additional dose as part of the primary series and a booster dose for those on immunosuppressive therapy.
- Ongoing work is clarifying the long-term impact of SARS-CoV-2 infection and postacute COVID-19 syndrome in IBD patients and the optimal timing for booster vaccine doses.

DISCLOSURE

K.C. Summa has no relevant commercial or financial conflicts of interest to disclose. S.B. Hanauer disclosures: AbbVie (consultant, lectures), Boehringer-Ingelheim (DSMB), BMS (consultant, lectures), Janssen (consultant, lectures), Pfizer (consultant, lectures, DSMB), Prometheus (Consultant, DSMB), and Takeda (consultant, lectures).

REFERENCES

1. Shivshankar P, Karmouty-Quintana H, Mills T, et al. SARS-CoV-2 infection: host response. Immunity, Ther Targets Inflamm 2022;45(4):1430–49.
2. Jackson CB, Farzan M, Chen B, et al. Mechanisms of SARS-CoV-2 entry into cells. Nat Rev Mol Cell Biol 2022;23(1):3–20.
3. Xiao F, Tang M, Zheng X, et al. Evidence for gastrointestinal infection of SARS-CoV-2. Gastroenterology 2020;158(6):1831–1833 e3.
4. Zou X, Chen K, Zou J, et al. Single-cell RNA-seq data analysis on the receptor ACE2 expression reveals the potential risk of different human organs vulnerable to 2019-nCoV infection. Front Med 2020;14(2):185–92.
5. Pan L, Mu M, Yang P, et al. Clinical characteristics of COVID-19 patients with digestive symptoms in Hubei, China: a descriptive, cross-sectional, multicenter study. Am J Gastroenterol 2020;115(5):766–73.

6. Han C, Duan C, Zhang S, et al. Digestive symptoms in COVID-19 patients with mild disease severity: clinical presentation, stool viral RNA testing, and outcomes. Am J Gastroenterol 2020;115(6):916–23.
7. Holshue ML, DeBolt C, Lindquist S, et al. First case of 2019 novel coronavirus in the United States. N Engl J Med 2020;382(10):929–36.
8. Solitano V, Facciorusso A, Jess T, et al. Comparative risk of serious infections with biologic agents and oral small molecules in inflammatory bowel diseases: a systematic review and meta-analysis. Clin Gastroenterol Hepatol 2022. https://doi.org/10.1016/j.cgh.2022.07.032.
9. Singh S, Facciorusso A, Dulai PS, et al. Comparative risk of serious infections with biologic and/or immunosuppressive therapy in patients with inflammatory bowel diseases: a systematic review and meta-analysis. Clin Gastroenterol Hepatol 2020;18(1):69–81 e3.
10. Aziz M, Fatima R, Haghbin H, et al. The incidence and outcomes of COVID-19 in IBD patients: a rapid review and meta-analysis. Inflamm Bowel Dis 2020;26(10): e132–3.
11. Allocca M, Chaparro M, Gonzalez HA, et al. Patients with inflammatory bowel disease are not at increased risk of COVID-19: a large multinational cohort study. J Clin Med 2020;9(11). https://doi.org/10.3390/jcm9113533.
12. Lukin DJ, Kumar A, Hajifathalian K, et al. Baseline disease activity and steroid therapy stratify risk of COVID-19 in patients with inflammatory bowel disease. Gastroenterology 2020;159(4):1541–1544 e2.
13. Macaluso FS, Giuliano A, Fries W, et al. Severe activity of inflammatory bowel disease is a risk factor for severe COVID-19. Inflamm Bowel Dis 2022. https://doi.org/10.1093/ibd/izac064.
14. Brenner EJ, Ungaro RC, Gearry RB, et al. Corticosteroids, but not TNF antagonists, are associated with adverse COVID-19 outcomes in patients with inflammatory bowel diseases: results from an international registry. Gastroenterology 2020; 159(2):481–491 e3.
15. Ungaro RC, Brenner EJ, Gearry RB, et al. Effect of IBD medications on COVID-19 outcomes: results from an international registry. Gut 2021;70(4):725–32.
16. Ungaro RC, Brenner EJ, Agrawal M, et al. Impact of medications on COVID-19 outcomes in inflammatory bowel disease: analysis of more than 6000 patients from an international registry. Gastroenterology 2022;162(1):316–319 e5.
17. Attauabi M, Seidelin J, Burisch J, et al. Association between 5-aminosalicylates in patients with IBD and risk of severe COVID-19: an artefactual result of research methodology? Gut 2021;70(10):2020–2.
18. Agrawal M, Brenner EJ, Zhang X, et al. Characteristics and outcomes of IBD patients with COVID-19 on tofacitinib therapy in the SECURE-IBD Registry. Inflamm Bowel Dis 2021;27(4):585–9.
19. Kramer A, Prinz C, Fichtner F, et al. Janus kinase inhibitors for the treatment of COVID-19. Cochrane Database Syst Rev 2022;6:CD015209.
20. Castanares-Zapatero D, Chalon P, Kohn L, et al. Pathophysiology and mechanism of long COVID: a comprehensive review. Ann Med 2022;54(1):1473–87.
21. Meringer H, Mehandru S. Gastrointestinal post-acute COVID-19 syndrome. Nat Rev Gastroenterol Hepatol 2022;19(6):345–6.
22. Freedberg DE, Chang L. Gastrointestinal symptoms in COVID-19: the long and the short of it. Curr Opin Gastroenterol 2022;38(6):555–61.
23. Choudhury A, Tariq R, Jena A, et al. Gastrointestinal manifestations of long COVID: a systematic review and meta-analysis. Therap Adv Gastroenterol 2022;15. 17562848221118403.

24. Zollner A, Koch R, Jukic A, et al. Postacute COVID-19 is characterized by gut viral antigen persistence in inflammatory bowel diseases. Gastroenterology 2022. https://doi.org/10.1053/j.gastro.2022.04.037.
25. Gaebler C, Wang Z, Lorenzi JCC, et al. Evolution of antibody immunity to SARS-CoV-2. Nature 2021;591(7851):639–44.
26. Weaver KN, Zhang X, Dai X, et al. Impact of SARS-CoV-2 vaccination on inflammatory bowel disease activity and development of vaccine-related adverse events: results from PREVENT-COVID. Inflamm Bowel Dis 2021. https://doi.org/10.1093/ibd/izab302.
27. Jena A, James D, Singh AK, et al. Effectiveness and durability of COVID-19 vaccination in 9447 patients with IBD: a systematic review and meta-analysis. Clin Gastroenterol Hepatol 2022;20(7):1456–1479 e18.
28. James D, Jena A, Bharath PN, et al. Safety of SARS-CoV-2 vaccination in patients with inflammatory bowel disease: a systematic review and meta-analysis. Dig Liver Dis 2022;54(6):713–21.
29. Li D, Debbas P, Cheng S, et al. Post-vaccination symptoms after a third dose of mRNA SARS-CoV-2 vaccination in patients with inflammatory bowel disease. medRxiv 2021. https://doi.org/10.1101/2021.12.05.21266089.
30. Chanchlani N, Lin S, Chee D, et al. Adalimumab and infliximab impair SARS-CoV-2 antibody responses: results from a therapeutic drug monitoring study in 11 422 biologic-treated patients. J Crohns Colitis 2022;16(3):389–97.
31. Kennedy NA, Goodhand JR, Bewshea C, et al. Anti-SARS-CoV-2 antibody responses are attenuated in patients with IBD treated with infliximab. Gut 2021; 70(5):865–75.
32. Kennedy NA, Lin S, Goodhand JR, et al. Infliximab is associated with attenuated immunogenicity to BNT162b2 and ChAdOx1 nCoV-19 SARS-CoV-2 vaccines in patients with IBD. Gut 2021;70(10):1884–93.
33. Siegel CA, Melmed GY, McGovern DP, et al. SARS-CoV-2 vaccination for patients with inflammatory bowel diseases: recommendations from an international consensus meeting. Gut 2021;70(4):635–40.
34. Alexander JL, Moran GW, Gaya DR, et al. SARS-CoV-2 vaccination for patients with inflammatory bowel disease: a British Society of Gastroenterology Inflammatory Bowel Disease section and IBD Clinical Research Group position statement. Lancet Gastroenterol Hepatol 2021;6(3):218–24.

The Impact of COVID-19 Infection on Miscellaneous Inflammatory Disorders of the Gastrointestinal Tract

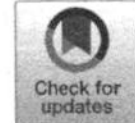

Mitchell S. Cappell, MD, PhD[a,*], Martin Tobi, MB, ChB[b], David M. Friedel, MD[c]

KEYWORDS

• COVID-19 • Pandemic • SARS • Gastrointestinal • Inflammation

KEY POINTS

- Clinicians should be aware that numerous inflammatory diseases of the gastroenterology tract may be somewhat modified in patients with active COVID-19 infection
- The clinical presentation of some gastrointestinal inflammatory diorders may be altered by acitve COVID-19 infection
- Management and treatment of some inflammatroy disorders of the gastrointestinal tract may have to be altered in patients with active COVID-19 infection

INTRODUCTION

The novel coronavirus pandemic with COVID-19 has caused immense morbidity and mortality, with more than one million deaths in the United States and more than 6 million deaths globally.[1] Mortality occurs in all groups but is disproportionately higher in the elderly, infirm, male gender, lower socioeconomic classes, and patients having significant comorbidities including those suffering from diabetes mellitus and obesity.[2] Moreover, the pandemic causes considerable morbidity and can persist in a chronic form as reviewed in another chapter in this monograph. Development of relatively effective vaccines, sporadically mandated public health measures such as masks, increasing herd immunity, moderately effective therapy, and perhaps less virulent

[a] Division of Gastroenterology, Department of Medicine, Aleda E. Lutz Veterans Hospital, Gastroenterology Service, Main Building, Room 3212, 1500 Weiss Street, Saginaw, MI 48602, USA; [b] Department of Research and Development, John D. Dingell Veterans Affairs Medical Center, 4747 John R. Street, Detroit, MI 48201, USA; [c] Division of Therapeutic Endoscopy, Division of Gastroenterology, Department of Medicine, NY of New York University Langone Hospital, 259 1st Street, Mineola, NY 11501, USA

* Corresponding author.

E-mail address: mitchell.cappell@va.gov

Gastroenterol Clin N Am 52 (2023) 115–138
https://doi.org/10.1016/j.gtc.2022.10.002
0889-8553/23/Published by Elsevier Inc.

emerging viral strains have significantly diminished COVID-19 infection severity and mortality, but the pandemic endures, with associated morbidity and mortality, especially in the unvaccinated and vulnerable populations. Long (chronic) COVID-19 can relatively frequently cause gastrointestinal (GI) infections or symptoms in some patients who had contracted symptomatic acute COVID-19 infection and is reviewed in another chapter in this monograph.

Organs, including the GI tract, that express angiotensin-converting enzyme 2 (ACE-2) are susceptible to local COVID-19 infection and associated inflammation. COVID-19 can affect the GI tract by direct infection and local inflammation or indirectly from GI ulcerations related to stress, particularly in mechanically ventilated patients or patients administered corticosteroids, and incidentally by deferred screening for GI neoplasms or malignancies such as Barrett's esophagus or colorectal neoplasms due to patient preference or inability of health systems to accommodate endoscopic screenings due to COVID exigencies.

METHODS

The medical and scientific community is generally aware of the nature and importance of systematic reviews. The essence of systematic reviews is that the method and particulars of the literature search are tabulated so that the reader could potentially reconstruct all the data (articles) used in the literature review if needed, including all the articles surveyed by the literature search using the computerized search terms of the literature review and all the articles excluded in the literature search with the listed reasons for every excluded article. The first task is an integral and essential part of a systematic review that requires little documentation, whereas the second task requires extensive documentation by compiling all individual articles excluded from the review article while specifying the reason for each exclusion. It is reasonable to separate these 2 distinct tasks and denote the accomplishment of the first task without the second task by creating a new term "semiquantitative review." By this term a review encompassing the first part of a systematic review, but not the second part, is denoted. This new term is useful because the first task of a systematic review provides one-half or more of the quality of a systematic review, while requiring much less documentation that is entailed in the second task.

This article inaugurates a "semiquantitative review" by declaring all the search terms used in the literature search (with the number of articles reviewed) without detailing the extensive list of excluded articles. This literature review was performed using PubMed and Ovid, independent literature search engines. The literature review was last conducted (and is up to date) as of August 26, 2022, when this article was submitted for publication, and included the following search terms or phrases (with number of identified articles per search term, as derived from PubMed listed in parenthesis): pharynx and COVID-19 (1514); oropharynx and COVID-19 (284); oropharyngeal involvement and COVID-19 (81); anosmia and COVID-19 (1662); dysgeusia and COVID-19 (406); olfactory dysfunction and COVID-19 (886); geographic tongue and COVID-19 (12); COVID tongue (217); gastroesophageal reflux (GERD) and COVID-19 (36); Barrett's epithelium and COVID-19 (13); proton pump inhibitor and COVID-19 (114); intestinal metaplasia and COVID-19 (6); laryngopharyngeal reflux and COVID-19 (3); esophagus, candida, and COVID-19 (1); esophagogastroduodenoscopy (EGD) and COVID-19 (13); nasal endoscopy (EGD) and COVID-19 (134); Barrett's ablation and COVID-19 (1); Barrett's esophagus screening and COVID-19 (7); Cytosponge and COVID-19 (2); high resolution manometry and COVID-19 (7); esophageal varices and COVID-19 (14); achalasia and COVID-19 (6); esophageal necrosis and COVID-19

(5); Boerhaave syndrome and COVID-19 (2); scleroderma and COVID-19 (94); pill esophagitis and COVID-19 (1); corrosive esophagitis and COVID-19 (1); eosinophilic esophagitis and COVID-19 (10); gastropathy and COVID-19 (115); gastroduodenitis and COVID-19; ulcers and COVID-19; *Helicobacter pylori* and COVID-19 (51); *H pylori* antigen and COVID-19 (12); GI hemorrhage and COVID-19 (134); GI bleeding and COVID-19 (262); melena and COVID-19 (35); hematemesis and COVID-19 (23); iron deficiency anemia and COVID-19 (39); fecal occult blood and COVID-19 (82); primary COVID ulcers (69); gastric ulcers and COVID-19 (20); duodenal ulcers and COVID-19 (15); celiac and COVID-19 (133); multisystem inflammatory syndrome and COVID-19 (2132); Crohn disease and COVID-19 (328); ulcerative colitis and COVID-19 (310); mesenteric ischemia and COVID-19 (94); pneumatosis intestinalis and COVID-19 (19); pneumatosis coli and COVID-19 (12); GI perforation and COVID-19 (75); GI obstruction and COVID-19 (110); intussusception and COVID-19 (56); mucormycosis and COVID-19 (747); microscopic colitis and COVID-19 (5); lymphocytic colitis and COVID-19 (3); collagenous colitis and COVID-19 (3); protein-losing enteropathy and COVID-19 (2); cytokine release syndrome and COVID-19 (2045); tocilizumab, perforation, and COVID-19 (19); *Clostridium difficile* and COVID-19 (131); Clostridiodes and COVID-19 (5); appendicitis and COVID-19 (403); diverticulitis and COVID-19 (41); colonic pseudo-obstruction and COVID-19 (5); irritable bowel syndrome (IBS) and COVID-19 (56); colon cancer and COVID-19 (215); colonic polyps and COVID-19 (11); colonoscopy and COVID-19 (218); enteroscopy and COVID-19 (2); capsule endoscopy and COVID-19 (29); balloon endoscopy and COVID-19 (5); computed tomography colonography (CTC) and COVID-19 (10); hemorrhoids and COVID-19 (105); anal fistula and COVID-19 (5); anal abscess and COVID-19 (2); anal fissure and COVID-19 (3); and long (chronic) COVID-19 and GI (77). This work illustrates the utility of a semiquantitative literature review that reviews so many articles, because a systematic review of this literature would encompass so many excluded articles, thereby encumbering such an article with an impractically long list.

PHARYNX

COVID-19 has been detected in oral and nasopharyngeal tissues and secretions, with implications for pathogenesis, transmissibility, and contamination. For example, chewing gum saturated with soluble ACE2 (ACE-2) proteins but lacking the virus may reduce viral transmission by 95%.[3] Oropharyngeal involvement most commonly pathologically produces erosions or ulcers.[4,5] Loss of smell (anosmia) and loss of taste (ageusia) or a taste disorder (dysgeusia) are commonly encountered with COVID-19 infection. For example, in a study of 322 patients with COVID-19 treated at a hospital in India from August through November 2020, 226 patients with COVID-19 (70.2%) experienced olfactory and gustatory disorders, including 165 (51.2%) patients with both olfactory and gustatory disorders, 34 (10.6%) patients with solely olfactory dysfunction, and 27 (8.4%) patients with solely gustatory dysfunction.[6] These symptoms usually present without gross oropharyngeal pathology of nasopharyngitis, nasal obstruction, or glossitis; without the symptom of rhinorrhea; and without zinc deficiency. The true mechanisms remain conjectural and unknown. It has been hypothesized that a decrease in the sensitivity of olfactory neurons and co-expression of ACE-2 and TMPRSS2 in alveolar epithelial cells may cause these olfactory-gustatory disorders.[7] These symptoms often are the first to appear with COVID-19 infection and the last to resolve.[8,9] Corticosteroids have been proposed as a therapy, but their efficacy is unproven.[10] Alternative therapies include nirmatrelvir/ritonavir (Paxlovid) and anticytokine monoclonals.[11] However, efficacy in clinical trials may not apply to the general population.[10]

Geographic tongue manifests as irregular loss of filiform papillae toward the rear of the tongue. This disorder affects about 1% to 2% of patients in the general population and is strongly related to psoriasis and is believed due to genetic and immunologic factors. In a Spanish study of 666 patients with COVID-19 infection, 3.9% had irregular depapillation of the distal lingual dorsum consistent with geographic tongue, also known as COVID tongue.[12] Geographic tongue has been linked with high expression of ACE-2 in epithelial cells at the back of the tongue, possibly leading to injury of infected papillae.[13] Candidiasis of the tongue[14] is reviewed under esophageal candidiasis. Oral manifestations and salivary duct abnormalities from acute COVID infection may persist for months.[15]

ESOPHAGUS

A database incorporating more than 26,000 COVID-19–infected patients reported 19% had symptoms of GERD (gastroesophageal reflux disease).[16] It is unknown whether COVID-19 increases the frequency of GERD symptoms because this study was performed without a control group for comparison. Moreover, GERD symptoms and those directly attributed to COVID-19 infection, such as cough and chest discomfort, may overlap, especially when mild, creating a diagnostic dilemma.[17] However, recent advancements in the rapidity and accuracy of COVID-19 testing generally permits differentiation of these 2 entities.[17] Conversely, patients presenting with predominantly or solely GI symptoms may still have COVID-19 infection in an endemic area.[18] Lastly, these 2 entities commonly coexist in obese subjects who are at high risk of GERD as well as at high risk of severely symptomatic COVID-19 infection. A genetic relationship between GERD and COVID-19 has been proposed, but obesity seems to be the most significant underlying cofactor.[19] Laryngopharyngeal reflux may be disproportionately increased with COVID-19 infection, and melatonin has been proposed as therapy for this condition.[20,21]

The relationship between medications to treat GERD and COVID-19 has been well analyzed. COVID-19 may preferentially infect Barrett's metaplastic epithelium (akin to small bowel epithelium) over normal esophageal columnar mucosa, thereby increasing susceptibility.[22] Proton pump inhibitor (PPI) therapy is associated with increased COVID-19 susceptibility[23] and worse COVID-19 outcomes.[24–26] Other investigators have refuted this association and advocated that other risk factors are more important in patient outcome.[27,28] Famotidine was previously touted as the preferred histamine-2 (H_2) receptor antagonist for hospitalized patients with COVID-19[29] possibly due to decreasing the risk of cytokine storm, but clinical trials unfortunately showed no therapeutic benefits of famotidine compared with other H_2 receptor antagonist therapies.[30,31]

Patients with severe COVID-19 infection are at high risk of developing invasive esophageal candidiasis, especially patients with acute respiratory distress syndrome, chronically receiving corticosteroid therapy, or undergoing prolonged endotracheal intubation.[32] Other proposed clinical risk factors for esophageal candidiasis include prolonged intensive care unit stays, central venous catheters, prolonged broad-spectrum antibiotic therapy, and prior bouts of esophageal candidiasis.[32] Patients with such risk factors are highly susceptible to candida infection because *Candida* species are frequent constituents of the human mycobiome. Deep-seated candida infections are associated with increased mortality. Esophageal candidiasis is associated with the profound immune dysregulation in COVID-19 infection, but the specific underlying immunologic defects are unknown. Esophageal candidiasis typically presents with dysphagia or odynophagia. At EGD esophageal candidiasis classically presents as a cheesy white superficial exudate. EGD with endoscopic brushings is usually diagnostic. Clinical awareness and screening are needed in the setting of severe COVID-19 infection. Echinocandins and azoles are the primary antifungals used to treat esophageal candidiasis. In patients with advanced COVID-19 infection, *Candida* spp may exhibit resistance to traditional antifungal agents.

The COVID-19 pandemic has greatly disrupted esophageal testing, especially EGD. Diversion of physician resources and endoscopy suite time to the COVID-19 pandemic crisis has decreased the use of screening and other routine endoscopic procedures, but it has spurred use of alternative testing modalities and innovations, especially regarding equipment. For example, one center substituted chest computed tomography (CT) for endoscopy to screen for esophageal varices.[33] A large US database reported that esophageal cancer diagnosis, as well as Barrett's esophagus screening and ablation, decreased during the peak of the pandemic, but the rate of performing esophagectomies did not change.[34] Unsedated nasal endoscopy using topical anesthetic agents such as benzocaine,[35] modified masks for esophageal function testing, and use of the Cytosponge device are notable innovations.[36–38] Fortunately, transmission of COVID-19 in the endoscopy suite to endoscopists, endoscopy staff, and noninfected patients has been exceedingly rare.[39] Practical triage permits optimal utilization of endoscopic resources. As with EGDs, the number of high-resolution manometries (HRMs) decreased by 17.2% from 1587 in 1999 to 1314 in 2020 attributed to the COVID pandemic that peaked in April and May 2020.[40] Notably, the rate of performing HRM hardly decreased in 2020 in areas of Japan relatively affected by the COVID-19 pandemic. One case of endoscopic variceal ligation was successfully performed with cessation of esophageal variceal hemorrhage in an intubated patient with COVID-19 infection.[41] The endoscopy staff successfully applied strict medical precautions to prevent spread of COVID-19 infection to medical personnel participating in the endoscopic procedure.

Uncommon esophageal diseases have been incidentally reported in patients with COVID-19, including achalasia,[42] esophageal necrosis,[43] esophageal rupture/Boerhaave syndrome,[44] and scleroderma esophagus/systemic sclerosis.[45] A patient with pneumonia and respiratory failure from COVID-19 infection had massive upper GI hemorrhage from prolonged nasogastric tube placement.[46] Pill-induced esophagitis was more prevalent in COVID-19–infected patients, partially related to doxycycline antibiotic therapy for treating COVID-19 infection.[47] Mental health issues may underlie the increased corrosive ingestion during the pandemic.[48] In one notable case, esophageal ulceration was detected at the site of COVID-19 virus infection, as detected by electron microscopy.[49]

Eosinophilic Esophagitis

Severity of COVID-19 infection and COVID-19–induced eosinophilic esophagitis (EoE) or eosinophilic GI disorder (EGID) flares was analyzed in a global registry incorporating 94 cases of patients with EoE and EGID who developed acute COVID-19 infection between March and April 2021 (median age, 21 years; range, 1.5–53 years; 73% men).[50] Most patients had a history of atopy (73%) and most had isolated EoE (80%). Before infection with COVID-19, the EoE/EGID activity was reported in clinical remission in 51 (54%) and as moderate in 20 (21%). EoE/EGID treatments at the time of COVID-19 infection included PPI in 49 (52%), swallowed or topical corticosteroids in 48 (51%), and dietary elimination therapy in 34 (36%). COVID-19 symptoms included cough (56%), pyrexia (49%), anosmia (21%), and ageusia (22%). Patients with COVID-19 infection typically had mild infection, with 15% asymptomatic, 70% with mild disease, 12% moderate disease, and only 2% with severe disease. Only 3 patients were hospitalized. No patients had intensive care unit admissions or deaths. Only one patient experienced an EGID flare during COVID-19 infection. Based on this global registry, patients with EoE do not seem to be at increased risk for severe COVID-19 infection or EoE/EGID flares during acute COVID-19 infection.

In a survey of 102 patients with EoE followed at The University of Salerno and Padua, one patient, a 23-year-old-man with a history of EoE for about 10 years, developed acute COVID-19 infection,[51] while chronically administered therapy with oral viscous budesonide, 15 mL twice daily, and following a legumes-free diet for a suspected dietary history of allergy to legumes. The patient developed acute symptoms of asthenia, headache, anosmia, and ageusia. At diagnosis of acute COVID-19 infection, therapy with budesonide was discontinued, and azithromycin therapy (500 mg/d) was initiated for 5 days. The patient never developed dysphagia, odynophagia, or other esophageal symptoms and never required respiratory assistance or oxygen therapy, findings consistent with moderate COVID-19 infection. He became COVID-19 free by nasal swab several weeks after diagnosis.

STOMACH

Common GI symptoms, such as nausea and vomiting or abdominal pain, may relate to COVID-19 affinity to the abundant ACE2 receptors in the GI tract, including the stomach and duodenum.[52] A large European study of endoscopic findings in COVID-19–infected patients noted common upper GI pathology, including ulcers (25%), erosive/superficial ulcerative gastroduodenitis (16%), and petechial/hemorrhagic gastropathy (9%).[53] A systematic review of EGD in COVID-19–infected patients reported upper GI ulcers in nearly half of subjects.[54] Gastric ulcers in patients with COVID-19 infection were associated with a poor prognosis in one small study.[55] An elderly COVID-19–infected patient died of emphysematous gastritis.[56] Gastric perforation has been reported in patients with COVID-19 infection.[57,58]

In a study conducted from June 1 to July 20, 2020, 108 patients diagnosed with COVID-19 infection underwent antigen screening tests to determine the presence of *H pylori* in stool samples. Thirty-one of the patients were *H pylori*-positive, including 8 women (25.8%), and 77 patients were *H pylori*-negative. The presence of *H pylori* infection was significantly associated with abdominal pain (19.4% vs 2.6%, $P = .007$) and diarrhea (32.3% vs 9.1%, $P = .006$). *H pylori* positivity was not significantly associated with hospital length of stay, severity of the course of COVID-19 infection, or the outcome of COVID-19 infection. This study suggests that *H pylori* does not affect the severity or outcome of COVID-19 infection but does increase the frequency of symptoms of abdominal pain and diarrhea.[59]

Gastrointestinal Hemorrhage

GI hemorrhage is uncommon in hospitalized patients with COVID-19 infection, especially relative to the frequency of other GI complaints. There is a paucity of endoscopic data reflecting prioritization of endoscopic resources and understandable reluctance to perform nonessential, elective endoscopies in COVID-19–infected patients. The spectrum of patient presentation parallels that expected for hospitalized patients with predominant pulmonary or multisystem pathology and prothrombotic tendency. Clinical presentations include progressive anemia, hemoccult-positive stool, hematemesis, melena, abdominal pain, and altered vital signs. Administration of anticoagulants, commonly administered to COVID-19–infected patients to prevent thrombosis, can exacerbate the bleeding. GI hemorrhage was reported in up to 13% of patients hospitalized with COVID-19 infection, but most studies reported a significantly lower prevalence.[60–63] Another global meta-analysis reported 9% of more than 25,000 COVID-19–infected patients presented with hematemesis.[64] The most common findings in this relatively sparse data set were peptic disease, including gastritis and gastroduodenal erosions/ulcers.[60–63] Pulmonary manifestations usually predominate in patients hospitalized with COVID-19 infection, but occasionally GI hemorrhage may be the presenting symptom.[65] GI hemorrhage can sometimes present with subtle symptoms and signs of GI bleeding and can sometimes present with subtle symptoms and signs of COVID-19 infection.[65] Several patients presented with GI bleeding from esophageal or GI ulcers presumably from primary COVID-19 infection, as evidenced by findings on electron microscopy.[66,67]

GI hemorrhage in COVID-19–infected patients may be self-limited and may be inferred without performing endoscopy, but sometimes the bleeding is severe or even life-threatening, mandating endoscopy.[68–71] Most, but not all, studies suggest a worse prognosis for COVID-19–infected patients with GI bleeding as compared with those without GI bleeding.[70–72] A meta-analysis of 123 patients with GI bleeding noted a reluctance to perform EGD for GI bleeding, with only 40% undergoing EGD and EGD reserved for patients with more severe GI bleeding.[65] This monograph has a chapter dedicated to GI bleeding in COVID-19–infected patients.

Similarly, a survey of 184 general surgeons reported that they operated on 7 or more cases on average per week before the COVID-19 pandemic compared with only 31 (8.5%) respondents reporting the same number of operations during the pandemic ($P < 0.001$). Two-hundred and nine respondents (57.6%) reported that at least 25% of their elective surgeries were canceled or postponed during the COVID-19 pandemic, whereas only 50 (13.8%) reported that at least 25% of their emergent surgeries were canceled or postponed ($P < 0.001$).[73]

SMALL INTESTINE

The vast small intestinal mucosal surface area, with a plethora of lymphatics, constitutes a battleground for host response to foreign antigens, including viruses. Both respiratory alveoli and enterocyte brush borders have abundant ACE-2 receptors, and viral RNA of SARS-CoV-19 has been detected in stool, sometimes persisting for many weeks.[74] Theoretically this can lead to immune-mediated pathology in both organs. Fecal-oral transmission of COVID-19 is likely.[75] There is burgeoning evidence for bidirectional crosstalk between the lungs and gut microbiome that has potential implications for COVID-19 dissemination and disruption of the microbiota by antibiotics.[75,76] Modulation of the gut microbiome by probiotics has a potential role in the prevention of COVID-19 infection and as an adjunctive therapy.[76,77]

Celiac patients do not seem to have increased susceptibility to COVID-19 infection, although one group noted an increased incidence of concomitant celiac disease and type I diabetes during the pandemic.[78,79] There is a concern about increased celiac cases in the future due to the pandemic.[80] Celiac patients do not have a worse outcome with acute COVID-19 infection.[81] One study suggested COVID-19 infection disproportionately disrupted amino acid absorption, with nutritional implications.[82] The mainstay of therapy for celiac disease in COVID-19–infected patients is strict maintenance of a gluten-free diet.[83]

Multisystem inflammatory syndrome, a newly described syndrome in children, mimics regional enteritis and has been found in pediatric patients with COVID-19 associated with viral cytopathic effects coupled with an abnormal immune response.[84] A similar presentation was noted in a young adult man,[85] who recovered from COVID-19 infection but presented later with small bowel obstruction, fistula, and contained perforation, deemed secondary to prior enteritis. COVID-19 may be associated with acute exacerbations of Crohn disease.[85,86]

The most severe small intestinal manifestations of COVID-19 infection are enteritis, hemorrhage, infarction, and perforation likely secondary to microcirculatory and sometimes large vessel thromboses. Histologic examination of intestinal ischemia in COVID-19–infected patients noted small vessel fibrin thrombi, submucosal vessels with fibrinous degeneration, and perivascular neutrophils.[87] Acute mesenteric ischemia in patients with COVID-19 may result from acute emboli, thrombi, and nonocclusive mesenteric ischemia, or combinations thereof.[88] A database of almost 3000 Italian patients hospitalized with COVID-19 infection noted 0.7% had mesenteric ischemia either at presentation or during the hospitalization, with almost 40% mortality reported in patients with mesenteric ischemia.[89] In a pooled database, 24% of patients with COVID-19 with mesenteric ischemia had small intestinal involvement.[90] Small series note small intestinal infarction.[91] Symptoms of early mesenteric ischemia are nonspecific, and CT findings are often only moderately specific, leading to frequent delayed diagnosis and delayed intervention, especially during the pandemic.[92] Large vessel thromboses have been reported in COVID-19–infected patients, including involvement of the superior mesenteric artery or the portal/mesenteric veins.[92–94]

Twenty-two percent of a series of COVID-19–infected patients with pneumatosis had isolated small intestinal involvement.[95] A child with multisystem inflammatory syndrome developed pneumatosis and small intestinal perforation but survived after undergoing surgery.[96] A Mexican series of COVID-19–infected patients included 10 patients with intestinal perforations, of whom 4 had perforations located in the proximal jejunum.[97] A case report described a child with both pneumatosis and protein losing enteropathy.[98] Two cases of severe enteritis necessitating small bowel resections were reported, including one COVID-19–infected patient without respiratory symptoms.[99,100]

COVID-19 infection may be associated with intussusception in infants or children due to bowel wall inflammation.[101,102] Two children had intussusception with COVID-19 infection with evidence of the virus causing inflammation in mesenteric and intestinal tissue.[103]

COVID-19–infected patients with underlying risk factors including uncontrolled diabetes, high-dose corticosteroid therapy, and exposure to mechanical ventilation have increasingly developed mucormycosis, sometimes with GI involvement.[104] Clinicians must by vigilant for invasive mucormycosis, complicating the therapy for advanced COVID-19 infection.[105]

COLON

A large study surveilling the incidence and severity of COVID-19 infection from February 1 through July 31, 2020 in 10,552 patients with microscopic colitis (MC), including 3237 with the MC type denoted collagenous colitis (CC) and 7315 with the MC type denoted lymphocytic colitis (LC), versus 52,624 matched controls without MC, as diagnosed by colonic biopsies in Sweden from 1989 through 2016 (using the Epidemiology Strengthened by histoPathology Reports in Sweden [ESPRESSO study]), reported that patients with the CC type had a significantly higher risk of developing COVID-19 infection (hazard ratio [HR] = 1.72; 95% confidence interval [CI], 1.29–2.28), a significantly higher risk of hospitalization for COVID-19 infection (HR = 3.40; 95% CI, 2.03–5.70), and a significantly higher risk of developing severe

COVID-19 infection (HR, 2.48; 95% CI, 1.33–4.63) compared with controls.[106] Severe COVID-19 infection was defined by hospitalization with laboratory-confirmed COVID-19 as the primary diagnosis or by intensive care unit admission or death within 30 days of hospital admission with COVID-19 infection regardless of whether COVID-19 was the primary diagnosis on admission. Individuals suffering from severe COVID-19 infection or death before July 31, 2020, were censured to further follow-up. These results were not due to potential confounders of immunosuppression from oral corticosteroid therapy (used to treat MC) or PPI use (associated with MC). Contrariwise, there were no associations between the LC type of MC and severe COVID-19 outcomes. This work strongly suggests an association between CC and COVID-19 infection and severe COVID-19 infection/poor patient outcome, but no such association between LC and these parameters of severe COVID-19 infection were observed. Although the precise biological mechanism for the observed association between CC and severe COVID-19 outcomes is unknown, the increased risk may relate to genetic factors that modify immune responses to viral pathogens, such as an extended HLA haplotype associated with CC (but unassociated with LC) that is associated with impaired immune responses to microbial and viral pathogens with CC. Interestingly, this study demonstrated an increased prevalence of the rs13071258 A variant on the genetic locus 3p21.31 in individuals with CC but not with LC. This locus harbors 6 genes potentially affecting immunologic defense to viral infections. This study provides important insight into the divergent response of CC versus LC to acute COVID-19 infection, but this study requires further confirmation of the postulated biological mechanisms.

Interestingly, this locus would be subject to chromosomal amplification in trisomy-21 (Down syndrome) because of the extra copy of this allele in this syndrome. This phenomenon may underlie the worse GI or other organ outcomes in patients with COVID-19 infection who have Down syndrome.[107] For example, patients with Down syndrome and COVID-19 infection have worse outcomes from chronic GERD than controls with COVID-19 infection without Down syndrome.[108]

In a case report, one patient with severe, chronic, CC had severe acute COVID-19 infection manifested by prolonged hospitalization.[109] Notably, this patient exhibited protein-losing enteropathy (PLE), attributed to collagenous duodenitis (CD) coexistent with advanced collagenous colitis from a pathologically thick microscopic collagen layer in the duodenum that likely prevented normal absorption of individual amino acids and small chains of amino acids in the small bowel. The reported novel association of CD (and CC) with PLE and their association with severe COVID-19 infection was potentially attributed to relative immunosuppression from hypoproteinemia, hypoalbuminemia, hypogammaglobulinemia, and severe malnutrition from PLE. This patient,[109] however, was not analyzed for the presence of the rs13071258 A variant on the genetic locus 3p21.31, which is potentially associated with severe COVID-19 infection in individuals with CC.[106]

A 62-year-old woman, with chronic GERD, but no administration of PPI or nonsteroidal antiinflammatory drugs (NSAIDs) for several years and no other GI symptoms or disorders, developed acute COVID-19 infection manifesting as acute onset of cough, severe headache, and low-grade pyrexia.[110] After 10 days of gradual improvement after instituting symptomatic therapy, the patient developed watery, nonbloody diarrhea, with up to 6 bowel movements daily, and rectal urgency, which persisted for 3 months despite symptomatic treatment with acetaminophen and loperamide. Stool microscopy and cultures were negative for standard enteric pathogens. Complete blood count, liver function tests, kidney function tests, thyroid function tests, and C-reactive protein levels were within normal limits. Tissue transglutaminase immunoglobulin A test was negative. Colonoscopy, performed for persistent diarrhea, revealed only scattered uncomplicated sigmoid diverticula. Histopathological analysis of sigmoid and descending colonic biopsies revealed increased chronic inflammatory cell infiltration of the lamina propria, lymphocytes extending into the surface epithelium and the epithelium lining the crypts, and findings typical for lymphocytic colitis without findings of collagenous colitis or inflammatory bowel disease. This case report suggests that lymphocytic colitis should be considered in the differential of chronic persistent watery diarrhea after acute COVID-19 infection, before diagnosing longCOVID, even though COVID-19 likely does not increase the risks of lymphocytic colitis.[106]

A 43-year-old man developed GI bleeding after treatment with tocilizumab, a monoclonal antibody against interleukon-6 (IL-6), for severe acute COVID-19 infection complicated by acute respiratory distress syndrome believed due to cytokine release syndrome (CRS).[111] Supportive investigations for CRS included highly elevated levels of IL-6, ferritin, and lactate dehydrogenase. Colonoscopy performed for GI bleeding revealed terminal ileal and cecal ulcers. The patient required surgical resection of the diseased terminal ileum and cecum because of cecal perforation. This patient had a history of potential confounders including lupus anticoagulant without receiving chronic anticoagulation therapy, chronic renal insufficiency, and the cytokine release syndrome itself, all of which could promote enteric ulcerations. Tocilizumab has been previously associated with lower GI perforation and colonic diverticular perforation during treatment of rheumatoid arthritis[112] but has not been previously associated with GI perforation during treatment of the cytokine release syndrome from severe COVID-19 infection.

In a study of 11 hospitals in New York City, the rate of Clostridiodes (Clostridium) difficile infection increased from the spring of 2019 to the spring of 2020 associated with the onset of the COVID-19 pandemic crisis in spring 2020.[113] Approximately one-third of cases of *C difficile* in spring of 2020 were in patients with COVID-19 infection, but two-thirds of cases were unassociated with COVID-19 infection. The increase in *C difficile* during the spring of 2020 correlated with a 20% increase in antibiotic usage in spring 2020 from the year earlier that was correlated with increased cephalosporin therapy to treat infections but was uncorrelated with increased use of other antibiotics. Cephalosporins are a known significant risk factor for *C difficile* infection. This correlation occurred in each of the 11 study hospitals, which used independent antibiotic protocols.

In a retrospective study of 6002 abdominal CT examinations conducted at 5 hospitals by investigators at the Massachusetts General Hospital, the rates of positive diagnoses of acute appendicitis and/or diverticulitis over the 6 weeks just before versus the 6 weeks just after the onset of the COVID-19 pandemic in March 2022 were 4% (144) versus 4%[100] for appendicitis and 8% versus 7% for diverticulitis ($P > 0.2$ for both).[114] For positive CT examinations, the rates of perforation, hospitalization, surgery, and catheter drainage changed minimally from before to after the pandemic onset by −2%, −3%, −2%, and −3%, respectively, for appendicitis (n = 244, $P > 0.3$ for all) and by +6% ($P = 0.2$), +9% ($P = 0.06$), +4% ($P = 0.01$), and +1% ($P = 0.6$), respectively, for diverticulitis (n = 443). CT examinations performed for suspected appendicitis or diverticulitis declined slightly after the pandemic onset most likely reflecting patients leaving urban centers due to the pandemic and altered triage of patients without COVID-19. However, the diagnostic rates, disease severity at presentation, and treatment approach otherwise remained mostly unchanged during the first 6 weeks of the COVID pandemic compared with the previous 6 weeks.

Several cases of acute colonic pseudoobstruction have been reported in patients with severe COVID-19–associated pneumonia.[115] Patients typically are elderly and

Table 1
Effect of COVID-19 infection on gastrointestinal disorders and diseases

Disease or Disorder	Clinical Characteristics	Mechanism
Anosmia & ageusia/ dysgeusia	Very common. Often the first symptom to manifest with COVID-19 infection and the last symptom to resolve. Bothersome symptoms but not life-threatening. Proposed, unproven therapies include corticosteroids and Paxlovid.	Not associated with nasopharyngitis, nasal obstruction, glossitis, zinc deficiency, or rhinorrhea. Postulated decreased sensitivity of olfactory neurons associated with expression of ACE-2 in alveolar epithelial cells.
Geographic (COVID) tongue	Affects about 4% of infected patients. Associated with minor symptoms.	Loss of filiform papillae in rear of tongue from damage caused by high expression of ACE-2 in epithelial cells.
GERD (gastroesophageal reflux disease)	Very common with COVID-19 infection but also very common without COVID-19 infection. GERD likely does not arise from acute COVID-19 infection but likely arises from shared risk factors, such as obesity.	COVID-19 may preferentially infect Barrett's epithelium over normal esophageal mucosa, and PPI therapy may be associated with increased COVID-19 susceptibility.
Esophageal candidiasis	Risk factors include acute respiratory distress syndrome, chronic corticosteroid therapy, and prolonged endotracheal intubation. Often associated with severe COVID-19 infection and has a high mortality due to this association. Typical symptoms are dysphagia and odynophagia. EGD classically demonstrates a cheesy exudate in esophagus. Endoscopic brushings are usually diagnostic. Primary therapies are echinocandins and azoles.	Associated with profound immune dysregulation with COVID-19 infection, but the specific underlying immunologic defects are unknown.
Pill-induced esophagitis	More prevalent in COVID-19 infected patients.	Partly related to increased use of doxycycline antibiotics to treat COVID-19 infection and increased corrosive ingestion due to COVID-19 pandemic–related stress.
Eosinophilic esophagitis	Apparently eosinophilic esophagitis does not increase the frequency or severity of COVID-19 infection. Acute COVID-19 infection does not apparently cause flares of eosinophilic esophagitis.	Patients with eosinophilic esophagitis typically have mild COVID-19 infection. COVID-19 esophageal infection might be related to oral corticosteroid therapy for eosinophilic esophagitis.

(*continued on next page*)

Table 1
(*continued*)

Disease or Disorder	Clinical Characteristics	Mechanism
Gastric ulcers	Gastric ulcers very common in patients with COVID-19 infection who are undergoing EGD.	*H pylori* does not apparently affect the severity of COVID-19 infection. Several patients had esophageal or gastric ulcers from primary COVID-19 infection, as demonstrated by electron microscopy.
GI hemorrhage	Occurs in about 9% or less of hospitalized COVID-19–infected patients. Often the GI bleeding is mild and does not mandate endoscopy. Patients with GI bleeding often have a worse prognosis from COVID-19 infection than nonbleeding COVID-19–infected patients. GI hemorrhage in patients with COVID-19 is often from gastric ulcers. GI bleeding may sometimes arise from anticoagulation used to treat a hypercoagulopathy associated with COVID-19 infection.	GI bleeding rarely due to ulcers associated with primary COVID-19 infection.
Celiac disease	Celiac patients do not have increased susceptibility to COVID-19 infection and do not have a worse outcome from COVID-19 infection. The mainstay of therapy in COVID-19–infected patients is maintenance of a gluten-free diet.	The 2 different diseases do not seem to significantly interact.
Multisystem inflammatory syndrome	Rare syndrome that occurs in children. Clinically can resemble regional enteritis. Can cause GI obstruction, fistula, or contained GI perforation.	Syndrome associated with an abnormal immune response due to viral cytopathic effects.
Mesenteric ischemia	COVID-19 infection likely increases the risk of mesenteric ischemia. Mesenteric ischemia has a high mortality in COVID-19–infected patients.	Most likely increased frequency of mesenteric ischemia due to microcirculatory thrombosis, but sometimes can occur from large vessel thrombosis. COVID-19 can produce a hypercoagulopathy. High mortality from mesenteric ischemia attributed to delayed diagnosis because symptoms can be confused with acute COVID-19 infection.

(*continued on next page*)

Table 1
(*continued*)

Disease or Disorder	Clinical Characteristics	Mechanism
Small bowel intussusception	Frequency may increase with COVID-19 infection.	Attributed to bowel wall or mesenteric lymph node inflammation, edema and thickening from local viral infection that forms a lead point for the intussusception.
GI infection with mucormycosis	Increased risk with advanced COVID-19 infection due to immunosuppression. Associated with high mortality.	Increased risk attributed to high-dose corticosteroid therapy, exposure to mechanical ventilation, and advanced COVID-19 infection.
Collagenous colitis	Significantly higher rate of contracting COVID-19 infection, having severe COVID-19 infection, and of being hospitalized for COVID-19 infection than patients with lymphocytic colitis or controls.	May relate to genetic factors associated with predisposition to developing collagenous colitis such as an extended HLA haplotype or the rs13071258 A variant on genetic locus 3p21.31 associated with collagenous colitis. This genetic locus harbors 6 genes potentially affecting the immune defense against viral infections.
Lymphocytic colitis	Has similar rate of contracting COVID-19 infection and developing severe infection as controls. Lymphocytic colitis should be considered in the differential of watery diarrhea after contracting acute COVID-19 infection.	Unlike collagenous colitis, lymphocytic colitis is not associated with genetic abnormalities affecting host defenses against viruses.
Tocilizumab-associated colonic perforation	Case report of developing terminal ileal and cecal ulcers that caused colonic perforation after initiating tocilizumab therapy for suspected cytokine release syndrome in a patient with COVID-19 infection.	Tocilizumab has previously been associated with lower GI perforation and colonic diverticular perforation after its use to treat rheumatoid arthritis.
Acute appendicitis and acute diverticulitis	COVID-19 infection does not affect the frequency of hospitalization, colonic perforation, or surgery from these 2 diseases.	COVID-19 infection does not seem to affect the natural history of these 2 diseases.
Irritable bowel syndrome	During pandemic patients with irritable bowel syndrome experienced more severe GI symptoms, more severe extraintestinal symptoms, and more sleep difficulties than	Patients likely experience more severe symptoms of irritable bowel syndrome due to anxiety related to the pandemic.

(*continued on next page*)

Table 1
(*continued*)

Disease or Disorder	Clinical Characteristics	Mechanism
	before the COVID-19 pandemic.	
Inflammatory bowel disease	COVID-19–infected patients have a worse outcome from inflammatory bowel disease when treated with corticosteroids but not when treated with tumor necrosis factor antagonists.	Corticosteroids may decrease immunologic defenses against COVID-19 infection. Another chapter in this monograph is devoted to COVID-19 infection in patients with inflammatory bowel disease.

have normal serum lactate levels, clinically obscure hypoxia, abdominal distension, sluggish bowel sounds, and colonic dilatation supported by radiographic findings at abdominal flat plate or abdominal CT. Acute colonic pseudoobstruction in patients admitted with COVID-19 pneumonia requires a high index of suspicion, as it warrants early mitigation by discontinuing offending agents, optimizing electrolytes, and therapeutic colonic decompression to decrease morbidity and mortality.

The COVID-19 pandemic has affected colonoscopy for screening or surveillance of colon cancer or colonic polyps. The COVID-19 pandemic has created a backlog of colonoscopy for such indications with attendant stricter application of colonoscopy indications due to potential risks to patients or endoscopy personnel from exposure to COVID-19 infection.[116] One approach to decrease exposure to COVID-19 infection is to offer some patients CTC. Indications for CTC in a study of 224 patients at 4 academic British hospitals included the following: change in bowel habits (116/224; 48%), positive fecal immunochemical test (69/224; 31%), iron deficiency anemia (50/224; 23%), weight loss (27/224; 7.6%), bleeding per rectum (27/224; 12%), polyp surveillance (25/224; 11%), and abdominal pain (20/224; 9%). Of 224 patients undergoing CT colonography in May to July 2020 at 4 British hospitals, 55 patients (24.6%), had a greater than or equal to 6 mm colonic polyp detected by CTC.[117] Of 169 patients contacted by telephone for follow-up, none reported any new symptoms of COVID-19 infection (cough, pyrexia, anosmia, ageusia) within 14 days of the CTC. None of the 86 staff performing CT colonography who were contacted developed COVID-19 infection after the procedure. These findings suggest that CT colonography can be performed relatively safely during the COVID-19 pandemic, with a relatively high yield of colonic polyps by expert GI radiologists. The risks of developing COVID-19 infection from CTC are low in patients and in the radiology staff.

In a study of 190 consecutive tertiary referrals for IBS, patients seen during the COVID-19 pandemic had greater IBS severity (IBS-SSS: 352 vs 318, $P = 0.03$), more severe extraintestinal symptoms (noncolonic score: 269 vs 225, $P = 0.03$), more frequent sleep difficulties ($P = 0.03$), and feelings of helplessness and loss of control ($P = 0.02$) compared with baseline patients before the pandemic.[118] However, patients during the pandemic had similar HAD-Anxiety ($P = 0.96$) and HAD-Depression ($P = 0.84$) scores (the HAD, or Hospital Anxiety and Depression score, is a 14-item self-administered anxiety and depression scale specifically designed for use in non-psychiatric settings to semiquantify feelings of anxiety and depression). During the pandemic, unmarried patients ($P = 0.03$) and workers in stressful jobs ($P = 0.0038$) had greater IBS severity. This study demonstrated that patients seen in tertiary care with refractory IBS during the COVID-19 pandemic had a

Table 2
Frequency of performing diagnostic and therapeutic GI tests during the COVID-19 pandemic (extensively reviewed in another chapter in this monograph on gastrointestinal endoscopy during the COVID-19 pandemic)

Test or Procedure	Effects Associated with COVID-19 Pandemic	Postulated Mechanism
EGD	The frequency of performing EGD during the acute pandemic peak (in March–April 2000) fell dramatically to just a few percentage of its baseline rate before the pandemic. The rate has recovered vigorously after March–April 2020 but still is lower than the baseline rate before the pandemic.	EGD is often deferred in patients with mild GI bleeding or other mild symptoms because of patient preference or concerns about transmission of COVID-19 infection to endoscopy suite personnel. EGD should be performed for urgent or emergent indications.
EGD for screening/surveillance of Barrett's esophagus and esophageal adenocarcinoma	Markedly decreased performance of EGDs for these indications during the pandemic	EGD often deferred or postponed due to these indications becauser EGD is considered a lower priority during pandemic compared with urgent indications for EGD. EGD should be performed urgently or emergently for suspected esophageal cancer.
CT of chest	Has been used as an alternative diagnostic test for EGD (eg, to detect esophageal varices)	CT, however, has limited applicability because it is rarely therapeutic. For example, CT, unlike EGD, cannot be used to band esophageal varices.
Cytosponge device	Recent innovation that permits acquiring esophageal tissue with less procedure time and at lower cost than EGD.	Experimental procedure that may soon provide a substitute for EGD that is less costly and less labor-intensive.
Unsedated nasal endoscopy	Can be used as an alternative to EGD. Does not require a nurse anesthetist.	Less costly than EGD. Requires less endoscopic resources, less endoscopic personnel, and less procedure time.
Screening and surveillance colonoscopy	Screening colonoscopy declined dramatically during the acute COVID-19 pandemic peak but has gradually recovered somewhat.	Screening colonoscopy is generally contraindicated in patients with acute COVID-19 infection. Screening colonoscopy is often deferred or postponed in favor of more urgent colonoscopy indications even in patients who are not positive for COVID-19 infection.

(*continued on next page*)

Table 2
(*continued*)

Test or Procedure	Effects Associated with COVID-19 Pandemic	Postulated Mechanism
Other colonoscopy indications	Colonoscopy for emergent or urgent indications usually performed. Colonoscopy may be deferred for elective indications depending on the indication and local practice patterns.	Colonoscopy may sometimes be deferred for elective indications due to perceived risk of contracting COVID-19 infection during colonoscopy to endoscopy staff or patients.
High-resolution manometry (HRM)	Number performed markedly decreased during pandemic.	Decrease attributed to risks of contracting or transmitting COVID-19 infection during the procedure. Also attributed to patient preference and strict endoscopy suite guidelines for performing procedures during the pandemic.

significantly higher symptom burden. These findings suggest the importance of the gut-brain axis in IBS and that lack of support and perceived loss of patient control during the COVID-19 pandemic may exacerbate the symptoms of IBS.

COVID-19–infected patients with inflammatory bowel disease as compared with patients without COVID-19 infection have a worse prognosis when treated with corticosteroids but not with tumor necrosis factor antagonists.[119,120] The management of patients with cancer receiving immune checkpoint inhibitor therapy may be affected by COVID-19 infection due to the occurrence of immune checkpoint inhibitor colitis.[121]

ANUS

Hemorrhoids are very common in both the general population and COVID-19–infected patients. Surgery for hemorrhoids should be prioritized according to symptoms and signs, with deferral of elective surgery. An e-consult may help in prioritizing patients for surgery.[122]

Anal fissures are very common during the pandemic and may be increased by COVID-19 infection, with a reported rate of 30% in patients with chronic COVID-19 attributed to sitting on a chair in front of a computer while working at home, and shared risk factors, especially obesity.[123]

In a survey of 45 office procedures performed by proctologists during the pandemic, the most common indication for surgery was anal abscesses and/or fistula (48.9%).[124]

SUMMARY

Although most of the morbidity and mortality of the COVID-19 pandemic involves the respiratory system, the virus also prominently affects the GI system in which it produces considerable symptoms and contributes to patient morbidity and occasionally mortality. The COVID-19 virus can directly infect GI mucosa due to the abundant ACE-2 receptors within these organs. This work describes the effect of COVID-19 on miscellaneous GI disorders (**Table 1**), thereby supplementing other chapters in this monograph reviewing individual GI symptoms or disorders in patients with COVID-

19 infection, inflammatory bowel disease, GI bleeding, GI endoscopy, surgical considerations with GI disorders, diagnostic and therapeutic GI radiology (**Table 2**), GI pathology, and chronic (long) COVID infection. Other chapters in this monograph review pancreatic and hepatic symptoms and disorders associated with COVID-19 infection.

CLINICS CARE POINTS

- It is important to consider gastrointestiunal inflammastory diseases because they may influence the inflammatory reactions to COVID-19 infection or in turn be influnced by inflammatory changes induced by the COVID-19 infection.
- The gastrointestinal tract, especially the stomach and small intestine, has as many ACE-2 (angiotensin converting enzyme-2) receptors to the COVID-19 virus as the respiratory tract, allowing for frequent local gastrointestinal mucosal infection, disruption, and inflammation by the virus.
- Clinicians must be aware of how the COVID-19 virus affects many gastrointestinal disorders to manage these disorders in patients with simultaneous COVID-19 infection.

ACKNOWLEDGEMENTS

Dr. Cappell is a full-time employee of the Aleda E. Lutz Hospital in Saginaw, a Veteran's Administration Hospital of the United States Government. All opinions expressed in this article are not necessarily that of the United States Government. Dr. Cappell thanks the administration of the hospital for allowing him to use time in which patient care or other hospital duties were not scheduled to work on this project.

REFERENCES

1. Schreiber M. What a million Covid dead means for the U.S.'s future. Scientific Am. Available at: www.scientificamerican.com March 29 2022. Accessed April 8, 2022.
2. Parohan M, Yaghoubi S, Seraji A, et al. Risk factors for mortality in patients with coronavirus disease 2019 (COVID-19) infection: a systematic review and meta-analysis of observational studies. Aging Male 2020;23(5):1416–24.
3. Daniell H, Nair SK, Esmaeili N, et al. Debulking SARS-CoV-2 in saliva using angiotensin converting enzyme 2 in chewing gum to decrease oral virus transmission and infection. Mol Ther 2022;30(5):1966–78.
4. de Sousa FACG, Paradella TC. Considerations on oral manifestations of COVID-19. J Med Virol 2021;93(2):667–8.
5. Barbato L, Bernardelli F, Braga G, et al. Surface disinfection and protective masks for SARS-CoV-2 and other respiratory viruses: A review by SIdP COVID-19 task force. Oral Dis 2020;18:10.
6. Manhas M, Koul D, Kalsotra G, et al. Incidence of olfactory and gustatory dysfunctions in the early stages of COVID-19: An objective evaluation. Int Arch Otorhinolaryngol 2022;26(2):e265–71. PMID: 35602269.
7. Neta FI, Fernandes ACL, Vale AJM, et al. Pathophysiology and possible treatments for olfactory-gustatory disorders in patients affected by COVID-19. Curr Res Pharmacol Drug Discov 2021;2:100035. Epub 2021 Jun 5. PMID: 34870148.

8. Benezit F, Le Turnier P, Declerck C, et al. Utility of hyposmia and hypogeusia for the diagnosis of COVID-19. Lancet Infect Dis 2020;20(9):1014–5.
9. Jalessi M, Barati M, Rohani M, et al. Frequency and outcome of olfactory impairment and sinonasal involvement in hospitalized patients with COVID-19. Neurol Sci 2020;41(9):2331–8.
10. Khani E, Khiali S, Beheshtirouy S, et al. Potential pharmacologic treatments for COVID-19 smell and taste loss: A comprehensive review. Eur J Pharmacol 2021; 5(912):174582.
11. Extance A. Covid-19: What is the evidence for the antiviral Paxlovid? BMJ 2022; 377:o1037. PMID: 35477536.
12. Nuño González A, Magaletskyy K, Martín Carrillo P, et al. Are oral mucosal changes a sign of COVID-19? A cross-sectional study at a field hospital. Actas Dermosifiliogr (Engl Ed.) 2021;112(7):640–4.
13. Iranmanesh B, Khalili M, Amiri R, et al. Oral manifestations of COVID-19 disease: A review article. Dermatol Ther 2021;34(1):e14578. https://doi.org/10.1111/dth.14578.
14. Bardellini E, Bondioni MP, Amadori F, et al. Non-specific oral and cutaneous manifestations of Coronavirus Disease 2019 in children. Med Oral Patol Oral Circ Bucal 2021;26(5):e549–53.
15. Gherlone EF, Polizzi E, Tetè G, et al. Frequent and persistent salivary gland ectasia and oral disease after COVID-19. J Dent Res 2021;100(5):464–71.
16. Wang L, Foer D, MacPhaul E, et al. PASCLex: A comprehensive post-acute sequelae of COVID-19 (PASC) symptom lexicon derived from electronic health record clinical notes. J Biomed Inform 2022;125:103951.
17. Kaulamo JT, Lätti AM, Koskela HO. Cough in the elderly during the COVID-19 pandemic. Lung 2022;17:1–8.
18. Saito H, Ozaki A, Mizuno Y, et al. Difficulty in diagnosing mild cases of COVID-19 without respiratory symptoms during the novel coronavirus pandemic: Careful monitoring needed for patients with persistent upper gastrointestinal symptoms. Clin Case Rep 2020;8(12):2787–90.
19. Ong JS, Gharahkhani P, Vaughan TL, et al. Assessing the genetic relationship between gastro-esophageal reflux disease and risk of COVID-19 infection. Hum Mol Genet. 2022;31(3):471–80.
20. Jiang G, Cai Y, Yi X, et al. The impact of laryngopharyngeal reflux disease on 95 hospitalized patients with COVID-19 in Wuhan, China: A retrospective study. J Med Virol 2020;92(10):2124–9.
21. Kow CS, Hasan SS. Could melatonin be used in COVID-19 patients with laryngopharyngeal reflux disease? J Med Virol 2021;93(1):92–3.
22. Jin RU, Brown JW, Li QK, et al. Tropism of severe acute respiratory syndrome coronavirus 2 for Barrett's esophagus may increase susceptibility to developing coronavirus disease 2019. Gastroenterology 2021;160(6):2165–8.e4.
23. Almario CV, Chey WD, Spiegel BMR. Increased risk of COVID-19 among users of proton pump inhibitors. Am J Gastroenterol 2020;115(10):1707–15.
24. Kim HB, Kim JH, Wolf BJ. Acid suppressant use in association with incidence and severe outcomes of COVID-19: a systematic review and meta-analysis. Eur J Clin Pharmacol 2022;78(3):383–91.
25. Ramachandran P, Perisetti A, Gajendran M, et al. Pre-hospitalization proton pump inhibitor use and clinical outcomes in COVID-19. Eur J Gastroenterol Hepatol 2022;34(2):137–41.

26. Lee SW, Ha EK, Yeniova AÖ, et al. Severe clinical outcomes of COVID-19 associated with proton pump inhibitors: a nationwide cohort study with propensity score matching. Gut 2021;70(1):76–84.
27. Israelsen SB, Ernst MT, Lundh A, et al. Proton pump inhibitor use is not strongly associated with SARS-CoV-2 related outcomes: A nationwide study and meta-analysis. Clin Gastroenterol Hepatol 2021;19(9):1845–54.e6.
28. Shafrir A, Benson AA, Katz LH, et al. The association between proton pump inhibitors and COVID-19 is confounded by hyperglycemia in a population-based study. Front Pharmacol 2022;4(13):791074.
29. Pahwani S, Kumar M, Aperna F, et al. Efficacy of oral famotidine in patients hospitalized with severe acute respiratory syndrome Coronavirus 2. Cureus 2022; 14(2):e22404. PMID: 35345695; PMCID: PMC8942052.
30. Malone RW. More than just heartburn: Does famotidine effectively treat patients with COVID-19? Dig Dis Sci 2021;66(11):3672–3.
31. Shoaibi A, Fortin SP, Weinstein R, et al. Comparative effectiveness of famotidine in hospitalized COVID-19 patients. Am J Gastroenterol 2021;116(4):692–9.
32. Arastehfar A, Carvalho A, Nguyen MH, et al. COVID-19-associated candidiasis (CAC): An underestimated complication in the absence of immunological predispositions? J Fungi (Basel) 2020;6(4):211.
33. Jothimani D, Danielraj S, Nallathambi B, et al. Optimal diagnostic tool for surveillance of oesophageal varices during COVID-19 pandemic. Clin Radiol 2021; 76(7):550.e1–7.
34. Trindade AJ, Zhang J, Hauschild J, et al. Impact of Coronavirus Disease 2019 on the diagnosis and therapy for Barrett's esophagus and esophageal cancer in the United States. Gastroenterology 2022;162(3):978–80.e6.
35. Darwin P, Zangara J, Heller T, et al. Unsedated esophagoscopy for the diagnosis of esophageal varices in patients with cirrhosis. Endoscopy 2000; 32(12):971–3.
36. Grant RK, Brindle WM, Robertson AR, et al. Unsedated transnasal endoscopy: A safe, well-tolerated and accurate alternative to standard diagnostic peroral endoscopy. Dig Dis Sci 2022;3:1–11.
37. Berté R, Arsié E, Penagini R. Safe esophageal function testing during the COVID-19 pandemic: A modified surgical mask for patients. Neurogastroenterol Motil 2020;32(9):e13979.
38. Pilonis ND, Killcoyne S, Tan WK, et al. Use of a cytosponge biomarker panel to prioritize endoscopic Barrett's oesophagus surveillance: a cross-sectional study followed by a real-world prospective pilot. Lancet Ocol 2022;23(2):270–8.
39. Elli L, Tontini GE, Filippi E, et al. Efficacy of endoscopic triage during the Covid-19 outbreak and infective risk. Eur J Gastroenterol Hepatol 2020;32(10):1301–4.
40. Ominami M, Sato H, Fujiyoshi Y, et al. Impact of the COVID-19 pandemic on high-resolution manometry and peroral endoscopic myotomy for esophageal motility disorder in Japan. Dig Endosc 2022;34(4):769–77.
41. El Kassas M, Al Shafie A, Abdel Hameed AS, et al. Emergency endoscopic variceal band ligation in a COVID-19 patient presented with hematemesis while on mechanical ventilation. Dig Endosc 2020;32(5):812–5.
42. Calì A, La Fortezza RF, Fusaroli P. An unexpected thoracic finding in a patient with COVID-19. Gastroenterology 2021;161(4):1111–2.
43. Deliwala SS, Gurvits GE. Acute esophageal necrosis in a patient with COVID-19. Am J Gastroenterol 2021;116(10):1977.

44. Rahman A, Alqasai S, Downing C. Unusual presentation of COVID pneumonia as esophageal rupture ended with successful management. Cureus 2021; 13(8):e17348.
45. Chandra A, Kahaleh B. Systemic sclerosis (SSc) after COVID-19: A case report. Cureus 2022;14(3):e23179, eCollection 2022 Mar.14(3):e23179.
46. Hlayhel A, Foran L, Trivedi A, et al. A case of esophageal ulcer and hemorrhage due to aberrant subclavian in a COVID positive patient. J Surg Case Rep 2022; 2022(1):rjab643. https://doi.org/10.1093/jscr/rjab643.
47. Panigrahi MK, Nayak HK, Samal SC. A recent surge of doxycycline-induced pill esophagitis during the corona virus disease 2019 (COVID-19) pandemic. Indian J Gastroenterol 2022;7:1–2.
48. Thongchuam C, Mahawongkajit P, Kanlerd A. The effect of the COVID-19 on corrosive ingestion in Thailand. Open Access Emerg Med 2021;13:299–304.
49. Binder L, Högenauer C, Langner C. Gastrointestinal effects of an attempt to avoid contracting COVID-19 by 'disinfection. Histopathology 2020;77(2):327–8.
50. Zevit N, Chehade M, Leung J, et al. Eosinophilic esophagitis patients are not at increased risk of severe COVID-19: A report from a global registry. Allergy Clin Immunol Pract 2022;10(1):143–9.e9. Epub 2021 Oct 22.PMID: 34688963.
51. Mennini M, Rea F, Riccardi C, et al. SARS-COV2 and eosinophilic esophagitis: a first case. Eur J Gastroenterol Hepatol 2021;33(8):1131–2. PMID: 34213509.
52. Xu J, Chu M, Zhong F, et al. Digestive symptoms of COVID-19 and expression of ACE2 in digestive tract organs. Cell Death Discov 2020;11(6):76.
53. Vanella G, Capurso G, Burti C, et al. Gastrointestinal mucosal damage in patients with COVID-19 undergoing endoscopy: an international multicentre study. BMJ Open Gastroenterol 2021;8(1):e000578.
54. Ashktorab H, Russo T, Oskrochi G, et al. Clinical and endoscopic outcomes in Coronavirus Disease-2019 patients with gastrointestinal bleeding. Gastro Hep Adv 2022;1(4):487–99.
55. Deb A, Thongtan T, Costilla V. Gastric ulcerations in COVID-19: an ominous sign? BMJ Case Rep 2021;14(7):e244059.
56. Garrosa-Muñoz S, López-Sánchez J, González-Fernández LM, et al. Could SARS-CoV-2 be associated with emphysematous gastritis? Dig Liver Dis 2021;53(5):540.
57. Poggiali E, Vercelli A, Demichele E, et al. Diaphragmatic rupture and gastric perforation in a patient with COVID-19 pneumonia. Eur J Case Rep Intern Med 2020;27(6):001738.
58. Gupta K, Thakur A, Kler N, et al. Gastric perforation and necrotizing enterocolitis associated with COVID antibodies. Indian J Pediatr 2022;89(1):93.
59. Balamtekin N, Artuk C, Arslan M, et al. The effect of Helicobacter pylori on the presentation and clinical course of coronavirus disease 2019 infection. J Pediatr Gastroenterol Nutr 2021;72(4):511–3.
60. Martin TA, Wan DW, Hajifathalian K, et al. Gastrointestinal bleeding in patients with coronavirus disease 2019: A matched case-control study. Am J Gastroenterol 2020;115(10):1609–16.
61. Marasco G, Maida M, Morreale GC, et al. Gastrointestinal bleeding in COVID-19 patients: A systematic review with meta-analysis. Can J Gastroenterol Hepatol 2021;2534975. https://doi.org/10.1155/2021/2534975.
62. Elshazli RM, Kline A, Elgaml A, et al. Gastroenterology manifestations and COVID-19 outcomes: A meta-analysis of 25,252 cohorts among the first and second waves. J Med Virol 2021;93(5):2740–68.

63. Melazzini F, Lenti MV, Maur A, et al. Peptic ulcer disease as a common cause of bleeding in patients with Coronavirus disease 2019. Am J Gastroenterol 2020; 115(7):1139–40. PMID: 32618672.
64. Goyal H, Sachdeva S, Perisetti A, et al. Management of gastrointestinal bleeding during COVID-19: less is more! Eur J Gastroenterol Hepatol 2021;33(9):1230–2.
65. Gulen M, Satar S. Uncommon presentation of COVID-19: Gastrointestinal bleeding. Clin Res Gastroenterol Hepatol 2020;44(4):e72–6.
66. Bisseling TM, van Laarhoven A, Huijbers A, et al. Coronavirus disease-19 presenting as esophageal ulceration. Am J Gastroenterol 2021;116(2):421–4. PMID: 33086224.
67. Li X, Huang S, Lu J, et al. Upper gastrointestinal bleeding caused by SARS-CoV-2 infection. Am J Gastroenterol 2020;115(9):1541–2.
68. Barrett LF, Lo KB, Stanek SR, et al. Self-limited gastrointestinal bleeding in COVID-19. Clin Res Hepatol Gastroenterol 2020;44(4):e77–80.
69. Mohamed M, Nassar M, Nso N, et al. Massive gastrointestinal bleeding in a patient with COVID-19. Arab J Gastroenterol 2021;22(2):177–9.
70. Trindade AJ, Izard S, Coppa K, et al. Gastrointestinal bleeding in hospitalized COVID-19 patients: a propensity score matched cohort study. J Intern Med 2021;289(6):887–94.
71. Hongxin C, Zhenhua T, Zhuang M, et al. Gastrointestinal bleeding, but not other gastrointestinal symptoms, is associated with worse outcomes in COVID-19 patients. Front Med (Lausanne) 2021;8:759152.
72. Iqbal U, Patel PD, Pluskota CA, et al. Outcomes acute Gastrointest bleeding patients COVID-19: A case-control Study. Gastroenterology Res 2022;15(1):13–8.
73. Wu XR, Zhang YF, Lan N, et al, On behalf of Chinese Society of Colorectal Surgery of China Medical Association. Pandemic. Practice patterns of colorectal surgery during the COVID-19 pandemic. Dis Colon Rectum 2020;63(12): 1572–4.
74. Ding S, Liang TJ. Is SARS-CoV-2 Also an enteric pathogen with potential fecal-oral transmission? A COVID-19 virological and clinical review. Gastroenterology 2020;159(1):53–61.
75. Konturek PC, Harsch IA, Neurath MF, et al. COVID-19 more than respiratory disease: a gastroenterologist's perspective. J Physiol Pharamacol 2020;71(2). https://doi.org/10.26402/jpp.2020.2.02.
76. Bottari B, Castellone V, Neviani E. Probiotics and Covid-19. Int J Food Sci Nutr 2021;72(3):293–9.
77. Tobi M, Talwar H, McVicker B. The celiac disease microbiome depends on the Paneth cells of the puzzle. Gastroenterology 2021;161(1):359. Epub 2021 Feb 11. PMID: 33581121.
78. Zhen J, Stefanolo JP, Temprano MP, et al. The risk of contracting COVID-19 is not increased in patients with celiac disease. Clin Gastroenterol Hepatol 2021;19(2):391–3.
79. Cakir M, Guven B, Issi F, et al. New-onset celiac disease in children during COVID-19 pandemic. Acta Paediatr 2022;111(2):383–8.
80. Trovato CM, Montuori M, Pietropaoli N, et al. COVID-19 and celiac disease: A pathogenetic hypothesis for a celiac outbreak. Int J Clin Pract 2021;75(9): e14452.
81. Lebwohl B, Larsson E, Söderling J, et al. Risk of severe Covid-19 in patients with celiac disease: A population-based cohort study. Clin Epidemiol 2021;13: 121–30.

82. Nisoli E, Cinti S, Valerio A. COVID-19 and Hartnup disease: an affair of intestinal amino acid malabsorption. Eat Weight Disord 2021;26(5):1647–51.
83. Samasca G, Lerner A. Celiac disease in the COVID-19 pandemic. J Transl Autoimmun 2021;4:100120. https://doi.org/10.1016/j.jtauto.2021.100120.
84. Sahn B, Eze OP, Edelman MC, et al. Features of intestinal disease associated with COVID-related multisystem inflammatory syndrome in children. J Pediatr Gastroenterol Nutr 2021;72(3):384–7.
85. Parigi TL, Bonifacio C, Danese S. Is It Crohn's disease? Gastroenterology 2020; 159(4):1244–6.
86. Abbassi B, Deb A, Costilla V, et al. Subacute enteritis two months after COVID-19 pneumonia with mucosal bleeding, perforation, and internal fistulas. Am Surg 2021;1. 31348211023461.
87. Zhang ML, Jacobsen F, Pepe-Mooney BJ, et al. Clinicopathological findings in patients with COVID-19-associated ischaemic enterocolitis. Histopathology 2021;79(6):1004–17.
88. Patel S, Parikh C, Verma D, et al. Bowel ischemia in COVID-19: A systematic review. Int J Clin Pract 2021;75(12):e14930.
89. Norsa L, Bonafinni PA, Caldato M, et al. Intestinal ischemic manifestations of SARS-CoV-2: Results from the ABDOCOVID multicentre study. World J Gastroenterol 2021;27(32):5448–59.
90. Serban D, Tribus LC, Vancea G, et al. Acute mesenteric Ischemia in COVID-19 Patients. J Clin Med 2022;11(1):200.
91. Ignat M, Philouze G, Aussenac-Belle L, et al. Small bowel ischemia and SARS-CoV-2 infection: An underdiagnosed distinct clinical entity. Surgery 2020; 168(1):14–6.
92. Ojha V, Mani A, Mukherjee A, et al. A Mesenteric ischemia in patients with COVID-19: An updated systematic review of abdominal CT findings in 75 patients. Abdom Radiol 2022;47(5):1565–602.
93. Abeysekera KW, Karteszi H, Clark A, et al. Spontaneous portomesenteric thrombosis in a non-cirrhotic patient with SARS-CoV-2 infection. BMJ Case Rep 2020; 13(12):e238906. PMID: 33371000.
94. Sukegawa M, Nishiwada S, Terai T, et al. Acute superior mesenteric artery occlusion associated with COVID-19 pneumonia: A case report. Surg Case Rep 2022;8(1):6. PMID: 35001200.
95. Wong K, Kim DH, Khanijo S, et al. Pneumatosis intestinalis in COVID-19: Case series. Cureus 2020;12(10):e10991. PMID: 33209547.
96. Heza L, Olive A, Miller J. Pneumatosis intestinalis and intestinal perforation in a case of multisystem inflammatory syndrome in children. BMJ Case Rep 2021; 14(4):e241688.
97. Estevez-Cerda SC, Saldaña-Rodríguez JA, Alam-Gidi AG, et al. Severe bowel complications in SARS-CoV-2 patients receiving protocolized care. Rev Gastroenterol Mex (English) 2021;86(4):378–86. PMID: 34400118.
98. Rohani P, Karimi A, Tabatabaie SR, et al. Protein losing enteropathy and pneumatosis intestinalis in a child with COVID 19 infection. J Pediatr Surg Case Rep 2021;64:101667. Epub 2020 Nov 5. PMID: 33173753.
99. Amarapurkar AD, Vichare P, Pandya N, et al. Haemorrhagic enteritis and COVID-19: causality or coincidence. J Clin Pathol 2020;73(10):686. PMID: 32482887.
100. Francese M, Ferrari C, Lotti M, et al. The thin red line: ileal angiodysplasia versus SARS-CoV-2-related haemorrhagic enteritis. J Clin Path 2022;2021:207754. PMID: 35039451.

101. Noviello C, Bollettini T, Mercedes R, et al. COVID-19 can cause severe intussusception in infants: Case report and literature review. Pediatr Infect Dis J 2021; 40(11):e437–8.
102. Athamnah MN, Masade S, Hamdallah H, et al. COVID-19 presenting as intussusception in infants: A case report with literature review. J Pediatr Case Rep 2021;66:101779.
103. Scottoni F, Giobbe GG, Zambaiti E, et al. Intussusception and COVID-19 in infants: Evidence for an etiopathologic correlation. Pediatrics 2022;149(6). e2021054644. 35322271.
104. Sannathimmappa MB, Nambiar V, Aravindakshan R. Storm of a rare opportunistic life threatening mucormycosis among post COVID-19 patients: A tale of two pathogens. Int J Crit Illn Inj Sci 2022;12(1):38–46. Epub 2022 Mar 24. PMID: 35433396.
105. Sharma A, Goel A. Mucormycosis: risk factors, diagnosis, treatments, and challenges during COVID-19 pandemic. Folia Microbiol (Praha) 2022;67(3):363–87.
106. Khalili H, Zheng T, Söderling J, et al, COVID-19 and microscopic colitis collaborators, Munch A, Sjoberg K, Almer S, Vigren L, Janczewska I, Ohlsson B, Bresso F, Mellander MR, Olén O, Roelstraete B, Franke A, Simon TG, D'Amato M, Ludvigsson JF. Association between collagenous and lymphocytic colitis and risk of severe coronavirus disease 2019. Gastroenterology 2021;160(7): 2585–7.e3. Epub 2021 Feb 19. PMID: 33610527.
107. Illouz T, Biragyn A, Frenkel-Morgenstern M, et al. Specific Susceptibility to COVID-19 in Adults with Down Syndrome. Neuromolecular Med 2021;23(4): 561–71.
108. Hüls A, Costa ACS, Dierssen M, et al. T21RS COVID-19 Initiative. Medical vulnerability of individuals with Down syndrome to severe COVID-19-data from the Trisomy 21 Research Society and the UK ISARIC4C survey. EClinicalMedicine 2021;33:100769. https://doi.org/10.1016/j.eclinm.2021.100769.
109. Gill I, Shaheen AA, Edhi AI, et al. Novel case report: A previously reported, but pathophysiologically unexplained, association between collagenous colitis and protein-losing enteropathy may be explained by an undetected link with collagenous duodenitis. Dig Dis Sci 2021;66(12):4557–64. PMID: 33537921.
110. Nassar IO, Langman G, Quraishi MN, et al. SARS CoV-2-triggered lymphocytic colitis. BMJ Case Rep 2021;14(8):e243003, 34429288.
111. Bruce-Hickman D, Sajeed SM, Pang YH, et al. Bowel ulceration following tocilizumab administration in a COVID-19 patient. BMJ Open Gastroenterol 2020; 7(1):e000484. PMID: 32816957.
112. Strangfeld A, Richter A, Siegmund B, et al. Risk for lower intestinal perforations in patients with rheumatoid arthritis treated with tocilizumab in comparison to treatment with other biologic or conventional synthetic DMARDs. Ann Rheum Dis 2017;76:504–10.
113. Maro A, Asrat H, Qiu W, et al. Trends in Clostridioides difficile infection across a public health system in New York City 2019-2021: A cautionary note. Am J Infect Control 2022;S0196–6553(22):00403–5. Online ahead of print. PMID: 35569616.
114. Kilcoyne A, Goiffon RJ, Anderson MA, et al. Impact of Covid-19 CT-diagnosed acute appendicitis and diverticulitis: Was there collateral damage? Clin Radiol 2022;S0009–9260(22):00170–82.
115. Samuel SV, Viggeswarpu S, Wilson BP, et al. Acute colonic pseudo-obstruction in two patients admitted with severe acute respiratory syndrome-coronavirus-2 pneumonia. ID Cases 2021;25:e01205. Epub 2021 Jun 24. PMID: 34189047.

116. Xiao AH, Chang SY, Stevoff CG, et al. Adoption of multi-society guidelines facilitates value-based reduction in screening and surveillance colonoscopy volume during COVID-19 pandemic. Dig Dis Sci 2021;66(8):2578–84.
117. Peprah D, Plumb A, Corr A, et al. Re-initiation of CT colonography services during the COVID-19 pandemic: Preliminary evaluation of safety. Br J Radiol 2021; 94(1121):20201316. Epub 2021 Apr 9. PMID: 33835838.
118. Noble H, Hasan SS, Whorwell PJ, et al. The symptom burden of irritable bowel syndrome in tertiary care during the COVID-19 pandemic. Neurogastroenterol Motil 2022;e14347. Epub ahead of print. PMID: 35238428.
119. Brenner EJ, Ungaro RC, Gearry RB, et al. Corticosteroids, but not TNF antagonists, are associated with adverse COVID-19 outcomes in patients with inflammatory bowel diseases: Results from an international registry. Gastroenterology 2020;159(2):481–91.e3. Epub 2020 May 18. PMID: 32425234.
120. Burke KE, Kochar B, Allegretti JR, et al. Immunosuppressive therapy and risk of COVID-19 infection in patients with inflammatory bowel diseases. Inflamm Bowel Dis 2021;27(2):155–61, 33089863.
121. Grover S, Bond SA, Mansour MK, et al. Management of immunotherapy colitis: Special considerations in the COVID-19 era. Cancer 2020;126(21):4630–3. Epub 2020 Aug 14. PMID: 32797685118.
122. Campennì P, Marra AA, Ferri L, et al. Impact of COVID-19 quarantine on advanced hemorrhoidal disease and the role of telemedicine in patient management. J Clin Med 2020;9(11):3416. https://doi.org/10.3390/jcm9113416.
123. Hassan SM, Jawad MJ, Jawad MJ, et al. Gastrointestinal and metabolic disturbances in post-COVID-19 disease outcomes. Wiad Lek 2021;74(12):3160–7. PMID: 35058383.
124. Giani I, Gallo G, Grossi U, et al. Resumption of proctology algorithm working group. the impact of COVID-19 pandemic on a tertiary referral proctology center: no one should be left behind. Minerva Surg 2022;77(1):30–4. Epub 2021 Jun 23. PMID: 34160175.

Gastrointestinal and Hepatobiliary Symptoms and Disorders with Long (Chronic) COVID Infection

Anam Rizvi, MD[a], Yonatan Ziv, MD[a], James M. Crawford, MD, PhD[b], Arvind J. Trindade, MD[c,*]

KEYWORDS

• Long COVID • Chronic COVID • COVID-19 infection • Pandemic • Gastrointestinal • Hepatobiliary

KEY POINTS

- Long (chronic) COVID syndrome is an evolving multisystem disease occurring 4 to 12 weeks after acute COVID-19 infection.
- Gastrointestinal (GI) and hepatobiliary manifestations of long COVID syndrome are common.
- Abdominal pain, nausea and vomiting, diarrhea, constipation, loss of taste, loss of appetite, weight loss, postinfectious irritable bowel syndrome, dyspepsia, and post-COVID cholangiopathy are GI and hepatobiliary sequelae of long COVID syndrome.
- Vaccination against COVID-19 is currently the best measure to prevent long COVID sequelae.
- Long COVID is likely to pose a significant strain on the health-care system in terms of outpatient care and economic costs in the future.

BACKGROUND

The COVID-19 pandemic has affected more than 590 million people with about 6 million deaths worldwide to date.[1] For many COVID-19 infection has been a transient

[a] Division of Gastroenterology, Donald and Barbara Zucker School of Medicine at Hofstra/Northwell, Northwell Health System, 270-05 76 th Avenue, New Hyde Park, NY 11040, USA; [b] Department of Pathology and Laboratory Medicine, Donald and Barbara Zucker School of Medicine at Hofstra/Northwell, 270-05 76th Avenue, New Hyde Park, NY 11040, USA; [c] Division of Gastroenterology, Long Island Jewish Medical Center, Donald and Barbara Zucker School of Medicine at Hofstra/Northwell, Northwell Health System, 270-05 76th Avenue, New Hyde Park, NY 11040, USA

* Corresponding author.

E-mail address: arvind.trindade@gmail.com

Gastroenterol Clin N Am 52 (2023) 139–156
https://doi.org/10.1016/j.gtc.2022.09.002
0889-8553/23/

and acute illness. However, some have experienced a persistence or new development of symptoms not attributable to alternative causes. This has created a new medical disease/syndrome to characterize a postacute COVID-19 syndrome now known as "long COVID," which is referred to throughout this review (other designations include post–COVID-19 syndrome, post-COVID conditions, postacute COVID-19, or chronic COVID).[2] Evidence is accumulating that long COVID is a multiorgan disease, involving the cardiopulmonary, neurologic, gastrointestinal (GI), nephrological, and other systems.[3,4] Substantial debate exists regarding the delineation of long COVID syndrome. The National Institute for Health and Care Excellence defines long COVID as sustained symptoms after acute COVID-19, not attributable to alternative diagnoses, including symptomatic COVID-19 from more than 4 to 12 weeks and post–COVID-19 syndrome more than 12 weeks postinfection.[5] The US Centers for Disease Control and Prevention (CDC) demarcates long COVID as prolonged sequelae greater than 4 weeks postinfection.[6] Due to varying definitions, the prevalence of long COVID syndrome is reported with a wide range from 10% to 87% of patients who were afflicted with COVID-19 infection.[3,7,8] If a 10% prevalence is selected more than 50 million patients would be afflicted with long-COVID.[9]

The associated risk factors and precipitants of long COVID syndrome remain abstruse. Although poor baseline health and severe acute COVID-19 illness have been associated with the development of long COVID,[10] puzzlingly it also frequently occurs in patients with mild-to-moderate disease not requiring critical care or respiratory support.[11–14]

It is apparent though that long COVID is likely to herald growing challenges to the health-care system.[6,15] Long COVID syndrome has extensive economic influence because residual symptoms can cause a loss of quality of life and earnings and an increase in medical spending. The incidence, costs, and impact of long COVID are continually being revised so the impact is difficult to estimate. Recent estimates suggest that long COVID syndrome could cost up to USD 3.7 trillion, with 59% of the total cost secondary to loss of quality of life. For perspective, the economic cost would rival the cost of the Great Recession.[16,17] This cost amounts to USD 11,000 per person, or approximately 17% of the pre-COVID US gross domestic product (GDP).[16,17] In this case, the increased health-care utilization alone would cost USD 528 billion in total.[16,17] Patient's self-reported experiences agree with these estimates as surveys from the COVID-19 Longhauler Advocacy Project suggest that more than 42% of patients with long COVID have medical bills more than USD 5000 and 51% are able to work fewer hours due to long COVID.[18]

This article reviews long-COVID syndrome in relation to the GI and hepatobiliary systems.

BRIEF OVERVIEW OF LONG COVID SYNDROME

Part of the difficulty in defining the incidence of long COVID syndrome is that it can affect almost all organ systems with various clinical presentations. Furthermore, for each long COVID sign and symptom, it is not clear if it is due to sequelae from the initial COVID infection or if it is a de novo pathologic process. This review emphasizes the manifestations of long COVID in the GI tract but first summarizes below some of the common manifestations occurring throughout the body (**Fig. 1**).

Cardiovascular

- Chest pain can occur in 21% of patients with symptoms persisting in 9% up to 6 months.[8,19,20] Palpitations can occur in 9% at 6 months.[19] The acute phase

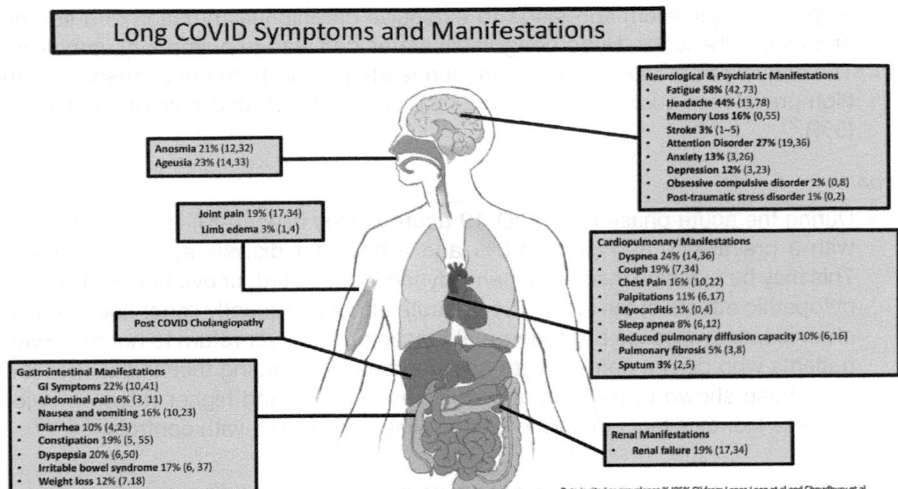

Fig. 1. Systemic manifestations of long COVID syndrome across multiple organ systems. (*Data* cited as prevalence % (95% CI) from Lopez-Leon S, Wegman-Ostrosky T, Perelman C, et al. More than 50 long-term effects of COVID-19: a systematic review and meta-analysis. Scientific Reports. 2021;11(1):16144; and Choudhury A, Tariq R, Jena A, et al. Gastrointestinal manifestations of long COVID: A systematic review and meta-analysis. Therap Adv Gastroenterol. 2022;15:17562848221118403).

of COVID-19 can be associated with acute myocardial infarction secondary to thrombosis, myocarditis, heart failure, and arrhythmia. Therefore, it is not surprising in a large study using national health-care databases from the US Department of Veterans Affairs estimated the risks and 1-year burdens of cardiovascular outcomes in patients who had COVID-19 was substantially increased for the spectrum of cardiovascular diseases versus controls, including inflammatory heart disease hazard ratio (HR) 2.02 (95%CI: 1.77, 2.30), ischemic heart disease 1.66 (95%CI: 1.52, 1.80), arrhythmia HR 1.69 (95%CI: 1.64, 1.75), thromboembolic disorders HR 2.39 (95%CI: 2.27, 2.51) and major adverse cardiovascular events HR 1.55 (95%CI: 1.50, 1.60).[15]

Neurologic/Psychiatric

- In a systematic review and meta-analysis, the authors identified a myriad of neurologic and psychiatric symptoms including memory loss (16%), anxiety (13%), headache (44%), fatigue (58%), sleep disorder (11%), and stroke (3%).[21] Much rarer symptoms include seizures, myelitis, and encephalopathy.[22,23] Despite the common neurologic symptoms being nonspecific and possibly multifactorial, there exists a strong biological plausibility of direct neurologic involvement of COVID-19 because SARS-CoV-2 RNA has been found in brain specimens as well as neuropathological abnormalities such as microgliosis, astrogliosis, edema, and hemorrhagic lesions. Whether these findings are due to neuroinvasion or a brain inflammatory lesion with hypoxic/ischemic injury is still currently debated but the latter is more likely.[24]

Pulmonary

- COVID-19 is primarily a respiratory virus and its respiratory effects and pathologic condition have been documented extensively. COVID-19 initially infects respiratory epithelium and leads to extensive chronic inflammation and fibrotic changes in the lungs. Hypercoagulable states can lead to pulmonary embolism. The sequela from the acute dysfunction leads to long-term consequences with high prevalence such as dyspnea (24%), cough (19%), and pulmonary fibrosis (5%).[21]

Renal

- During the acute phase of COVID-19 acute kidney injury (AKI) is quite common with a prevalence as high as 28% and a need for dialysis as high as 9%.[25] This may be cytokine mediated, hemodynamic mediated, or even possibly direct cytopathic effects of the virus. These acute effects frequently linger and result in chronic kidney disease because renal function may never return to normal. Even patients who do not demonstrate any degree of AKI during their initial infection have been shown to have greater declines in eGFR and higher rates of major adverse kidney events during follow-up when compared with controls.[19,26,27]

POTENTIAL MECHANISMS OF LONG-COVID IN GASTROINTESTINAL TRACT

The mucosal layer of the GI tract is a protective barrier composed of intestinal epithelial cells and mucin-producing goblet cells.[28,29] A virus that could systematically dismantle this protective barrier in the GI tract can precipitate GI symptoms and produce inflammatory changes with attendant consequences.

The pathophysiological mechanisms of long COVID remain poorly understood. Hypotheses to explain ongoing sequelae of long COVID include the following[2]:

1. Direct viral toxicity, vessel injury, microthrombosis, or macrothrombosis resulting in tissue damage, as occurring in acute COVID-19 infection,[28–32]
2. Persistent low-level replication of the virus or of viral antigens resulting in inadequate viral clearance,[14,33]
3. Perpetuating inflammation and autoimmune responses to COVID-19 infection resulting in ongoing tissue injury,[34]
4. Dysbiosis,[35–38]
5. Increased awareness and reporting of symptoms diffusely associated with COVID-19, and
6. Consequences of therapies of COVID-19 infection, particularly aggressive therapies in the setting of critical COVID-19 infection with prolonged recovery.

Direct Viral Toxicity, Vessel Injury, Microthrombosis, Macrothrombosis

COVID-19 infection results from the SARS-CoV-2 virus, which infects host cells by binding viral spike glycoprotein to the angiotensin converting enzyme 2 (ACE2) receptor. The integration of the SARS-CoV-2 virus into the host cell then allows for viral replication, shedding, and release of downstream inflammatory cytokines.[28,29] Notably ACE2 receptors, or the entry gates for SARS-CoV-2 virus, are present in a myriad of organ systems located throughout the human body including the lungs, heart, brain, kidneys, GI tract, and liver.[39] These are often the same systems implicated in long COVID. Direct viral injury via ACE2 receptors may be predictive of the downstream organ-specific symptomology occurring in this syndrome. GI and hepatobiliary systems are susceptible to severe acute respiratory infection (SARS-CoV2) as host intestinal epithelial cells and cholangiocytes show high levels of expression of the virus's entry receptor, ACE2.[40–42] Studies with human intestinal organoids, or a cultured "mini-gut" in a dish, demonstrated direct viral injury by showing that SARS-CoV-2 replicates robustly within enterocytes and subsequently produces large amounts of infective virus particles in the intestine.[43]

Furthermore, endothelial cell damage due to direct viral entry can trigger inflammatory and prothrombotic pathways, including increased thrombin production, inhibition of fibrinolysis, complement pathway activation, and precipitating thromboinflammation, which causes microthrombi deposition and microvascular dysfunction. This endothelial injury triggered by COVID-19 infection has been found in the vascular beds of multiple organs, including small intestine, liver, lungs, kidney, and heart.[30–32]

Inadequate Viral Clearance

Considering that fecal shedding of viral SARS-CoV-2 RNA can outlast oropharyngeal shedding and has been shown to persist in fecal samples 7 months after initial infection, the GI tract may be particularly predisposed to long COVID-19 sequelae.[33] Studies have shown associations between fecal SARS-CoV-2 RNA viral shedding and increased incidence of GI symptoms such as abdominal pain, nausea, vomiting, and diarrhea,[44] providing a potential explanation for the persistence of long-COVID GI symptoms. This is further advanced by new data showing viral antigen presence, even in the absence of fecal viral RNA shedding, up to 7 months after initial COVID-19 infection in 52% to 70% patients with inflammatory bowel disease (IBD) who had colonic biopsies performed; in this cohort, the presence of postacute COVID-19 symptoms were associated with viral antigen persistence ($P = .001$).[14]

Inflammation, Autoimmune Responses

Secondary or downstream proinflammatory state propagation as a consequence of COVID-19 infection may provide another explanation for long COVID syndrome GI sequelae. In intestinal epithelial cells, ACE2 receptors stabilize amino acid transporters and their subsequent metabolic products that uphold gut immunity and beneficial microbiota.[39,45] ACE2 receptor deficiency or decreased production causes a proinflammatory state with upregulation of interleukin-6 and fecal calprotectin and epithelial cell injury.[39,45,46] Patients with long COVID syndrome have shown prolonged immunologic dysfunction up to 8 months after infection, with lack of native T and B cells and elevated levels of interferons.[34]

Dysbiosis

Changes in the diversity of the native GI microbiome, or dysbiosis, has been noted in patients with acute COVID-19 infection.[35,47,48] Oral cavity and fecal studies have found less butyric acid-producing bacteria and more lipopolysaccharide-producing bacteria in patients with COVID-19 infection.[35,36] After acute COVID-19 infection, patients have been found to deplete commensal anti-inflammatory gut bacteria, such as *Faecalibacterium prausnitzii*, *Eubacterium rectale*, and bifidobacteria, which remained low in fecal microbiota samples collected up to 30 days after diagnosis suggesting a long-term role in causing dysbiosis. This reduction in gut commensal bacteria correlated with increased concentration of inflammatory markers (inflammatory cytokines, C reactive protein [CRP], lactate dehydrogenase, aspartate aminotransferase [AST], and gamma-glutamyl transferase).[37] This is also supported by another study in which fecal microbiota samples of COVID-19 patients were followed postdischarge at 2 weeks and at 6 months; at 6 months, patients with COVID-19 infection continued to have decreased microbiome diversity and higher levels of CRP, correlated with an increased proinflammatory state with dysbiosis.[38] The pathophysiological mechanism by which SARS-CoV-2 initiates dysbiosis is largely unknown. It is postulated that downregulation of ACE2 disrupts gut immunity and promotes inflammation, increasing the propensity for invasion by opportunistic gut bacteria and downstream cytokine storms.[49,50]

It is evident that further robust studies are needed to establish the molecular mechanisms of long COVID syndrome.

GASTROINTESTINAL AND HEPATOBILIARY MANIFESTATIONS OF LONG COVID SYNDROME

Abdominal Pain, Nausea and Vomiting, Diarrhea, Constipation

GI sequelae of acute COVID-19 infection include symptoms of abdominal pain (pooled prevalence 2.7%), nausea and vomiting (pooled prevalence 4.6%–10.3%), and diarrhea (pooled prevalence 7.4%–13.2%).[51–53] The respective pooled frequencies of abdominal pain, nausea and vomiting, and diarrhea occurring in long COVID syndrome are 7% (95%CI: 0.03–0.11), and 5% (95%CI: 0.03–0.10).[54] In a case-control study of 46,857 outpatients diagnosed with COVID-19 matched 1:1 with patients without COVID-19, patients with COVID-19 infection were 1.3 times more likely to experience abdominal pain or nausea and vomiting at 31 to 60 days after initial outpatient encounter.[55] Most initial abdominal pain, nausea, vomiting, and diarrhea symptoms resolve by 3 to 6 months, at rates of 90.5% and 89.4%, respectively.[56] More limited data exist regarding constipation as a GI manifestation of long COVID syndrome. Constipation has been shown to be a long COVID GI manifestation after acute COVID-19 infection; in a study of 147 patients without preexisting GI manifestations 6.8% developed new onset of constipation at a median follow-up of 106 days (IQR 78–141).[57]

Dyspepsia, Postinfectious Irritable Bowel Syndrome

Long COVID disorders of the gut–brain axis or functional GI disorders (FGID), including irritable bowel syndrome (IBS) and dyspepsia, are now being acknowledged.[58] The development of FGID after episodes of viral gastroenteritis has been previously supported.[59] Longer lasting symptoms of FGID are shown to occur after episodes of GI inflammation and dysbiosis, both of which occur after COVID-19 infection.[49,59,60] Furthermore, mood disturbances are strongly and bidirectionally linked to FGID such as IBS,[61,62] and patients commonly meet diagnostic criteria for depression, anxiety, and posttraumatic stress disorder after COVID-19 infection.[63] Limited studies have examined the frequency of postinfectious IBS or dyspepsia; a meta-analysis reported 17% (95% CI, 0.06–0.37) for postinfectious IBS and 20% (95% CI 0.06–0.50) for dyspepsia.[54] Postinfectious IBS, postinfectious functional dyspepsia, or both, were found at rates of 5.3%, 2.1%, and 1.8%, respectively, at 6 months in a case-control study of 280 patients.[64] It is hypothesized that more patients will subsequently develop long COVID FGIDs based on the characteristic biological nature of COVID-19 infection that causes intestinal inflammation and dysbiosis in conjunction with environmental and psychological stressors.[65]

Loss of Taste

Dysgeusia is a common symptom occurring in acute COVID-19 infection. Research has shown high expression of ACE2 receptors in taste receptor cells and salivary glands.[66,67] Regarding loss of taste in long COVID, a meta-analysis found a frequency of 17% (95% CI, 0.10–0.27).[54] In Denmark, 49 patients found, after COVID-19 hospitalization, that taste impairment increased from 17% at baseline to 33% and 31% at 6 and 12 weeks, respectively.[68] Another retrospective observational study of 74 patients reported 10.8% had persistent ageusia at 6 months; loss of taste occurred more commonly in women and in those who reported facial headaches early on during the infection course.[69] Loss of taste up to 3 months in a study of 83 participants was weakly correlated with low IgA levels at 6 weeks and 6 months; IgA is known to play a role in mucosal immunity by providing most of neutralizing antibodies to SARS-CoV-2.[70,71]

Weight Loss, Anorexia, Malnutrition

Weight loss to the extent of cachexia, or more than 5% body weight loss, has been associated with COVID-19 infection at rates ranging from 29% to 52% among hospitalized cohorts.[72–75] The frequency of anorexia occurring in patients with long COVID has been estimated at 20% (95% CI, 0.08–0.43).54 In a study that followed patients who required artificial nutrition during acute COVID-19 infection (82.3% with anorexia during acute illness with mean weight loss of 10.9 $\pm$ 6 kg, $P \leq .001$), at 6 months, 6.8% patients experienced ongoing anorexia with global mean weight gain remaining less than half at baseline (4.03 $\pm$ 6.2 kg, $P \leq .0001$).[76] This was supported by other studies showing that in COVID-19 patients with malnutrition, inability to gain weight may persist at 3 and 6 months; 59.1% of patients with malnutrition were unable to gain weight at 3 months (median weight loss −14.7 lbs [IQR: −26.6 to −7.9]) and 56.4% were unable to gain weight at 6 months (median weight loss −17.8 lbs [IQR: −35.2 to −6.5]).[56] In a survey of more than 1000 patients who developed COVID-19 infection in the general population, 3.3% reported ongoing weight loss at a median interval of 20 weeks.[77]

Liver Enzyme Elevations

Elevated liver enzymes commonly occur in acute COVID-19 infection at pooled incidence rates of 23.1% (95%CI: 19.3–27.3) at initial presentation and at 24.4% (95% CI: 13.5–40) during the illness (n = 20,874 patients).[78] Alanine aminotransferase and AST elevations are more common in severe COVID-19 infection,[79] and retrospective studies demonstrate worse morbidity and mortality in patients with abnormal liver enzymes.[78] Aside from hepatotoxicity from direct viral injury during COVID-19 infection, data regarding liver enzyme elevations during this period may be complicated by drug-induced liver injury secondary to COVID-19 therapies (such as acetaminophen, hydroxychloroquine, lopinavir, ritonavir, remdesivir, and baricitinib).[80] Most liver enzyme elevations resolve within 2 months postdischarge from COVID-19 hospitalization.[81] Notably viral antigens have been found in hepatic tissue up to 180 days after acute infection.[82] However, further population-based studies will need to be performed to elucidate liver injury in relation to long COVID syndrome.

Post–COVID-19 Cholangiopathy

Severe prolonged cholestasis and liver injury may occur during critically ill COVID-19 infection, leading to a novel disease state now called post-COVID cholangiopathy (PCC).[83] A retrospective review of 2047 patients found 0.59% (n = 12) had prolonged cholestatic injury (defined as ALP > 3$\times$ the upper limit of normal) at a mean time interval of 118 days.[84] The condition of PCC occurs, in contrast to "secondary sclerosing cholangitis of critically ill patients" (SSC-CIP),[85] which develops after critical illness in patients who experience respiratory failure at a rate of approximately 1 in 2000 patients requiring intensive care unit hospitalizations.[86–88] Although surviving patients with COVID-19 may develop a severe SSC-CIP-like clinical syndrome with prolonged and severe elevations in serum alkaline phosphatase in the months following prolonged hospitalization for severe illness, there are distinct histopathologic features in post-COVID patients not reported in patients with SSC-CIP 83. On liver biopsy of PCC patients, an unprecedented degree of cholangiocyte vacuolization is accompanied by severe regenerative and degenerative changes of the bile duct and ductular epithelial layer (**Fig. 2** A and B). A microangiopathy affecting all 3 microvascular compartments is also observed (**Fig. 2**C and D). Hepatic artery muscular hypertrophy and endothelial swelling can obliterate the lumina; portal vein endophlebitis may be ongoing, and endothelial damage with features of sinusoidal obstructive syndrome (veno-occlusive disease) is observed in terminal hepatic veins. In these patients with postacute COVID-19, viral protein or RNA are not detected in liver biopsies. One must posit an ongoing pathobiology of microvascular and biliary injury in these patients with post-COVID. However, whether COVID cholangiopathy constitutes a condition distinct from SSC-CIP remains debatable.[89] In terms of recovery from severe cholestatic injury after COVID-19 infection, a small case series of 7 patients were followed-up to 400 days after initial infection and demonstrated normalization or improvement in liver enzymes in the majority.[89] Rarely PCC causes end-stage liver disease requiring liver transplantation.[90]

Gastrointestinal Bleeding

GI bleeding has been associated with acute COVID-19 infection at rates of 0.5% to 3% or more.[91–93] When examining long-term follow-up of patients with GI bleeding in the setting of COVID-19 infection, GI bleeding resolved without recurrent episodes at rates of 92% at 3 months and 94.7% at 6 months and endoscopic intervention was rarely required for successful resolution.[56]

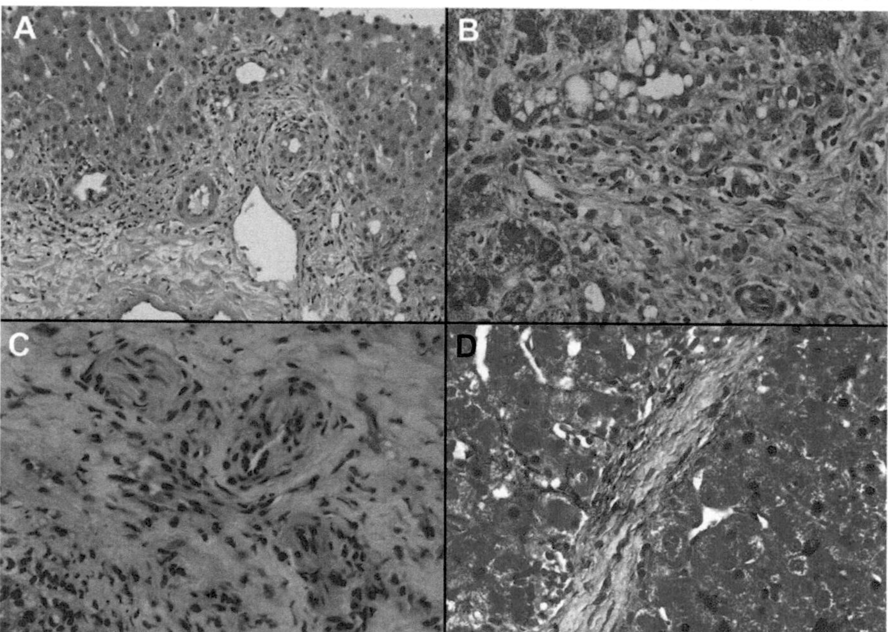

Fig. 2. COVID cholangiopathy, in liver biopsies of postacute COVID-19–infected patients with severe acute COVID-19. (*A*) Portal tract showing ductular reaction at interface, and vacuolization of cholangiocytes in both ductules and interlobular bile duct (H&E stain, 200×). (*B*) Reactive ductule at portal tract interface, showing profound cholangiocyte vacuolization (Trichrome stain, 400×). (*C*) Portal tract hepatic arteries showing muscular hypertrophy and near-total occlusion by endothelial cells (H&E stain, 400×). (*D*). Terminal hepatic vein showing total fibrotic occlusion (Trichrome stain, 400×).

Acute Pancreatitis

The prevalence of SARS-CoV-2 infection presenting as acute pancreatitis has ranged between 0.27% and 0.5% among patients hospitalized with COVID-19.[56,94] At this time, recurrence of pancreatitis does not seem to be a significant GI manifestation of long COVID. The limited data available regarding long-term follow-up of patients with acute pancreatitis secondary to acute COVID-19 infection showed resolution without recurrence at 3 and 6 months.[56]

Acute Abdominal Diseases

Other acute and rare abdominal diagnoses associated with acute COVID-19 infection include bowel ischemia and acute cholecystitis.[95,96] Due to the often urgent or emergent nature of these conditions requiring surgical intervention, these diseases lend themselves to be more likely associated with acute COVID-19 infection and associations with long COVID are currently lacking.

Associations with Gastrointestinal Manifestations of Long COVID

Recent survey data from patients after COVID-19 infection with at least 6 months of follow-up found that mental health symptoms before and after infection were associated with post–COVID-19 chronic GI symptoms. The survey had a 42% response rate (N = 749), of whom 29% (N = 220) reported GI symptoms. The presence of post–COVID-19 mental health symptoms (adjusted odds ratio (OR) 6.16 [95% CI, 4.21–9.01]) as well as both pre–COVID-19 and post–COVID-19 mental health symptoms (adjusted OR 16.5 [95% CI 6.97–38.9]) were significantly associated with post–COVID-19 GI symptoms. Hospitalized patients were more likely to report post–COVID-19 GI symptoms compared with nonhospitalized counterparts ($P < .01$). No associations between sex or ethnicity and GI symptoms were found. More than 10% of this cohort also reported having "any GI symptom" because their most bothersome COVID-19–related problem.[57]

DISEASE BURDEN OF LONG COVID SYNDROME AND GI HEALTH

In analyzing data from Veteran's Health Association (VHA) users beyond 30 days of initial illness, individuals with COVID-19 infection (n = 73,435) had higher risk of death (HR 1.59 [1.46–1.73]) and required more outpatient care (HR 1.20 [1.19–1.21]). The study showed 1 in every 10 patients discharged after COVID-19 hospitalization had a new and disabling clinical condition following hospital discharge, of which GI disorders were noted at a hazard ratio of 3.58 [95%CI: 2.15–4.88]. Accompanying the higher risk of developing new GI symptoms was the increased utilization of medications to alleviate these symptoms including, laxatives (9.22 [95%CI: 6.99–11.31]), antiemetic agents (9.22 [95%CI: 6.99–11.31]), histamine antagonists (4.83 [95%CI: 3.63–5.91]), other antacids (1.07 [95%CI: 0.62–1.42]), and antidiarrheal agents (2.87 [95% CI: 1.70–3.91]).[15] Similarly, in a Danish cohort of patients followed-up to 6 months after COVID-19 infection, higher rates of general practitioner and outpatient care utilization were reported and attributed to postacute COVID-19 symptoms. However, long COVID symptoms in this cohort generally did not require hospitalization.[97]

VACCINATION AND LONG COVID SYNDROME

Vaccines seem to reduce the risk of long COVID but the degree of protection varies among studies. In a large prospective, community-based, nested, case-control study of 2370 patients who had confirmed after vaccination COVID infections those receiving 2 vaccine doses had approximately half the risk of continuing symptoms 28 days later.[98] In a longitudinal observational study, the prevalence of long COVID in the unvaccinated group was 41.8% versus 16% in the triple-vaccinated group.[99] However, in a case-control study using US Department of Veterans Affairs national health-care databases, the risk of long-term COVID was only reduced by 15% in individuals who were vaccinated.[15] Because vaccination clearly reduces the incidence of developing COVID-19 infection, coupled with the fact those with breakthrough infections after vaccination have a lower risk of developing long COVID, vaccination is likely currently the best available intervention to prevent long COVID.

POTENTIAL THERAPIES FOR LONG COVID SYNDROME

Currently, no approved therapy exists to prevent long COVID and its multiorgan system sequelae.[58] Because the ACE2 receptor is the means for SARS-CoV-2 viral entry, conceivably medications targeting these receptors may be promising to prevent the initial host cell invasion and the subsequent consequences that result in long COVID. Because of this molecular mechanism, clinical trials are investigating recombinant human ACE2, angiotensin 1 to 7 agonists, monoclonal antibodies targeting ACE2 receptor, and a TMPRSS2 inhibitor, camostat mesylate, which could block the SARS-CoV-2 entry into primary lung cells. [39,50]

Probiotic treatment is another avenue of potential therapy for long COVID syndrome under investigation.[100] The rationale is that dysbiosis during long COVID syndrome may be mitigated by curated probiotics producing antiviral metabolites that support adaptive immunity.[100,101] China's National Health Commission recommended probiotics for severe COVID-19 to potentially protect against secondary infections by fostering gut immunity.[102] Limited prospective data regarding probiotic use for long COVID management exist. A randomized control trial of 200 patients reporting post-COVID fatigue showed 14-day probiotic supplementation could reduce fatigue symptoms and improve functional status.[103] More robust data regarding the therapeutic potential of probiotics is necessary before widespread adoption.

The management of GI sequelae of long COVID syndrome is currently based on supportive care and symptom management on an individual basis. One study showed new GI symptoms after COVID-19 infection correlated with higher usage of medications such as laxatives, antiemetic agents, histamine antagonists, other antacids, and antidiarrheal agents.[15] Despite the higher use of medications for symptomatic management, there is inadequate evidence to support overarching medical guidelines for these agents. For example, a case of diarrhea after COVID-19 infection was reported to be successfully alleviated with a regimen containing lopinavir–ritonavir[104] but a clinical trial of 199 patients showed no reduction in diarrhea or other COVID-19 symptoms with lopinavir–ritonavir therapy.[105]

Considering weight loss and malnutrition can persist for months beyond the initial COVID-19 illness,[56] it would be prudent to consider nutritional supplementation and medical consultation with a nutritionist to develop an individualized plan of care to target these sequelae. The European Society for Clinical Nutrition and Metabolism provided practical recommendations for patients at risk of malnutrition and weight loss from COVID-19 infection, including diet counseling, advocating nutritional screening for high-risk individuals such as older adults and those with multiple comorbidities as well as oral nutritional supplementation. To prevent malnutrition, oral nutritional supplementation of at least 400 kcal/d, including 30g or more of protein per day was recommended for at least 1 month. For post-ICU patients after COVID-19 infection, the recommended length of high-intensity oral nutritional supplementation is expanded to 2 months.[106]

DISCUSSION

Long COVID is now a recognized and evolving syndrome. The definition is centered on symptoms as a result of COVID-19 infection, which either persist from the original infection or new symptoms not attributable to alternative causes other than COVID-19 infection. Data have shown a significantly higher burden of post–COVID-19 infection sequelae in individuals hospitalized with COVID-19 compared with seasonal influenza, distinguishing the unique nature of long COVID syndrome.[15] The time interval after which long COVID syndrome can be characterized varies from 4 weeks to 12 weeks after acute infection.[5,6] Current GI and hepatobiliary manifestations of long COVID include abdominal pain, nausea and vomiting, diarrhea, constipation, weight loss, postinfectious IBS, dyspepsia, and PCC. Some GI manifestations of acute COVID-19 infection do not seem to be significantly associated with a chronic ongoing syndrome such as acute pancreatitis, bowel ischemia, and acute cholecystitis.

Accurate epidemiologic reporting of the GI and hepatobiliary manifestations of long COVID (and long COVID generally) is convoluted likely due to multiple factors including the evolution of definitions, accuracy of diagnosis, accuracy of reporting symptoms, and differences in health-care systems. In a recent meta-analysis, GI manifestations of long COVID were estimated at 22% (N = 12 studies, 158,731 patients).[54] As the body of knowledge regarding cases of patients with COVID-19 infection expands, so too the epidemiologic understanding of long COVID and its GI sequelae will expand. Working toward a standard, recognized global criteria for long COVID is essential.

The molecular mechanisms and pathophysiological pathways underlying the development of long COVID remain to be investigated. Prolonged fecal shedding of viral SARS-CoV-2 RNA occurring in IBD and general population cohorts months after COVID-19 infection is shown to correlate with GI symptomatology,[14,33] offering an interesting insight regarding the persistence of long COVID GI manifestations. The ability to endoscopically sample GI tissue of patients with GI manifestations of long COVID relatively easily can possibly provide further avenues to study molecular mechanisms that precipitate ongoing GI symptoms of this syndrome.[2] Novel technology using "mini-guts" to study cell-specific viral replication provide a reliable experimental model to study SARS-CoV-2.[43]

Finally, it is imperative to continue studying the pathogenesis of long COVID because of the substantial health-care burden it poses. As alluded to previously, even at the lower end of reported prevalence at 10%, long COVID syndrome would potentially affect 50 million people globally.[9] Patients with long COVID syndrome have been shown to have higher rates of outpatient health-care utilization, physician visits, medication use for symptomatic management, burden of health loss, and mental health symptoms.[10,15,57,97] These findings reflect that long COVID represents a growing health-care challenge, which will likely necessitate multidisciplinary health-care system planning to develop strategies to reduce the chronic health burden among such patients.

SUMMARY

Long COVID is an evolving disease involving symptoms and sequelae from multiple organ systems occurring weeks after acute COVID-19 infection. Due to varying definitions and accumulating data, the prevalence of long COVID has wide-ranging estimates from 10% to 87%[3,7,8]; these estimates reveal that many millions are and will be affected by long COVID. Limited data regarding the risk factors and precipitants of long COVID exist in many patients even without severe or pulmonary involvement of COVID-19.[11–14] The pathophysiological basis by which long COVID occurs after acute infection resolves requires further investigation but interesting molecular evidence is accumulating such as widespread location of ACE2 receptors throughout the body supporting direct viral injury and persistence of virus in fecal and hepatic samples months after infection.[33,82] GI and hepatobiliary manifestations of long COVID include abdominal pain, nausea and vomiting, diarrhea, constipation, loss of taste, loss of appetite, involuntary weight loss, postinfectious IBS, dyspepsia, and PCC. Likely a bidirectional relationship exists between mental health symptoms and GI manifestations of long COVID.[57] Patients suffering with long COVID are found to have increased outpatient care, physician visits, medications for symptomatic relief, and overall loss of health compared with the baseline.[15] Ongoing symptoms of long COVID can result in a loss of quality of life, earnings, and increased medical spending.[16–18] Further studies are needed to understand the molecular basis, prevalence, risk factors, preventative measures, and therapeutic options for long COVID and its GI and hepatobiliary manifestations.

CLINICS CARE POINTS

- Long COVID definitions vary: CDC defines occurrence beginning at 4 weeks after acute infection, whereas NIH defines occurrence beginning at 12 weeks after acute infection.
- Long COVID symptoms often occur without severe COVID-19 infection.
- Molecular mechanisms by which long COVID is propagated involve direct viral injury and endothelial damage, inadequate viral clearance, creating an inflammatory state, and dysbiosis.
- Most common long COVID GI symptoms of abdominal pain, nausea and vomiting, and diarrhea usually resolve by 3 to 6 months and liver enzyme abnormalities resolve by 2 months.
- FGIDs such as postinfectious IBS and dyspepsia occur in long COVID.
- PCC is a novel condition involving chronic cholestasis and liver injury with a characteristic predominant cholangiocyte injury and accompanying microvascular changes. PCC rarely progresses to end-stage liver disease that requires liver transplantation.
- Weight loss and malnutrition may be prolonged in long COVID and may require management of dietary counseling, nutritional screening, and oral nutritional supplementation.
- GI manifestations of long COVID syndrome are associated with mental health symptoms.
- Vaccination remains the most effective current measure to prevent long COVID because no other therapies are currently proven to prevent or treat long COVID.
- Patients with long COVID syndrome have increased utilization of outpatient visits, medications for symptomatic management, and overall health compared with controls.
- Recent estimates suggest that long COVID could cost up to USD 3.7 trillion, with 59% of the total due to loss of quality of life.

DISCLOSURE

A J. Trindade is a consultant to Boston Scientific, Pentax Medical, Exact Sciences, and Lucid Diagnostics. He receives research support from Lucid Diagnostics. A Rizvi, Y Ziv, and J Crawford have no COI to disclose.

REFERENCES

1. COVID-19 Dashboard Global Map. Available at: https://coronavirus.jhu.edu/. Accessed July 30 2022.
2. Leppkes M, Neurath MF. Rear Window-What Can the Gut Tell Us About Long-COVID? Gastroenterology 2022;163(2):376–8.
3. Taquet M, Dercon Q, Luciano S, et al. Incidence, co-occurrence, and evolution of long-COVID features: A 6-month retrospective cohort study of 273,618 survivors of COVID-19. Plos Med 2021;18(9):e1003773.
4. Crook H, Raza S, Nowell J, et al. Long covid-mechanisms, risk factors, and management. BMJ 2021;374:n1648.
5. COVID-19 rapid guideline: managing the long-term effects of COVID-19 (NG188): Evidence reviews 6 and 7: monitoring and referral. London: National Institute for Health and Care Excellence (NICE); 2020 Dec. (NICE Guideline, No. 188.) Available from: https://www.ncbi.nlm.nih.gov/books/NBK567265/.
6. Datta SD, Talwar A, Lee JT. A Proposed Framework and Timeline of the Spectrum of Disease Due to SARS-CoV-2 Infection: Illness Beyond Acute Infection and Public Health Implications. JAMA 2020;324(22):2251–2.
7. Greenhalgh T, Knight M, A'Court C, et al. Management of post-acute covid-19 in primary care. BMJ 2020;370:m3026.
8. Carfi A, Bernabei R, Landi F, et al. Persistent Symptoms in Patients After Acute COVID-19. JAMA 2020;324(6):603–5.
9. Altmann DM, Boyton RJ. Decoding the unknowns in long covid. BMJ 2021;372: n132.
10. Xie Y, Bowe B, Al-Aly Z. Burdens of post-acute sequelae of COVID-19 by severity of acute infection, demographics and health status. Nat Commun 2021;12(1):6571.
11. Dennis A, Wamil M, Alberts J, et al. Multiorgan impairment in low-risk individuals with post-COVID-19 syndrome: a prospective, community-based study. BMJ Open 2021;11(3):e048391.
12. Miyazato Y, Morioka S, Tsuzuki S, et al. Prolonged and Late-Onset Symptoms of Coronavirus Disease 2019. Open Forum Infect Dis 2020;7(11):ofaa507.
13. Townsend L, Dowds J, O'Brien K, et al. Persistent Poor Health after COVID-19 Is Not Associated with Respiratory Complications or Initial Disease Severity. Ann Am Thorac Soc 2021;18(6):997–1003.
14. Zollner A, Koch R, Jukic A, et al. Postacute COVID-19 is Characterized by Gut Viral Antigen Persistence in Inflammatory Bowel Diseases. Gastroenterology 2022;163(2):495–506.e8.
15. Al-Aly Z, Xie Y, Bowe B. High-dimensional characterization of post-acute sequelae of COVID-19. Nature 2021;594(7862):259–64.
16. Cutler DM, Summers LH. The COVID-19 Pandemic and the $16 Trillion Virus. JAMA 2020;324(15):1495–6.
17. Cutler DM. The Economic Cost of Long COVID: An Update. 2022. Available at: https://scholar.harvard.edu/cutler/news/long-covid. Accessed Aug 31, 2022.
18. Calculations & Formulas. Available at: https://www.longhauler-advocacy.org/calculations-formulas. Accessed Aug 31, 2022.
19. Huang C, Huang L, Wang Y, et al. 6-month consequences of COVID-19 in patients discharged from hospital: a cohort study. Lancet 2021;397(10270): 220–32.
20. Satterfield BA, Bhatt DL, Gersh BJ. Cardiac involvement in the long-term implications of COVID-19. Nat Rev Cardiol 2022;19(5):332–41.

21. Lopez-Leon S, Wegman-Ostrosky T, Perelman C, et al. More than 50 long-term effects of COVID-19: a systematic review and meta-analysis. Scientific Rep 2021;11(1):16144.
22. Cavallieri F, Sellner J, Zedde M, et al. Neurologic complications of coronavirus and other respiratory viral infections. Handb Clin Neurol 2022;189:331–58.
23. Maury A, Lyoubi A, Peiffer-Smadja N, et al. Neurological manifestations associated with SARS-CoV-2 and other coronaviruses: A narrative review for clinicians. Rev Neurol (Paris) 2021;177(1–2):51–64.
24. Cosentino G, Todisco M, Hota N, et al. Neuropathological findings from COVID-19 patients with neurological symptoms argue against a direct brain invasion of SARS-CoV-2: A critical systematic review. Eur J Neurol 2021;28(11):3856–65.
25. Silver SA, Beaubien-Souligny W, Shah PS, et al. The Prevalence of Acute Kidney Injury in Patients Hospitalized With COVID-19 Infection: A Systematic Review and Meta-analysis. Kidney Med 2021;3(1):83–98 e81.
26. Copur S, Berkkan M, Basile C, et al. Post-acute COVID-19 syndrome and kidney diseases: what do we know? J Nephrol 2022;35(3):795–805.
27. Bowe B, Xie Y, Xu E, et al. Kidney Outcomes in Long COVID. J Am Soc Nephrol 2021;32(11):2851–62.
28. Ma C, Cong Y, Zhang H. COVID-19 and the Digestive System. Am J Gastroenterol 2020;115(7):1003–6.
29. Galanopoulos M, Gkeros F, Doukatas A, et al. COVID-19 pandemic: Pathophysiology and manifestations from the gastrointestinal tract. World J Gastroenterol 2020;26(31):4579–88.
30. Gupta A, Madhavan MV, Sehgal K, et al. Extrapulmonary manifestations of COVID-19. Nat Med 2020;26(7):1017–32.
31. Ackermann M, Verleden SE, Kuehnel M, et al. Pulmonary Vascular Endothelialitis, Thrombosis, and Angiogenesis in Covid-19. N Engl J Med 2020;383(2):120–8.
32. Leppkes M, Knopf J, Naschberger E, et al. Vascular occlusion by neutrophil extracellular traps in COVID-19. EBioMedicine 2020;58:102925.
33. Natarajan A, Zlitni S, Brooks EF, et al. Gastrointestinal symptoms and fecal shedding of SARS-CoV-2 RNA suggest prolonged gastrointestinal infection. Med (N Y). 2022;3(6):371–387 e379.
34. Phetsouphanh C, Darley DR, Wilson DB, et al. Immunological dysfunction persists for 8 months following initial mild-to-moderate SARS-CoV-2 infection. Nat Immunol 2022;23(2):210–6.
35. Ren Z, Wang H, Cui G, et al. Alterations in the human oral and gut microbiomes and lipidomics in COVID-19. Gut 2021;70(7):1253–65.
36. Gu S, Chen Y, Wu Z, et al. Alterations of the Gut Microbiota in Patients With Coronavirus Disease 2019 or H1N1 Influenza. Clin Infect Dis 2020;71(10):2669–78.
37. Yeoh YK, Zuo T, Lui GC, et al. Gut microbiota composition reflects disease severity and dysfunctional immune responses in patients with COVID-19. Gut 2021;70(4):698–706.
38. Chen Y, Gu S, Chen Y, et al. Six-month follow-up of gut microbiota richness in patients with COVID-19. Gut 2022;71(1):222–5.
39. Hoffmann M, Kleine-Weber H, Schroeder S, et al. SARS-CoV-2 Cell Entry Depends on ACE2 and TMPRSS2 and Is Blocked by a Clinically Proven Protease Inhibitor. Cell 2020;181(2):271–280 e278.
40. Xiao F, Tang M, Zheng X, et al. Evidence for Gastrointestinal Infection of SARS-CoV-2. Gastroenterology 2020;158(6):1831–1833 e1833.

41. Harmer D, Gilbert M, Borman R, et al. Quantitative mRNA expression profiling of ACE 2, a novel homologue of angiotensin converting enzyme. FEBS Lett 2002; 532(1–2):107–10.
42. Zhao B, Ni C, Gao R, et al. Recapitulation of SARS-CoV-2 infection and cholangiocyte damage with human liver ductal organoids. Protein Cell 2020;11(10): 771–5.
43. Lamers MM, Beumer J, van der Vaart J, et al. SARS-CoV-2 productively infects human gut enterocytes. Science 2020;369(6499):50–4.
44. Cheung KS, Hung IFN, Chan PPY, et al. Gastrointestinal manifestations of SARS-CoV-2 infection and virus load in fecal samples from a hong kong cohort: systematic review and meta-analysis. Gastroenterology 2020;159(1):81–95.
45. Penninger JM, Grant MB, Sung JJY. The role of angiotensin converting enzyme 2 in modulating gut microbiota, intestinal inflammation, and coronavirus infection. Gastroenterology 2021;160(1):39–46.
46. Hashimoto T, Perlot T, Rehman A, et al. ACE2 links amino acid malnutrition to microbial ecology and intestinal inflammation. Nature 2012;487(7408):477–81.
47. Petersen C, Round JL. Defining dysbiosis and its influence on host immunity and disease. Cell Microbiol 2014;16(7):1024–33.
48. Singh R, Zogg H, Wei L, et al. Gut Microbial Dysbiosis in the Pathogenesis of Gastrointestinal Dysmotility and Metabolic Disorders. J Neurogastroenterol Motil 2021;27(1):19–34.
49. Marasco G, Lenti MV, Cremon C, et al. Implications of SARS-CoV-2 infection for neurogastroenterology. Neurogastroenterol Motil 2021;33(3):e14104.
50. Jin B, Singh R, Ha SE, et al. Pathophysiological mechanisms underlying gastrointestinal symptoms in patients with COVID-19. World J Gastroenterol 2021; 27(19):2341–52.
51. Sultan S, Altayar O, Siddique SM, et al. AGA Institute Rapid Review of the Gastrointestinal and Liver Manifestations of COVID-19, Meta-Analysis of International Data, and Recommendations for the Consultative Management of Patients with COVID-19. Gastroenterology 2020;159(1):320–334 e327.
52. Parasa S, Desai M, Thoguluva Chandrasekar V, et al. Prevalence of Gastrointestinal Symptoms and Fecal Viral Shedding in Patients With Coronavirus Disease 2019: A Systematic Review and Meta-analysis. JAMA Netw Open 2020;3(6): e2011335.
53. Elshazli RM, Kline A, Elgaml A, et al. Gastroenterology manifestations and COVID-19 outcomes: A meta-analysis of 25,252 cohorts among the first and second waves. J Med Virol 2021;93(5):2740–68.
54. Choudhury A, Tariq R, Jena A, et al. Gastrointestinal manifestations of long COVID: A systematic review and meta-analysis. Therap Adv Gastroenterol 2022;15. 17562848221118403.
55. Chevinsky JR, Tao G, Lavery AM, et al. Late Conditions Diagnosed 1-4 Months Following an Initial Coronavirus Disease 2019 (COVID-19) Encounter: A Matched-Cohort Study Using Inpatient and Outpatient Administrative Data-United States, 1 March-30 June 2020. Clin Infect Dis 2021;73(Suppl 1):S5–16.
56. Rizvi A, Patel Z, Liu Y, et al. Gastrointestinal Sequelae 3 and 6 Months After Hospitalization for Coronavirus Disease 2019. Clin Gastroenterol Hepatol 2021; 19(11):2438–2440 e2431.
57. Blackett JW, Wainberg M, Elkind MSV, et al. Potential Long Coronavirus Disease 2019 Gastrointestinal Symptoms 6 Months After Coronavirus Infection Are Associated With Mental Health Symptoms. Gastroenterology 2022;162(2):648–650 e642.

58. Houston KV, Yoo B-S, D'Souza SM, et al. Post-COVID-19 GI Manifestations: Are We in for the "Long Haul". Americal J Gastroenterol Hepatol 2021;2:01–5.
59. Barbara G, Grover M, Bercik P, et al. Rome Foundation Working Team Report on Post-Infection Irritable Bowel Syndrome. Gastroenterology 2019;156(1): 46–58 e47.
60. Gurusamy SR, Shah A, Talley NJ, et al. Small Intestinal Bacterial Overgrowth in Functional Dyspepsia: A Systematic Review and Meta-Analysis. Am J Gastroenterol 2021;116(5):935–42.
61. Margolis KG, Cryan JF, Mayer EA. The Microbiota-Gut-Brain Axis: From Motility to Mood. Gastroenterology 2021;160(5):1486–501.
62. Zamani M, Alizadeh-Tabari S, Zamani V. Systematic review with meta-analysis: the prevalence of anxiety and depression in patients with irritable bowel syndrome. Aliment Pharmacol Ther 2019;50(2):132–43.
63. Mazza MG, De Lorenzo R, Conte C, et al. Anxiety and depression in COVID-19 survivors: Role of inflammatory and clinical predictors. Brain Behav Immun 2020;89:594–600.
64. Ghoshal UC, Ghoshal U, Rahman MM, et al. Post-infection functional gastrointestinal disorders following coronavirus disease-19: A case-control study. J Gastroenterol Hepatol 2022;37(3):489–98.
65. Schmulson M, Ghoshal UC, Barbara G. Managing the Inevitable Surge of Post-COVID-19 Functional Gastrointestinal Disorders. Am J Gastroenterol 2021; 116(1):4–7.
66. Doyle ME, Appleton A, Liu QR, et al. Human Type II taste cells express angiotensin-converting enzyme 2 and are infected by severe acute respiratory syndrome coronavirus 2 (SARS-CoV-2). Am J Pathol 2021;191(9):1511–9.
67. Song J, Li Y, Huang X, et al. Systematic analysis of ACE2 and TMPRSS2 expression in salivary glands reveals underlying transmission mechanism caused by SARS-CoV-2. J Med Virol 2020;92(11):2556–66.
68. Leth S, Gunst JD, Mathiasen V, et al. Persistent symptoms in patients recovering from COVID-19 in Denmark. Open Forum Infect Dis 2021;8(4):ofab042.
69. Messin L, Puyraveau M, Benabdallah Y, et al. COVEVOL: natural evolution at 6 Months of COVID-19. Viruses 2021;13(11):2151.
70. Rank A, Tzortzini A, Kling E, et al. One year after mild COVID-19: the majority of patients maintain specific immunity, but one in four still suffer from long-term symptoms. J Clin Med 2021;10(15).
71. Wheatley AK, Juno JA, Wang JJ, et al. Evolution of immune responses to SARS-CoV-2 in mild-moderate COVID-19. Nat Commun 2021;12(1):1162.
72. Allard L, Ouedraogo E, Molleville J, et al. Malnutrition: percentage and association with prognosis in patients hospitalized for coronavirus disease 2019. Nutrients 2020;12(12):3679.
73. Pironi L, Sasdelli AS, Ravaioli F, et al. Malnutrition and nutritional therapy in patients with SARS-CoV-2 disease. Clin Nutr 2021;40(3):1330–7.
74. Di Filippo L, De Lorenzo R, D'Amico M, et al. COVID-19 is associated with clinically significant weight loss and risk of malnutrition, independent of hospitalisation: A post-hoc analysis of a prospective cohort study. Clin Nutr 2021;40(4): 2420–6.
75. Anker MS, Landmesser U, von Haehling S, et al. Weight loss, malnutrition, and cachexia in COVID-19: facts and numbers. J Cachexia Sarcopenia Muscle 2021;12(1):9–13.

76. Ramos A, Joaquin C, Ros M, et al. Impact of COVID-19 on nutritional status during the first wave of the pandemic. Clin Nutr 2021. https://doi.org/10.1016/j.clnu.2021.05.001.
77. Kayaaslan B, Eser F, Kalem AK, et al. Post-COVID syndrome: A single-center questionnaire study on 1007 participants recovered from COVID-19. J Med Virol 2021;93(12):6566–74.
78. Kulkarni AV, Kumar P, Tevethia HV, et al. Systematic review with meta-analysis: liver manifestations and outcomes in COVID-19. Aliment Pharmacol Ther 2020;52(4):584–99.
79. Guan WJ, Ni ZY, Hu Y, et al. Clinical Characteristics of Coronavirus Disease 2019 in China. N Engl J Med 2020;382(18):1708–20.
80. Olry A, Meunier L, Delire B, et al. Drug-Induced Liver Injury and COVID-19 Infection: The Rules Remain the Same. Drug Saf 2020;43(7):615–7.
81. An YW, Song S, Li WX, et al. Liver function recovery of COVID-19 patients after discharge, a follow-up study. Int J Med Sci 2021;18(1):176–86.
82. Cheung CCL, Goh D, Lim X, et al. Residual SARS-CoV-2 viral antigens detected in GI and hepatic tissues from five recovered patients with COVID-19. Gut 2022; 71(1):226–9.
83. Roth NC, Kim A, Vitkovski T, et al. Post-COVID-19 Cholangiopathy: A Novel Entity. Am J Gastroenterol 2021;116(5):1077–82.
84. Faruqui S, Okoli FC, Olsen SK, et al. Cholangiopathy After Severe COVID-19: Clinical Features and Prognostic Implications. Am J Gastroenterol 2021; 116(7):1414–25.
85. Yeh M, Crawford J. Vascular Disorders of the Liver. In: RD O JR G, editor. Pathology of the gastrointestinal tract, pancreas, liver and biliary tree. 4th Edition edition. Philadelphia, PA: WB Saunders; 2022. p. 1595–696.
86. Scheppach W, Druge G, Wittenberg G, et al. Sclerosing cholangitis and liver cirrhosis after extrabiliary infections: report on three cases. Crit Care Med 2001;29(2):438–41.
87. Brooling J, Leal R. Secondary Sclerosing Cholangitis: a Review of Recent Literature. Curr Gastroenterol Rep 2017;19(9):44.
88. Leonhardt S, Veltzke-Schlieker W, Adler A, et al. Secondary Sclerosing Cholangitis in Critically Ill Patients: Clinical Presentation, Cholangiographic Features, Natural History, and Outcome: A Series of 16 Cases. Medicine (Baltimore) 2015;94(49):e2188.
89. Shih AR, Hatipoglu D, Wilechansky R, et al. Persistent Cholestatic Injury and Secondary Sclerosing Cholangitis in COVID-19 Patients. Arch Pathol Lab Med 2022;146(10):1184–93.
90. Durazo FA, Nicholas AA, Mahaffey JJ, et al. Post-Covid-19 Cholangiopathy-A New Indication for Liver Transplantation: A Case Report. Transplant Proc 2021;53(4):1132–7.
91. Trindade AJ, Izard S, Coppa K, et al. Gastrointestinal bleeding in hospitalized COVID-19 patients: a propensity score matched cohort study. J Intern Med 2021;289(6):887–94.
92. Mauro A, De Grazia F, Lenti MV, et al. Upper gastrointestinal bleeding in COVID-19 inpatients: Incidence and management in a multicenter experience from Northern Italy. Clin Res Hepatol Gastroenterol 2021;45(3):101521.
93. Marasco G, Maida M, Morreale GC, et al. Gastrointestinal Bleeding in COVID-19 Patients: A Systematic Review with Meta-Analysis. Can J Gastroenterol Hepatol 2021;2021:2534975.

94. Inamdar S, Benias PC, Liu Y, et al. Prevalence, Risk Factors, and Outcomes of Hospitalized Patients With Coronavirus Disease 2019 Presenting as Acute Pancreatitis. Gastroenterology 2020;159(6):2226–2228 e2222.
95. Zhang ML, Jacobsen F, Pepe-Mooney BJ, et al. Clinicopathological findings in patients with COVID-19-associated ischaemic enterocolitis. Histopathology 2021;79(6):1004–17.
96. Balaphas A, Gkoufa K, Meyer J, et al. COVID-19 can mimic acute cholecystitis and is associated with the presence of viral RNA in the gallbladder wall. J Hepatol 2020;73(6):1566–8.
97. Lund LC, Hallas J, Nielsen H, et al. Post-acute effects of SARS-CoV-2 infection in individuals not requiring hospital admission: a Danish population-based cohort study. Lancet Infect Dis 2021;21(10):1373–82.
98. Antonelli M, Penfold RS, Merino J, et al. Risk factors and disease profile of post-vaccination SARS-CoV-2 infection in UK users of the COVID Symptom Study app: a prospective, community-based, nested, case-control study. Lancet Infect Dis 2022;22(1):43–55.
99. Azzolini E, Levi R, Sarti R, et al. Association Between BNT162b2 Vaccination and Long COVID After Infections Not Requiring Hospitalization in Health Care Workers. JAMA 2022;328(7):676–8.
100. Sundararaman A, Ray M, Ravindra PV, et al. Role of probiotics to combat viral infections with emphasis on COVID-19. Appl Microbiol Biotechnol 2020; 104(19):8089–104.
101. Marazzato M, Ceccarelli G, d'Ettorre G. Dysbiosis in SARS-CoV-2-Infected Patients. Gastroenterology 2021;160(6):2195.
102. Diagnosis and Treatment Protocol for Novel Coronavirus Pneumonia (Trial Version 7). Chin Med J (Engl) 2020;133(9):1087–95.
103. Rathi A, Jadhav SB, Shah N. A Randomized Controlled Trial of the Efficacy of Systemic Enzymes and Probiotics in the Resolution of Post-COVID Fatigue. Medicines (Basel) 2021;8(9):47.
104. Song Y, Liu P, Shi XL, et al. SARS-CoV-2 induced diarrhoea as onset symptom in patient with COVID-19. Gut 2020;69(6):1143–4.
105. Cao B, Wang Y, Wen D, et al. A Trial of Lopinavir-Ritonavir in Adults Hospitalized with Severe Covid-19. N Engl J Med 2020;382(19):1787–99.
106. Barazzoni R, Bischoff SC, Breda J, et al. ESPEN expert statements and practical guidance for nutritional management of individuals with SARS-CoV-2 infection. Clin Nutr 2020;39(6):1631–8.

Gastrointestinal Endoscopy in Patients with Coronavirus Disease 2019

Indications, Findings, and Safety

Shahnaz Sultan, MD, MHSc

KEYWORDS

- COVID-19 • Endoscopy • Transmission risk • Personal protective equipment
- Gastrointestinal manifestations

KEY POINTS

- SARS-CoV-2 transmission seems to mainly occur via *respiratory particles* (respiratory droplets and smaller aerosols that are expelled from the respiratory tract during speaking, breathing, and coughing) and close contact with infected persons.
- WHO and CDC advise using respirator masks, such as N95s, when performing procedures that might pose higher risk for transmission if the patient has SARS-CoV-2 infection (eg, that generate potentially infectious aerosols or involving anatomic regions where viral loads might be higher, such as the nose and throat, oropharynx, and respiratory tract).
- Endoscopic findings in patients with COVID-19 suggest that SARS-CoV-2 does not seem to behave as a highly invasive and injurious pathogen to gastrointestinal mucosa.

INTRODUCTION

The spread of coronavirus disease 2019 (COVID-19), caused by the severe acute respiratory syndrome coronavirus 2 (SARS-CoV-2), was declared a pandemic by the World Health Organization (WHO) on March 11, 2020.[1] Since the outbreak was first identified in December 2019 in Wuhan, China, the public health and social impact of the disease and the cumulative morbidity and mortality across the world has been enormous. As with any new or emerging pathogen, early in the pandemic, there was limited evidence and understanding of how SARS-CoV-2 was transmitted, limited testing capability, and resource constraints, especially in the availability of personal protective equipment (PPE).[2] Endoscopy centers shut down and the volume of endoscopic procedures plummeted save for only urgent, lifesaving, or time-sensitive procedures. In line with international consensus statements and guidelines as well as

Division of Gastroenterology, Hepatology and Nutrition, University of Minnesota, 420 Delaware Street Southeast, MMC 36, Minneapolis, MN 55455, USA
E-mail address: ssultan@umn.edu

Gastroenterol Clin N Am 52 (2023) 157–172
https://doi.org/10.1016/j.gtc.2022.11.002
0889-8553/23/Published by Elsevier Inc.

local state- and health system-level policies, endoscopy centers slowly opened up and increased their volume of procedures with the paramount goal of reducing the potential risk of infection for patients and health care workers (HCWs).[3–6] Many studies showed drastic reductions in endoscopy volumes during the onset of the pandemic and persistent reductions in procedural volumes for sustained periods thereafter.[7–9] This article summarizes the evolution of our understanding of SARS-CoV-2 infection, the performance of safe endoscopy, as well as indications and endoscopic findings in patients with COVID-19.

Understanding Modes of Transmission of Respiratory Viruses

A critical aspect of managing any pandemic from a respiratory virus requires a clear understanding of how an infectious pathogen is transmitted and the equipment or protection that is therefore needed to minimize transmission. Respiratory viruses are transmitted between individuals when the virus is released from the respiratory tract of an infected person and is transferred through the environment, to infect the respiratory tract of an exposed and susceptible person. The major modes of transmission of a respiratory virus from one person to another include large droplets, aerosols, direct contact, or indirect contact (fomites).[10] Often, the relative contributions of different modes to a successful transmission and the relative effects of each mode, as well as modifications of risk by viral, host, and environmental factors, are unknown[10] (**Table 1**).

Understanding Modes of Transmission of Severe Acute Respiratory Syndrome Coronavirus 2

Our current understanding of SARS-CoV-2 transmission has shifted and evolved since the beginning of the pandemic. According to the WHO, SARS-CoV-2 transmission seems to occur mainly via *respiratory particles* and close contact with infected symptomatic cases.[11] These particles not only include respiratory droplets but also droplets as small as 5 μm, and smaller aerosols that are expelled from the respiratory tract during speaking, breathing, and coughing.[12]

The risk of transmission via aerosols is influenced by many factors including the concentration and mass of particles emitted, the viral load, the proximity and duration of exposure, and the circulation of air in the environment.[10] The relative contribution according to particle size in virus transmission, however, is unknown. Epidemiologic evidence suggests that the risk of transmission is predominantly from short-range exposure from a person who generates significant amounts of virus. The SARS-CoV-2 virus has been detected in the air with a half-life of just more than 1 hour, and this evidence was offered as proof of "viable" virus that could be transmitted via aerosolization. However, this study was significantly limited in that it was conducted in a laboratory setting under an artificially created environment and not representative of real-world data.[13] Human-to-human transmission can also occur from unknown infected persons (eg, asymptomatic carriers or individuals with mild symptoms), as well as individuals with virus shedding during the preincubation period before symptoms develop.[14]

A potentially compounding factor for transmission events is the contagiousness and transfer of SARS-CoV-2 infectious particles from fomites or contaminated surfaces (eg, door handles). As other coronaviruses and respiratory viruses are known to be transmitted this way, spread through fomites may be an additional source of transmission. In early studies of hospitalized patients with COVID-19 positive SARS-CoV-2 samples were identified in various locations around patients' rooms, including the bed, sink, bathroom, light switches, and doors.[15] In addition, positive samples were

Table 1
Transmission patters of respiratory viruses, such as coronavirus

Definition	Key Attributes of Transmission
Large droplets originate in the upper respiratory system and vary in size between 5 and 60 μm	• Contain epithelial cells from the lining of the airways, immune cells as well as electrolytes present in mucus and saliva, and infectious agents that reside in the upper respiratory systems (bacteria, fungi, and viruses). • Large droplets are expelled from the mouth and the nose in multiple ways, including sneezing, coughing, talking, breathing, and singing. • Once expelled, large droplets greater than 5 μm can deposit by falling on surfaces (generally within 3 feet of their source) and cause propagation through fomites. • During normal breathing, aerosol particles smaller than 5 μm can disperse farther by airborne transmission • Large droplets evaporate at rates depending on temperature and relative humidity
Aerosols are generated in a similar way as large droplets but are smaller	• Aerosols also originate in the upper respiratory system and they have the same contents as large droplets • Their small size, however, allows them to remain suspended in the air for longer periods and thus travel much farther than 3 feet
Fomites are the surfaces on which infectious particles cling once deposited	• Droplets and aerosols expelled from the upper respiratory tract can survive for hours or days once attached to a fomite, depending on the microbe and the environment • Fomites facilitate indirect transmission from person to person

found on the shoes and stethoscopes of staff exiting patient rooms, but no contamination was found in the anteroom or corridor outside the room. These studies raised concerns about environmental contamination by patients with SARS-CoV-2 through respiratory droplets and fecal shedding.[16] Despite the consistent evidence of SARS-CoV-2 contamination and survival of the virus on certain surfaces, there have been no specific reports demonstrating direct fomite transmission and the risk is generally thought to be small.[17] People who come into contact with potentially infectious surfaces often also have close contact with the infectious person, thus making the distinction between respiratory droplet and fomite transmission difficult to differentiate.

Viral SARS-CoV-2 particles have been isolated from various bodily fluids, including feces, urine, saliva, semen, and tears, raising concerns about possible transmission through these routes; however, the presence of viral particles in these fluids has not been shown to correlate with clinical symptoms.[18,19] The detection of viral particles in the stool was of particular importance because coronaviruses can have direct pathogenicity in the gastrointestinal (GI) tract and cause enteric diseases; this raised concerns about fecal-oral spread as well as safety of endoscopy because aerosolization and increased exposure to fecal material may pose additional infectious risk. According to one systematic review of 35 studies that included 1636 patients with laboratory-confirmed COVID-19 who received fecal, anal, and/or rectal swab SARS-CoV-2 RNA examinations, the pooled prevalence of fecal SARS-CoV-2 was 43% with about half of these patients demonstrating persistent shedding even after respiratory samples turned negative, and shedding was found more commonly in patients with GI symptoms.[20] Despite these data, no cases of direct fecal-oral transmission were reported thereby questioning the viability and infectivity of SARS-CoV-2 virus found in fecal matter. Importantly, wastewater evaluation has been a useful surveillance strategy for tracking and predicting rates of prevalent COVID-19 for health care utilization.[21]

The Role of Personal Protective Equipment in Minimizing Risk of Infection from Severe Acute Respiratory Syndrome Coronavirus 2

PPE includes gowns gloves, eye protection (eg, face shield or goggles), and surgical/medical or respirator masks. Surgical masks (also known as medical masks) are fluid resistant and often used for droplet precautions, because they are designed to block large particles, but are less effective in blocking small particle aerosols (<5 μm). Surgical masks provide a barrier to prevent droplets reaching the wearer's nose, mouth, and respiratory tract. Most masks are not designed to fit closely to the face, which means that airborne particles (aerosols <100 microns) could potentially pass though the gap between the mask and the face. In contrast, respirator masks are designed to block aerosols. Respiratory protection for airborne precautions in health care commonly follows 2 filtering device paths, N95 or N99 masks/respirators or filtering facepiece respirators (such as FFP2 or FFP3) and powered air-purifying respirators (PAPRs). The N95 masks filter at least 95% of aerosols (<5 μm) and droplet-size (5–50 μm) particles and are not resistant to oil. Lightweight, no-hose PAPRs are a highly effective alternative to face masks that force air through a large, multilayer filter housed in the helmet and provide positive pressure within the face-shield compartment. These devices are approved by US National Institute for Occupational Safety and Hazard and can provide high-level protection from common airborne viruses that exceeds that for N95 face masks without the need for "fit-testing" and also have the advantage of providing head and neck protection.[22] Maximum protection is achieved only with proper donning and doffing techniques.

Requirements for Personal Protective Equipment During Endoscopy

Owing to the high risk of human-to-human transmission and the potential for transmission of infection with SARS-CoV-2 during routine performance of endoscopy, there was a lack of clarity regarding the necessity of PPE.[23] Since the initial SARS infection in the early 2000s, there was ongoing recognition that certain medical interventions, labeled aerosol-generating procedures (AGPs), increased the risk of potential infection due to aerosol generation.[24] According to the WHO, an AGP is any medical or patient care procedure that results in the production of airborne particles, or aerosols that are "associated with an increased risk of pathogen transmission" and therefore require enhanced precautions.[25] Per the WHO, the following procedures were considered AGPs: open airway suction, sputum induction, cardiopulmonary resuscitation, endotracheal intubation and extubation, noninvasive ventilation such as bilevel positive airway pressure and continuous positive airway pressure, bronchoscopy, and manual ventilation. The quantitative evidence to support this categorization was, however, limited to retrospective cohort/case-control studies that were all deemed as very low quality.[26]

The gastroenterology community had a significant controversy as to whether upper or lower endoscopy qualified as AGPs.[27] AGP classification was critical in informing infection prevention and control policies, specifically the requirements for respiratory protective devices, such as N95 or N99 masks/respirators or filtering facepiece respirators (such as FFP2 or FFP3) or masks at endoscopy.[28] In the context of COVID-19, a classification of a procedure as an AGP necessitated a higher grade of PPE to protect against aerosolized virus and potential airborne transmission risk. Although certain interventions such as intubation and bronchoscopy were acknowledged as high risk, there was a lot more uncertainty about endoscopic procedures. Possible sources of aerosolization during endoscopy include intubation and removal of the endoscope, coughing, belching during endoscopy, heavy breathing from sedation, patient expulsion of gas and liquid, and dispersion of contaminated fluid during insertion and removal of tools through the working channel of the endoscope, adjustment of the air/water button, retrieval of tissue from a biopsy channel, and during precleaning of the endoscope.[29] Our knowledge of the role of aerosol generation during endoscopy has expanded during the course of the pandemic. Several investigators, using various techniques, have studied this phenomenon to help us better understand the degree and quantity of aerosolization that is generated during routine endoscopy. These newer studies are summarized in **Table 2**.

A major criticism of this approach to categorizing AGPs into discrete dichotomous categories (AGP vs non-AGP and high-risk vs low-risk AGPs) is that this categorization does not consider the continuum of procedure-related aerosol generation and the different levels of transmission risks. Thus, there is likely a hierarchy of AGPs with each intervention conveying a different degree of transmission risk.[34] Further

Table 2
Recent studies that have aimed to assess the possibility and quantity of aerosol generation during upper and lower gastrointestinal endoscopy

Particle-counting approach: aerosols from patients undergoing upper gastrointestinal endoscopy were measured by a handheld optical particle counter before, during, and after the procedure. Particle sizes were reported to be in the range of 0.3 to 10 μm.[10–12]	
Sagami et al,[30] 2021	• A significant increase in the number of particles during and after the procedure was noted in the upper endoscopy group with conscious sedation compared with the nonendoscopy control group
Chan et al,[31] 2020	• A significant increase in particles of all sizes was noted during upper gastrointestinal endoscopy when measured at 10 cm from the patient's mouth
Air sampling approach: *aerosols were measured in a sample of air*	
Gregson et al,[32] 2022	• An uneventful upper endoscopy (without coughing or burping) does not generate aerosol above that associated with tidal breathing • Insertion and removal of an endoscope for esophagogastroduodenoscopy (EGD) does not generate an increase in aerosol concentration. • High aerosol concentrations were noted when endoscopy triggered coughing or belching by the patient
Phillips et al,[33] 2022	• Upper endoscopy (per oral and transnasal) as well as lower endoscopy generate aerosols (increased over background levels) • Lower endoscopy generates less aerosols than upper endoscopy, thus upper endoscopy should be classified as an AGP, whereas lower endoscopy depends on the definition of AGP used • Most significant contributing events for aerosol particle generation: local anesthetic throat spray application followed by extubation. which is the second-most particle-generating event (but the particles generated were in the droplet range with less propensity for airborne transmission) and then coughing or gagging • For lower endoscopy the absolute number of particles produced was higher (because of longer procedure duration) but the risk from lower procedures is likely to be considerably lower than equivalent aerosols generated by upper procedures • No statistically significant particle production from rectal insufflation or injection of water through the scope

complicating this issue is that numerous studies have shown that certain respiratory events, such as coughing, can generate vastly greater numbers of droplets and aerosols, considerably more aerosol particles than aerosols generated from currently classified AGPs.[35–39] In addition, some studies have found that traditional AGPs pose no greater risk than talking or breathing.[40] It is difficult to infer risk of infection from these studies because aerosols may not necessarily contain viable virus material, and the amount and quantity of aerosol generation does not equate to infectivity from endoscopy.

In summary, aerosol generation occurs as a continuum and endoscopy is associated with variable degrees of aerosolization. Risk of infection from aerosolized viral particles is, however, associated not only with the degree of aerosolization but also with other factors such as quantity of infective virus, proximity to source, and room ventilation. Based on these studies, however, there is increasing consensus that upper GI endoscopy should be classified as an AGP and periprocedural management including PPE recommendations should follow the AGP protocols to minimize transmission.

Current recommendations by the WHO and Centers for Disease Control and Prevention (CDC) advise the use of respirator masks, such as N95s or N99s, when performing surgical procedures that might pose higher risk for transmission if the patient has SARS-CoV-2 infection. These procedures generate potentially infectious aerosols or involve anatomic regions where viral loads might be higher, such as the nose and throat, oropharynx, or respiratory tract. Respirator masks are warranted in caring for individuals with COVID-19 or when community transmission levels increase, but standard surgical masks are adequate for routine care not involving aerosol-generating procedures.[25,41] A systematic review of 172 observational studies on COVID-19, SARS-CoV-1, and Middle East respiratory syndrome coronavirus indicated that people, including HCWs, are strongly protected by wearing surgical face masks (adjusted odds ratio, 0.15 95% confidence interval, 0.07–0.34), with eye protection potentially conferring additional benefit.[42]

Early Impact of the Coronavirus Disease 2019 Pandemic on Endoscopy Units

In March 2020 when the COVID-19 outbreak was declared a global pandemic all endoscopy services came to a virtual halt.[1] Considering the escalating rates of hospitalizations and deaths, limited PPE availability, limited COVID-19 test availability, and the burden on the health care system, routine elective endoscopy services were temporarily discontinued. HCWs, physicians, and nursing staff were redeployed, and protocols were developed for triaging of endoscopies to identify and perform only endoscopic procedures for urgent or emergent indications. Although there were variations in how procedures were prioritized, many centers limited procedures for the following indications: active GI bleeding, acute cholangitis, food impactions, GI obstructions, and cancer diagnosis/staging/treatment. This strategy was aimed to reduce the risk of spreading infection, reducing use of limited PPE supplies, and reducing use of hospital resources.

Numerous studies from the United States, United Kingdom, The Netherlands, Canada, China, Spain, Japan, and Taiwan reporting on endoscopy volumes during the initial 3 to 4 months of the pandemic demonstrated reductions in total number of upper endoscopies and colonoscopies of 51% to 72% and 59% to 85%, respectively (compared with the same period from prior years).[43–49] After the initial phase, many centers resumed limited endoscopy services with the implementation of stringent infection prevention and control policies and worked to reduce the backlog of colonoscopies by offering patients noninvasive stool-based tests for colorectal cancer screening.[50,51]

Resumption of Endoscopy with a Focus on Safety During the Coronavirus Disease 2019 Pandemic

An important framework for managing health and safety interventions used by the CDC to develop infection control policies was the Hierarchy of Controls, which recommended using strategies to reduce risks of exposure to the virus in addition to the use of PPE.[52] Such strategies included eliminating hazards by avoiding admission/treatment of people with active infection and using COVID-19 testing to segregate patients with the infection. Engineering controls such as physical barriers, and administrative controls to facilitate physical distancing, were also included in the hierarchy. And finally given the physical proximity required to deliver many elements of care, the use of PPE was also a required control measure within the health care environment.

Following the hierarchy of controls framework, various operational changes were implemented across endoscopy suites and centers to safely reopen endoscopy units while mitigating the risk of infection.[53] These changes were implemented based on local factors such as availability of resources, local prevalence of COVID-19, patient demographics, procedure indication, and hospital/endoscopy unit policies. The common goals of these changes were to maintain endoscopic volume and efficiency, while minimizing risk of transmission and infection to patients, staff, and HCWs. Sources of human-to-human transmission could occur from unknown infected persons (eg, asymptomatic carriers or individuals with mild symptoms), as well as individuals with virus shedding during the presymptomatic incubation period. Sources of risk during endoscopy included aerosols generated during endoscopy, which could increase the potential for subsequent airborne transmission, infection from respiratory secretions from patients, and potential contamination from other sources of bodily fluid (stool and patient saliva). Many authorities issued guidance on how to safely restart routine endoscopy and advocated for stringent infection control policies that included universal masking of patients, symptom screening before endoscopy, COVID testing before endoscopy, and use of high-level PPE[54–60] (**Box 1**).

Endoscopy Room and Endoscope Cleaning

Enhanced cleaning procedures with cleaning of all horizontal surfaces, especially frequently touched surfaces, with particular emphasis on areas within a few feet of the patent (using standard hospital-grade disinfectant solution with viricidal agents) were implemented by most endoscopy units.[6,53,61] Endoscope cleaning and decontamination processes remained unchanged; as per guidelines, mechanical and detergent cleaning followed by high-level disinfection (a process that eliminates or kills all vegetative bacteria, mycobacteria, fungi, and viruses, except for small numbers of bacterial spores, and reduces the number of microorganisms and organic debris by 4 logs, or 99.99%).[62]

Preprocedure Testing: Changing Recommendations Through the Course of the Pandemic

The use of preprocedure testing in asymptomatic individuals became a common path to triage for risk stratification. A critical aspect of resuming endoscopy services included providing reassurance to patients and importantly to reassure HCWs, including endoscopists, nurses, and staff. At the pandemic onset, in the absence of available diagnostic tests and knowledge of treatments for COVID-19, one of the earliest evidence-based guidelines was developed by the American Gastroenterological Association (AGA); the guideline panel members made a strong recommendation to use N95 (or N99 or PAPR) masks (along with gowns, shoe covers, goggles, and face

Box 1

Overview of modifications implemented across various endoscopy centers during various stages of the pandemic before the availability of vaccines

Preprocedure modifications

Triage and risk stratification used a screening questionnaire for (1) symptoms of COVID-19 (such as cough, shortness of breath, and persistent fever), (2) known history of contact with a patient with COVID-19, and (3) travel to high risk areas. These were performed in all cases at least 24 to 72 hours before endoscopy

Preprocedure SARS-CoV-2 testing: individualized protocols for outpatient preprocedural testing of patients 24 to 72 hours before the scheduled appointment depending on local prevalence rates and institutional policies. Reverse transcription-polymerase chain reaction testing was performed in all asymptomatic patients before endoscopic procedures to risk stratify and determine PPE needs (see section later).

- Patient reassurance about safety precautions taken to decrease transmission from patient to patient

Procedural modifications for patients

All patients required to wear surgical masks and keep at least 1 to 2 m distance from others.

Arrangements made in advance to reduce patient congestion in the waiting area.

Chairs and beds spaced to avoid the transmission of viral particles to noninfected patients.

Informed consent includes informing individuals about the possible risk of nosocomial infection (COVID-19 infection) during endoscopy

Patients informed to report back if experiencing any de novo symptoms postprocedure.

Triage and screening questionnaire: at the time of presentation to the endoscopy, questions asked again regarding (1) symptoms of COVID-19 (such as cough, shortness of breath, and persistent fever), (2) known history of contact with a patient with COVID-19, and (3) travel to high-risk areas. These were performed in all cases at least 24 to 72 hours before endoscopy

High-risk patients, classified by the presence of respiratory tract symptoms, previous travel to COVID-19 locations in the past 14 days, and close contact with COVID-19-positive patients, prompted procedure cancellation and self-quarantine

Temperature measurements before entering the endoscopy unit

Patient's relative/caregiver or driver required to wait offsite and return after the procedure is completed.

If this is not feasible, the waiting area should be appropriately distanced.

Procedural modifications for HCWs

Barriers such as glass or plastic walls/shields set up in check-in areas

Safe distancing in the preoperative area as well as decreased numbers of patients that nursing staff can receive for preprocedure care.

Endoscopy staff with preexisting conditions at higher risk of contracting COVID-19 have been assigned nonclinical duties

Use of PPE mandated by all health care systems to minimize the risk of transmission

All endoscopy team members required to wear surgical masks, gloves, hair coverings, face shields or goggles, water-proof disposable gowns, and shoe covers or boots.

Initially use of highest level of PPE mandated by all health care systems to minimize the risk of transmission

Eventually PPE for endoscopy personnel adjusted according to patient risk stratification with full PPE required for high-risk or confirmed COVID-19-positive patients.

In low-resource settings, reusable respirators, face shields, goggles, and boots deemed acceptable after appropriate sterilization and decontamination methods

Training and adherence to strict precautions of properly donning and doffing

Staff required to complete questionnaire about symptoms before their daily work. Similar distances should be maintained between individuals.

Staff required to keep at least 1 to 2 m of distance from staff and patients

For COVID-19-positive (or suspected) cases, procedures performed in a negative pressure endoscopic unit, if available, or portable industrial-grade high-efficiency particulate air filters placed in endoscopy rooms

In low-resource situations, adequate ventilation of the room was acceptable

As much as possible, all required documentation should be performed outside the endoscopy room.
Minimal number of workers should be in procedure room to minimize risk
Team switching during procedures discouraged to minimize PPE usage and decrease contamination risks

Postprocedure modifications
Procedural downtime and room turnover time needed to allow for dispersion of potential virus-laden aerosols depends on rate of air changes per hour. The precise time needed for closure of the room depends on the use of negative pressure and air-exchange rate
Patients with COVID-19: some centers used only negative pressure rooms (room maintained under negative pressure for at least 30 minutes, and in the absence of negative pressure, for 60 minutes, before the next patient)
Initially patients are monitored in the recovery area, with no family available in the waiting room
Eventually limited family available in the waiting room with adequate spacing between seats and requirement of face masks
Postprocedure telephone follow-ups with patients used to enquire about developing any new COVID-19-related symptoms (traced and contacted after 7 and 14 days)

shields) instead of surgical masks for all HCWs performing upper endoscopies. Recommendations also included wearing double gloves and using negative pressure rooms, placing a high value on minimizing risks to HCWs, despite having low or very low certainty of evidence for risk of transmission of infection, because of documented community spread during a pandemic. In addition to limited resources for testing, limitations of PPE availability necessitated reuse or prolonged use of N95 masks. Finally, the decision to extend the recommendation to lower GI tract procedures was based on limited evidence of possible aerosolization during colonoscopy and the uncertain risks associated with evidence of the presence of SARS-CoV-2 RNA in fecal samples. These recommendations assumed the absence of widespread reliable testing for the diagnosis of COVID-19 infection or immunity and unclear data on prevalence.

As the number of COVID tests that received Emergency Use Authorization approval increased, preprocedure testing became more readily available, and questions arose regarding the role of routine preprocedure testing of all individuals to minimize risk for patients and HCWs. At the individual patient level, testing in symptomatic patients helped identify individuals who could be isolated to prevent the spread of disease. At the population level, widespread testing of individuals (symptomatic and asymptomatic) was critical to determine the true prevalence of disease and the provision of health care services, and to reintroduce endoscopy across health care systems and ambulatory care centers. Recommendations developed by the AGA provided a framework for routine preprocedure testing before endoscopy (for all asymptomatic persons) that accounted for local contextual factors such as the local prevalence of SARS-CoV2 and availability of PPE and weighed the pros and cons of a pretesting strategy. Based on a systematic review and meta-analysis of the tests (available at that time), the authors of this guideline conducted and made conditional recommendations against endoscopy centers adopting routine preprocedural testing to triage patients into low- and high-prevalence settings because of concerns about the accuracy of test results and the potential downsides for individuals with false-positive or false-negative test results. It was suggested that all HCWs wear N95s (or higher) masks, if available, and forego testing. For endoscopy centers where the prevalence of asymptomatic SARS-CoV-2 infection was intermediate (0.5%–2%), the AGA suggested implementing a pretesting strategy, if tests were available, to determine the type of PPE (such as use of surgical masks in individuals who tested negative). Alternatively, in settings where the logistics of testing were challenging and the downsides outweighed the benefits, HCWs could choose to wear N95 (or higher) masks and again forego testing. The changing prevalence of COVID-19 was an important factor as new variants emerged and created documented new waves of infection.

The rapid development of vaccines and the widespread implementation of vaccination programs worldwide helped decrease morbidity and mortality from COVID-19. Another important positive change was the availability of relatively effective treatments. Furthermore, within the GI community, as our understanding of disease transmission increased and data on infection rates from endoscopy and universal screening and testing became available, and PPE became widely available, many endoscopy centers again revised their testing policies. In contrast to early reports of high rates of HCW infections early in the pandemic (in the setting of limited PPE) accumulating evidence demonstrated low rates of COVID-19 infections among HCWs performing endoscopy.[60] This evidence along with data demonstrating the relative effectiveness of vaccines in decreasing rates of transmission of infection prompted a recommendation against routine preprocedure testing emphasizing the downsides of testing at the patient level (of burden, cost, and access) and at the population level (low rates of screening and surveillance endoscopies leading to lower rates of screening, surveillance, and diagnosis of various GI cancers).

Endoscopic Indications and Findings

In patients with COVID-19, several systematic reviews and meta-analyses have described the prevalence of GI symptoms including diarrhea (8%–17%), nausea or vomiting (4%–20%), loss of appetite (2%–21%), abdominal pain (3%–20%), anorexia (8%–10%), abdominal distension (1%) and loss of taste (1%–3%).[63–70] Most GI symptoms associated with COVID-19 are mild. Diarrhea caused by SARS-CoV-2 may be the initial symptom in patients with COVID-19. A small subset of patients with COVID-19 may develop isolated GI symptoms throughout the disease (2.9%–16%).[71]

Our understanding of the endoscopic findings in COVID-19 is limited. Several case series and retrospective and prospective cohort studies have helped us to understand the direct and indirect effects of COVID-19 on the GI tract.[72–75] GI endoscopy for GI bleeding in patients with COVID-19 is reviewed in the article by Cappell and Friedel in this issue. Mechanistically, viruses in the GI tract, including coronaviruses, can contribute to disease by interacting with the mucous layer, epithelial cells, and potentially lamina propria immune cells. SARS-CoV-2 infection can disrupt the tight and adherent junctions of the endothelium and intestinal epithelium, which may lead to a leaky gut, local and systemic invasion of normal microbiota, and consequent immune activation.[76]

In one retrospective, single-center study of 95 laboratory-confirmed cases of SARS-CoV-2 infection from Zhuhai, China, 6 patients with GI symptoms underwent upper endoscopy and 2 underwent proctoscopy. Biopsies were taken from the esophagus, stomach, duodenum, and rectum for viral RNA detection. One patient with severe symptoms of GI bleeding localized to the esophagus and attributed to multiple round herpetic erosions and ulcers, each with a diameter of 4 to 6 mm. SARS-CoV-2 RNA was detected in the esophageal erosions and bleeding site, as well as in the stomach, duodenum, and rectum. In the other 5 patients (cases 2–6) no erosions, ulcers, or bleeding was noted. SARS-CoV-2 RNA could also be detected in the esophagus, stomach, duodenum, and rectum of another patient with severe COVID-19 infection (case 2). In contrast, the virus was only detected in the duodenum of the nonsevere case 3 and could not be detected in any GI specimens of the nonsevere cases 4 to 6.[73]

In a case report of a patient with COVID-19 who underwent endoscopy, biopsies revealed no damage to the epithelium of the esophagus, stomach, duodenum, and rectum, but infiltrates of occasional lymphocytes were observed in esophageal squamous epithelium and numerous infiltrating plasma cells and lymphocytes with interstitial edema were observed in the lamina propria of the stomach, duodenum, and rectum.[75]

In a retrospective study from Lombardy, Italy, 38 patients with confirmed SARS-CoV-2 underwent endoscopic evaluation (24 EGDs, 20 colonoscopies). Endoscopic lesions were observed in 18 of 24 EGDs (75%) and in 14 of 20 colonoscopies (70%). The main findings were esophagitis (20.8%), bulbar ulcer (20.8%), erosive gastritis (16.6%), neoplasm (8.3%), and Mallory-Weiss tear (4.1%). Colonoscopy revealed segmental colitis associated with diverticulosis (25%), colonic ischemia (20%), diffuse hemorrhagic colitis (5%), and colonic neoplasms (5%).[74]

Finally, in a multicenter cohort of ~2000 hospitalized patients with COVID-19 across a geographically diverse network of medical centers in North America, only 1.2% of patients (n = 24) underwent endoscopy despite a high prevalence of GI symptoms and substantial burden of critical or prolonged illness. Most endoscopic procedures were performed for either emergency cases (eg, ongoing GI bleeding or biliary obstruction) or for placement of enteral access tubes. Among those who underwent endoscopy, the indications and findings were judged more likely to reflect overall systemic illness or related to prolonged hospitalization rather than direct viral injury from COVID-19. The investigators did not observe inflammatory pathology and concluded that SARS-CoV-2 did not seem to behave as a highly invasive and injurious pathogen to GI mucosa.[72]

SUMMARY

In summary, the unprecedented COVID-19 pandemic led to significant disruptions in gastroenterology practice necessitating endoscopy centers to be adaptive, reactive, and innovative. With the emergence of new variants and the ever-present threat of new pandemics, lessons learned during these past few years will help maintain the safe practice of endoscopy and prepare for new and emerging pathogens. Although mechanistically SARS-CoV-2 may contribute to enteric disease, endoscopic findings in patients with COVID-19 are likely to reflect the underlying critical illness rather than the direct effect of the virus.

CLINICS CARE POINTS

- Aerosolization during upper and lower endoscopy occurs along a continuum, and respirator masks, such as N95s, along with eye protection, gowns, and gloves are an important strategy to minimize risk of viral transmission
- Endoscopy centers should incorporate several strategies based on the Hierarchy of Controls Model to reduce the risk of viral transmission
- The role of preprocedure testing should be based on local prevalence, testing availability, PPE availability, and patient burden
- Although SARS-CoV2 can be detected in stool, there have been no reports of infection via the fecal-oral route
- Endoscopic and histologic findings in patients with COVID-19 are more consistent with prolonged and severe systemic illness and suggest no direct viral or inflammatory pathogenic effects

DISCLOSURE

The author has nothing to disclose.

REFERENCES

1. WHO Director-General's opening remarks at the media briefing on COVID-19 – 11. WHO; 2020. Available at: https://www.who.int/director-general/speeches/detail/who-director-general-s-opening-remarks-at-the-media-briefing-on-covid-19. Accessed November 2022.
2. Cohen J, Rodgers YVM. Contributing factors to personal protective equipment shortages during the COVID-19 pandemic. Prev Med 2020;141:106263.
3. Chiu PWY, Ng SC, Inoue H, et al. Practice of endoscopy during COVID-19 pandemic: position statements of the Asian Pacific Society for Digestive Endoscopy (APSDE-COVID statements). Gut 2020;69:991–6.
4. Gralnek IM, Hassan C, Beilenhoff U, et al. ESGE and ESGENA Position Statement on gastrointestinal endoscopy and the COVID-19 pandemic. Endoscopy 2020; 52:483–90.
5. Lui RN, Wong SH, Sanchez-Luna SA, et al. Overview of guidance for endoscopy during the coronavirus disease 2019 pandemic. J Gastroenterol Hepatol 2020; 35:749–59.
6. Sultan S, Lim JK, Altayar O, et al. AGA Rapid Recommendations for Gastrointestinal Procedures During the COVID-19 Pandemic. Gastroenterology 2020;159: 739–758 e4.
7. Forbes N, Smith ZL, Spitzer RL, et al. Changes in Gastroenterology and Endoscopy Practices in Response to the Coronavirus Disease 2019 Pandemic: Results From a North American Survey. Gastroenterology 2020;159:772–774 e13.
8. Parasa S, Reddy N, Faigel DO, et al. Global Impact of the COVID-19 Pandemic on Endoscopy: An International Survey of 252 Centers From 55 Countries. Gastroenterology 2020;159:1579–1581 e5.
9. Repici A, Pace F, Gabbiadini R, et al. Endoscopy Units and the Coronavirus Disease 2019 Outbreak: A Multicenter Experience From Italy. Gastroenterology 2020;159:363–366 e3.
10. Leung NHL. Transmissibility and transmission of respiratory viruses. Nat Rev Microbiol 2021;19:528–45.
11. World Health Organization. Infection prevention and control of epidemic-and pandemic prone acute respiratory infections in health care. Available at: https://www.who.int/publications/i/item/infection-prevention-and-control-of-epidemic-and-pandemic-prone-acute-respiratory-infections-in-health-care. Accessed November 2022.
12. Shiu EYC, Leung NHL, Cowling BJ. Controversy around airborne versus droplet transmission of respiratory viruses: implication for infection prevention. Curr Opin Infect Dis 2019;32:372–9.
13. van Doremalen N, Bushmaker T, Morris DH, et al. Aerosol and Surface Stability of SARS-CoV-2 as Compared with SARS-CoV-1. N Engl J Med 2020;382:1564–7.
14. Cai J, Sun W, Huang J, et al. Indirect Virus Transmission in Cluster of COVID-19 Cases, Wenzhou, China, 2020. Emerg Infect Dis 2020;26:1343–5.
15. Ong SWX, Tan YK, Chia PY, et al. Air, Surface Environmental, and Personal Protective Equipment Contamination by Severe Acute Respiratory Syndrome Coronavirus 2 (SARS-CoV-2) From a Symptomatic Patient. JAMA 2020;323:1610–2.

16. Knowlton SD, Boles CL, Perencevich EN, et al. Bioaerosol concentrations generated from toilet flushing in a hospital-based patient care setting. Antimicrob Resist Infect Control 2018;7:16.
17. Centers for Disease Control and Prevention. Scientific Brief: SARS-CoV-2 Transmission. Available at: https://www.cdc.gov/coronavirus/2019-ncov/science/science-briefs/sars-cov-2-transmission.html. Accessed November 2022.
18. Peng L, Liu J, Xu W, et al. SARS-CoV-2 can be detected in urine, blood, anal swabs, and oropharyngeal swabs specimens. J Med Virol 2020;92:1676–80.
19. Kutti-Sridharan G, Vegunta R, Vegunta R, et al. SARS-CoV2 in Different Body Fluids, Risks of Transmission, and Preventing COVID-19: A Comprehensive Evidence-Based Review. Int J Prev Med 2020;11:97.
20. Zhang Y, Cen M, Hu M, et al. Prevalence and Persistent Shedding of Fecal SARS-CoV-2 RNA in Patients With COVID-19 Infection: A Systematic Review and Meta-analysis. Clin Transl Gastroenterol 2021;12:e00343.
21. Wang H, Churqui MP, Tunovic T, et al. The amount of SARS-CoV-2 RNA in wastewater relates to the development of the pandemic and its burden on the health system. iScience 2022;25:105000.
22. The use and effectiveness of powered air purifying respirators in health care. Washington (DC): Workshop Summary; 2015.
23. Jackson T, Deibert D, Wyatt G, et al. Classification of aerosol-generating procedures: a rapid systematic review. BMJ Open Respir Res 2020;7.
24. Hamilton GS. Aerosol-generating procedures in the COVID era. Respirology 2021;26:416–8.
25. World Health Organizatiion. Infection prevention and control of epidemic-and pandemic prone acute respiratory infections in health care. available at: https://www.who.int/publications/i/item/infection-prevention-and-control-of-epidemic-and-pandemic-prone-acute-respiratory-infections-in-health-care. Accessed November 2022.
26. Tran K, Cimon K, Severn M, et al. Aerosol-generating procedures and risk of transmission of acute respiratory infections: a systematic review. CADTH Technol Overv 2013;3:e3201.
27. Nampoolsuksan C, Chinswangwatanakul V, Methasate A, et al. Management of aerosol generation during upper gastrointestinal endoscopy. Clin Endosc 2022;55(5):588–93.
28. Centers for Disease Prevention and Control. Coronavlrus 2019. Available at: https://www.cdc.gov/coronavirus/2019-ncov/index.html. Accessed November 2022.
29. Johnston ER, Habib-Bein N, Dueker JM, et al. Risk of bacterial exposure to the endoscopist's face during endoscopy. Gastrointest Endosc 2019;89:818–24.
30. Sagami R, Nishikiori H, Sato T, et al. Aerosols Produced by Upper Gastrointestinal Endoscopy: A Quantitative Evaluation. Am J Gastroenterol 2021;116:202–5.
31. Chan SM, Ma TW, Chong MK, et al. A Proof of Concept Study: Esophagogastroduodenoscopy Is an Aerosol-Generating Procedure and Continuous Oral Suction During the Procedure Reduces the Amount of Aerosol Generated. Gastroenterology 2020;159:1949–1951 e4.
32. Gregson FKA, Shrimpton AJ, Hamilton F, et al. Identification of the source events for aerosol generation during oesophago-gastro-duodenoscopy. Gut 2022;71:871–8.
33. Phillips F, Crowley J, Warburton S, et al. Aerosol and droplet generation in upper and lower GI endoscopy: whole procedure and event-based analysis. Gastrointest Endosc 2022;96:603–611 e0.

34. Harding H, Broom A, Broom J. Aerosol-generating procedures and infective risk to healthcare workers from SARS-CoV-2: the limits of the evidence. J Hosp Infect 2020;105:717–25.
35. Bourouiba L. Turbulent Gas Clouds and Respiratory Pathogen Emissions: Potential Implications for Reducing Transmission of COVID-19. JAMA 2020;323: 1837–8.
36. Dhand R, Li J. Coughs and Sneezes: Their Role in Transmission of Respiratory Viral Infections, Including SARS-CoV-2. Am J Respir Crit Care Med 2020;202: 651–9.
37. Lindsley WG, King WP, Thewlis RE, et al. Dispersion and exposure to a cough-generated aerosol in a simulated medical examination room. J Occup Environ Hyg 2012;9:681–90.
38. Noti JD, Lindsley WG, Blachere FM, et al. Detection of infectious influenza virus in cough aerosols generated in a simulated patient examination room. Clin Infect Dis 2012;54:1569–77.
39. Wilson NM, Marks GB, Eckhardt A, et al. The effect of respiratory activity, non-invasive respiratory support and facemasks on aerosol generation and its relevance to COVID-19. Anaesthesia 2021;76:1465–74.
40. Hamilton F, Arnold D, Bzdek BR, et al. Aerosol generating procedures: are they of relevance for transmission of SARS-CoV-2? Lancet Respir Med 2021;9:687–9.
41. Infection Control Recommendations. CDC 2019. Available at: https://www.cdc.gov/coronavirus/2019-ncov/hcp/infection-control-recommendations.html. Accessed Nov 2022.
42. Chu DK, Akl EA, Duda S, et al. Physical distancing, face masks, and eye protection to prevent person-to-person transmission of SARS-CoV-2 and COVID-19: a systematic review and meta-analysis. Lancet 2020;395:1973–87.
43. Cheng SY, Chen CF, He HC, et al. Impact of COVID-19 pandemic on fecal immunochemical test screening uptake and compliance to diagnostic colonoscopy. J Gastroenterol Hepatol 2021;36:1614–9.
44. Lantinga MA, Theunissen F, Ter Borg PCJ, et al. Impact of the COVID-19 pandemic on gastrointestinal endoscopy in the Netherlands: analysis of a prospective endoscopy database. Endoscopy 2021;53:166–70.
45. Leeds JS, Awadelkarim B, Dipper C, et al. Effect of the SARS-CoV2 Pandemic on Endoscopy Provision - The Impact of Compliance with National Guidance. Expert Rev Gastroenterol Hepatol 2021;15:459–64.
46. Lui TKL, Leung K, Guo CG, et al. Impacts of the coronavirus 2019 pandemic on gastrointestinal endoscopy volume and diagnosis of gastric and colorectal cancers: a population-based study. Gastroenterology 2020;159:1164–1166 e3.
47. Markar SR, Clarke J, Kinross J, et al. Practice patterns of diagnostic upper gastrointestinal endoscopy during the initial COVID-19 outbreak in England. Lancet Gastroenterol Hepatol 2020;5:804–5.
48. Rutter CM, Inadomi JM, Maerzluft CE. The impact of cumulative colorectal cancer screening delays: A simulation study. J Med Screen 2022;29:92–8.
49. Tinmouth J, Dong S, Stogios C, et al. Estimating the backlog of colonoscopy due to coronavirus disease 2019 and comparing strategies to recover in Ontario, Canada. Gastroenterology 2021;160:1400–1402 e1.
50. Huang Q, Liu G, Wang J, et al. Control measures to prevent Coronavirus disease 2019 pandemic in endoscopy centers: Multi-center study. Dig Endosc 2020;32: 914–20.
51. Moraveji S, Thaker AM, Muthusamy VR, et al. Protocols, personal protective equipment use, and psychological/financial stressors in endoscopy units during

the COVID-19 pandemic: a large survey of hospital-based and ambulatory endoscopy centers in the United States. Gastroenterology 2020;159: 1568–1570 e5.
52. Winkler ML, Hooper DC, Shenoy ES. Infection prevention and control of severe acute respiratory syndrome coronavirus 2 in health care settings. Infect Dis Clin North Am 2022;36:309–26.
53. Perisetti A, Goyal H, Sharma N. Gastrointestinal Endoscopy in the Era of COVID-19. Front Med (Lausanne) 2020;7:587602.
54. Antonelli G, Karsensten JG, Bhat P, et al. Resuming endoscopy during COVID-19 pandemic: ESGE, WEO and WGO Joint Cascade Guideline for Resource Limited Settings. Endosc Int Open 2021;9:E543–51.
55. Gralnek IM, Hassan C, Ebigbo A, et al. ESGE and ESGENA Position Statement on gastrointestinal endoscopy and COVID-19: Updated guidance for the era of vaccines and viral variants. Endoscopy 2022;54:211–6.
56. Hennessy B, Vicari J, Bernstein B, et al. Guidance for resuming GI endoscopy and practice operations after the COVID-19 pandemic. Gastrointest Endosc 2020;92:743–747 e1.
57. Leddin D, Armstrong D, Raja Ali RA, et al. Personal protective equipment for endoscopy in low-resource settings during the COVID-19 pandemic: guidance from the world gastroenterology organisation. J Clin Gastroenterol 2020;54: 833–40.
58. Siddique SM, Sultan S, Lim JK, et al. Spotlight: COVID-19 PPE and endoscopy. Gastroenterology 2020;159:759.
59. Sultan S, Siddique SM, Altayar O, et al. AGA institute rapid review and recommendations on the role of pre-procedure SARS-CoV-2 testing and endoscopy. Gastroenterology 2020;159:1935–1948 e5.
60. Sultan S, Siddique SM, Singh S, et al. AGA rapid review and guideline for SARS-CoV2 testing and endoscopy post-vaccination: 2021 Update. Gastroenterology 2021;161:1011–1029 e11.
61. Calderwood AH, Day LW, Muthusamy VR, et al. ASGE guideline for infection control during GI endoscopy. Gastrointest Endosc 2018;87:1167–79.
62. Chu NS, McAlister D, Antonoplos PA. Natural bioburden levels detected on flexible gastrointestinal endoscopes after clinical use and manual cleaning. Gastrointest Endosc 1998;48:137–42.
63. Bolia R, Dhanesh Goel A, Badkur M, et al. Gastrointestinal manifestations of pediatric coronavirus disease and their relationship with a severe clinical course: a systematic review and meta-analysis. J Trop Pediatr 2021;67:fmab051.
64. Mao R, Qiu Y, He JS, et al. Manifestations and prognosis of gastrointestinal and liver involvement in patients with COVID-19: a systematic review and meta-analysis. Lancet Gastroenterol Hepatol 2020;5:667–78.
65. Parasa S, Desai M, Thoguluva Chandrasekar V, et al. Prevalence of gastrointestinal symptoms and fecal viral shedding in patients with coronavirus disease 2019: a systematic review and meta-analysis. JAMA Netw Open 2020;3: e2011335.
66. Shehab M, Alrashed F, Shuaibi S, et al. Gastroenterological and hepatic manifestations of patients with COVID-19, prevalence, mortality by country, and intensive care admission rate: systematic review and meta-analysis. BMJ Open Gastroenterol 2021;8:e000571.
67. Wang J, Yuan X. Digestive system symptoms and function in children with COVID-19: A meta-analysis. Medicine (Baltimore) 2021;100:e24897.

68. Zarifian A, Zamiri Bidary M, Arekhi S, et al. Gastrointestinal and hepatic abnormalities in patients with confirmed COVID-19: A systematic review and meta-analysis. J Med Virol 2021;93:336–50.
69. Zeng W, Qi K, Ye M, et al. Gastrointestinal symptoms are associated with severity of coronavirus disease 2019: a systematic review and meta-analysis. Eur J Gastroenterol Hepatol 2022;34:168–76.
70. Sultan S, Altayar O, Siddique SM, et al. AGA institute rapid review of the gastrointestinal and liver manifestations of COVID-19, Meta-analysis of international data, and recommendations for the consultative management of patients with COVID-19. Gastroenterology 2020;159:320–334 e27.
71. Megyeri K, Dernovics A, Al-Luhaibi ZII, et al. COVID-19-associated diarrhea. World J Gastroenterol 2021;27:3208–22.
72. Kuftinec G, Elmunzer BJ, Amin S, et al. The role of endoscopy and findings in COVID-19 patients, an early North American Cohort. BMC Gastroenterol 2021;21:205.
73. Lin L, Jiang X, Zhang Z, et al. Gastrointestinal symptoms of 95 cases with SARS-CoV-2 infection. Gut 2020;69:997–1001.
74. Massironi S, Vigano C, Dioscoridi L, et al. Endoscopic findings in patients infected with 2019 novel coronavirus in Lombardy, Italy. Clin Gastroenterol Hepatol 2020;18:2375–7.
75. Xiao F, Tang M, Zheng X, et al. Evidence for gastrointestinal infection of SARS-CoV-2. Gastroenterology 2020;158:1831–1833 e3.
76. Chen TH, Hsu MT, Lee MY, et al. Gastrointestinal involvement in SARS-CoV-2 Infection. Viruses 2022;14:1188.

Surgical Implications of Coronavirus Disease-19

Ander Dorken-Gallastegi, MD, Dias Argandykov, MD, Anthony Gebran, MD, Haytham M.A. Kaafarani, MD, MPH*

KEYWORDS

• COVID • SARS-CoV-2 • Surgery • Operative • Risk • Anesthesia

KEY POINTS

- All preoperative patients should be screened for (1) history of exposure to someone with known COVID-19 within the last 14 days and (2) symptoms suspicious of COVID-19.
- Perioperative COVID-19 increases the risk of postoperative morbidity and mortality. Surgical risk calculators may underestimate postoperative risk in COVID-19 patients.
- A multicenter international study suggests that elective surgery should be delayed for 7 weeks following COVID-19 diagnosis, at which time perioperative risk becomes comparable to the non-COVID-19 population.
- There are no data comparing operative versus nonoperative management of COVID-19 patients for emergency surgical conditions that can also be managed medically; decision to operate should be made judiciously considering clinical acuity, patient comorbidities, and local resources.
- COVID-19 patients seem to have higher rates of postoperative thrombotic and pulmonary complications, and potentially a lower rate of bleeding complications. Telemedicine appointments could be a viable approach to minimize ambulatory hospital visits.

INTRODUCTION

Coronavirus disease-19 (COVID-19), caused by the severe adult respiratory syndrome coronavirus-2 (SARS-CoV-2), was first reported in late 2019 and quickly developed into a global pandemic in the first few months of 2020.[1] COVID-19 strained health care systems and resulted in unprecedented challenges to health care providers around the world. For surgical patients, COVID-19 complicates perioperative risk and subsequently the benefits versus risks balance of any invasive operation. In addition, it quickly became evident that surgery plays a central role in the treatment of severe COVID-19 (eg, tracheostomy and gastrostomy tube placement) as well as COVID-19 complications (eg, bowel ischemia).[2] In addition, health care providers

Trauma, Emergency Surgery, and Surgical Critical Care, Massachusetts General Hospital, Harvard Medical School, Boston, MA, USA
* Corresponding author. 165 Cambridge Street, Suite 810, Boston, MA.
E-mail address: hkaafarani@mgh.harvard.edu

Gastroenterol Clin N Am 52 (2023) 173–183
https://doi.org/10.1016/j.gtc.2022.10.003
0889-8553/23/© 2022 Published by Elsevier Inc.

involved in the perioperative care of patients are at a significant risk of contracting the disease, especially those involved in airway management. Finally, COVID-19 poses a major logistical challenge for the surgical service, as the strain on health care systems led to widespread cancellations of elective surgery and difficulties in maintaining even basic surgical services.

As the COVID-19 pandemic continues to evolve with the surge of novel virus variants such as the delta and omicron, it is important for physicians to understand and appreciate the surgical implications of COVID-19 (**Box 1**). This review provides an overview of the implications of the ongoing COVID-19 pandemic on surgical care

Box 1
Surgical implications of coronavirus disease-19

Preoperative Screening and Testing

All preoperative patients should be screened for (1) history of exposure to someone with known COVID-19 within the last 14 days and (2) symptoms suspicious of COVID-19 (eg, fever, cough, dyspnea, and chills). Patients who answer "yes" to at least one of these questions should undergo PCR testing for SARS-CoV-2.

Surgical Risk Assessment

Patients with perioperative COVID-19 seem to have higher risk of postoperative morbidity and mortality compared with patients without COVID-19. Surgical risk calculators may underestimate postoperative risk in COVID-19 patients.

Timing of Surgery after SARS-CoV-2 Infection

A multicenter international study suggests that elective surgery should be delayed for 7 weeks following COVID-19 diagnosis, at which time perioperative risk becomes comparable to the non-COVID-19 population

Risk of Contracting SARS-CoV-2 Perioperatively

The risk of contracting SARS-CoV-2 perioperatively is low (<2%), and the use of COVID-19-free surgical pathways reduce the risk of postoperative infection.

Emergency Surgery

There are no data comparing operative versus nonoperative management of COVID-19 patients for emergency surgical conditions that can also be managed medically; decision to operate should be made judiciously considering clinical acuity, patient comorbidities, and local resources.

Elective Surgery

An estimated 28.5 million elective surgical cases were cancelled worldwide during the peak 3-month period of the pandemic, resulting in a significant backlog in surgical care. Hospitals and health care systems should prepare to address the backlog in surgical care despite the ongoing disruptions in the health care supply chain.

Oncological Surgery

Cancer surgeries are frequently time-sensitive and are considered essential operations. Cooperation between surgical centers could help maintain the regional quality of surgical cancer care, despite capacity issues or other problems at individual hospitals

Anesthesia Considerations

The type of anesthesia should be primarily dictated by the individual operation and patient characteristics. The number of personnel in the operating room during intubation and extubation should be minimized and high-level PPE should be used for aerosol-producing procedures on COVID-19 patients.

Postoperative Follow-up

COVID-19 patients seem to have higher rates of postoperative thrombotic and pulmonary complications, and potentially a lower rate of bleeding complications. Telemedicine appointments could be a viable approach to minimize ambulatory hospital visits.

and provides recommendations for the perioperative management of all patients during the pandemic.

Preoperative Evaluation

A joint statement by the American Society of Anesthesiologists (ASA) and the Anesthesia Patient Safety Foundation (APSF) recommends screening all patients preoperatively for (1) history of exposure to someone with known COVID-19 within the last 14 days and (2) symptoms suspicious of COVID-19 (fever, cough, dyspnea, chills, muscle pain, headache, sore throat, and/or new loss of taste or smell, nausea, vomiting, or diarrhea) not explained by other causes.[3,4] Patients who screen positive for one of these criteria should be referred for further evaluation. Careful screening of symptoms can also be important for risk stratification of COVID-19 positive patients, as a multicenter retrospective observational study from the United States showed that the presence of such symptoms increased patient risks, COVID-19 patients who had preoperative respiratory symptoms were at higher risk of pulmonary complications than asymptomatic COVID-19 patients, following emergency general surgery.[5] Owing to the highly variable presentation of COVID-19, screening for symptoms and viral exposure can yield false negative results in a subset of infected patients. During the peak of the pandemic, many institutions implemented universal testing protocols for all patients undergoing surgery or other aerosol-producing procedure (eg, esophagogastroduodenoscopy). If resources allow, universal testing less than 3 days before the operation could help to identify asymptomatic patients, and such testing has been supported by major organizations.[6–9] An international multicenter study of 8784 patients undergoing elective cancer surgery during the first peak of the pandemic found that routine polymerase chain reaction (PCR) testing from a nasopharyngeal swab sample was associated with lower rates of pulmonary complications in regions with high prevalence of COVID-19 and before major surgery, but not in regions with a low disease prevalence performing minor surgery.[10] The efficacy of universal testing in fully vaccinated patients and in communities with high vaccination rates remains unclear. As such, we recommend that institutional policies for preoperative testing be tailored to the local prevalence of COVID-19 and to available local resources. Testing may be deferred if a patient has tested positive within the last 90 days and meets the criteria for Ending Isolation and Precautions for People with COVID-19, as described by the Centers for Disease Control.[11]

Surgical Risk in Patients with Perioperative Coronavirus Disease-19

Surgical patients with COVID-19 represent a distinct population requiring special consideration to assess perioperative risk. A growing body of evidence shows a substantially higher risk of morbidity and mortality in patients undergoing surgery with perioperative COVID-19.[12–14] SARS-CoV-2 status should be considered in the decision for operative management, carefully weighing the expected operative benefits versus the postoperative risk associated with COVID-19. The precise prediction of surgical risk can be challenging in COVID-19 patients because it is unclear whether the established risk calculators for postoperative mortality and morbidity such as the Predictive OpTimal Trees in Emergency Surgery Risk Calculator and the American College of Surgeons (ACS)-Natiional Surgical Quality Improvement Program (NSQIP) Surgical Risk Calculator are applicable in the setting of SARS-CoV-2 infection.[15,16]

An early study evaluating the outcome of patients with perioperative COVID-19 (defined as the presence of SARS-CoV-2 infection within 7 days before or within 30 days after an operation) reported a remarkably high 30-day mortality rate of 23.8%.[14] In this international observational study including 1126 patients, 51.2% developed pulmonary complications in the postoperative period. A similar trend was observed in another prospective multicenter study assessing the impact of COVID-19 on outcomes in 70 US hospitals across 27 states: rates of 30-day mortality and postoperative pulmonary complications were 11.0% and 39.5%, respectively.[17] Other cohort studies demonstrated substantial variability in mortality from 5.4% to 42.8%.[18,19] This heterogeneity in mortality should be carefully interpreted as several studies were subject to selection bias in comparing outcomes between patients with COVID-19 versus without COVID-19. Patients in the COVID-19 arm were potentially sicker at baseline BECAUSE many centers had a higher threshold to operate on patients with COVID-19.[12,20] To address this potential selection bias, an observational study compared the surgical outcomes of COVID-19-positive patients to a propensity score-matched controls who underwent surgery during the same period and were COVID-19-negative.[21] Although this study did not find a statistically significant difference in 30-day mortality between the matched cohorts, patients with COVID-19 had higher 90-day mortality, a higher rate of complications (primarily pulmonary), and a higher rate of failure to rescue (mortality in patients who develop complications).[21] This study compared COVID-19-negative patients treated during the pandemic period (2020) to propensity score-matched patients treated before the pandemic (2019). Interestingly, patients undergoing surgery during the pandemic had a higher rate of failure to rescue events, suggesting that the perioperative risk associated with COVID-19 may not be solely related to the biological effects of SARS-CoV-2 infection, but also to the strain on health care systems. Based on these data suggesting an association between perioperative COVID-19 and a higher risk of postoperative morbidity and mortality, most studies recommended delaying nonessential surgical interventions and carefully weighing the benefits versus risks of all operative interventions in patients with current COVID-19 infection.[12,14,20]

Timing of Surgery After Severe Adult Respiratory Syndrome Coronavirus-2 Infection

The first large study examining the optimal timing of surgery following COVID-19 infection was an international, prospective, cohort study that enrolled more than 140,000 patients in October 2020.[22] Among them, 3127 patients were preoperatively diagnosed with COVID-19. This study demonstrated that patients operated within 7 weeks following COVID-19 diagnosis had a significantly increased risk of 30-day postoperative mortality and pulmonary complications compared with COVID-19-negative patients. In addition, there was a gradual and consistent relationship between the precise timing of surgery within 7 weeks of diagnosis and the risk of mortality, with the following odds ratios for specific time periods within 7 weeks: 0 to 2 weeks = 4.1 (95% CI, 3.3–4.8), 3 to 4 weeks = 3.9 (95% CI, 2.6–5.1), and 5 to 6 weeks = 3.6 (95% CI, 2.0–5.2). In contrast, there was no significant difference in mortality between patients who were operated at ≥7 weeks following COVID-19 diagnosis (and were asymptomatic at the time of surgery) and COVID-19-negative patients. However, patients with ongoing COVID-19-related symptoms at the time of surgery (even after 7 weeks following diagnosis) had significantly higher 30-day mortality. It should be noted that most studies evaluating outcomes of COVID-19 patients undergoing surgery were conducted before widespread vaccination and the emergence of novel virus variants (eg, delta, omicron). The APSF and ASA 2022 joint statement, on the timing of elective surgery after COVID-19 infection,[23] suggests the following waiting times between the COVID-19 diagnosis and surgery:

- Four weeks for an asymptomatic patient or a patient recovering from only mild, non-respiratory symptoms

- Six weeks for a symptomatic patient (eg, cough, dyspnea) who did not require hospitalization
- Eight to ten weeks for a symptomatic patient who is diabetic, immunocompromised, or hospitalized
- Twelve weeks for a patient who was admitted to an intensive care unit due to COVID-19 infection

Surgical and anesthesia societies from the United Kingdom similarly provided an updated multidisciplinary statement pertaining to the timing of elective surgery, which also recommended postponing elective surgery for 7 weeks following COVID-19 diagnosis, unless the benefits of immediate surgery clearly outweigh the risks of operation.[24] This statement also highlights the importance of preoperative vaccination and suggests that the last dose should be administered at least 2 weeks before the operation.

Risk of Contracting Severe Adult Respiratory Syndrome Coronavirus-2 Perioperatively

The risk of contracting COVID-19 perioperatively seems to be low. An international multicenter study, including 9171 patients from 447 hospitals and 55 countries, conducted during the first peak of the pandemic (Spring 2020) found that the rate of postoperative COVID-19 infection was as low as 3.2%.[25] The rates of postoperative COVID-19 infection, pulmonary complications, and mortality were lower in patients treated at hospitals implementing a COVID-19–free surgical pathway, defined as complete segregation of operating rooms, intensive care units, and inpatient ward areas used in the treatment of elective surgical patients versus patients with COVID-19.[25] In a single-center study from the United States during the initial peak of the pandemic (March 15–May 15, 2020), the rate of postoperative SARS-CoV-2 infection was reported at 1.8%.[26] Preoperative and intraoperative variables associated with postoperative SARS-CoV-2 infection were history of diabetes mellitus, cardiovascular disease, use of angiotensin receptor blockers, and surgery for liver transplantation.[26]

Trauma and Emergency Surgery

The COVID-19 pandemic has had a profound impact on acute care surgery including emergency general surgery and trauma surgery as well as on surgical critical care. During the first wave of the pandemic, and with the overwhelming number of critically ill COVID-19 patients and the need for critical care experts, most acute and critical care surgeons assumed the role of medical intensivists, caring for severely ill COVID-19 patients. Acute care surgeons also played a critical role in the management of devastating COVID-19 complications, such as COVID-19-related bowel ischemia (ie, COVID bowel).[27,28] One of the earliest studies evaluating the outcomes of patients undergoing emergency operations was conducted at two hospitals in New York City.[13] The findings revealed a substantially elevated risk of perioperative morbidity and mortality in this patient population which was later confirmed by several other large multicenter studies.[5,21,29] These studies recommended judicious consideration of nonoperative management for certain "emergent" surgical conditions or possibly delaying operative intervention. These data should be interpreted carefully as these studies did not evaluate outcomes after nonoperative management in COVID-19 patients. The results of the World Society of Emergency Surgery COVID-19 survey conducted in June 2020 on surgical specialists in emergency surgery revealed alarming results.[30] Respondents reported fewer emergency surgical patients, and an increased number of patients with more severe abdominal sepsis which might be associated with delayed presentation, potentially due to strains on health care systems and fear of contracting SARS-CoV-2 among patients.

Trauma teams similarly experienced reallocation of resources toward the treatment of COVID-19.[31] Following the implementation of stay-at-home orders, several studies, across different geographic locations, reported decreased overall trauma volume.[32–34] In the United States, several studies reported alterations in injury patterns: a markedly increased proportion of penetrating trauma potentially associated with increased gun violence or possibly a relative increase in the ratio due to decreased blunt trauma.[35,36] Despite lower patient volume, the pandemic presented significant challenges to trauma care. The contemporary management of the massively bleeding patient, largely based on early and balanced blood product transfusions while minimizing crystalloid infusions,[37] and most trauma centers had to adopt stringent transfusion practices because of critical blood shortage related to the pandemic.[38,39] Rehabilitation and physical therapy post-injury, which are associated with improved outcomes following injury, were limited to minimize hospital length of stay and ambulatory hospital visits.[40] A retrospective study evaluating the overall impact of COVID-19 on the outcomes of patients admitted to trauma centers across Pennsylvania between March and July 2020 reported an elevated risk of morbidity and mortality associated with COVID-19.[41]

Elective Surgery

Elective surgery was severely disrupted during the COVID-19 pandemic. During the initial peak, elective surgery came to a near-complete halt as hospitals were overwhelmed by the influx of severely ill patients and available resources were directed to the care of COVID-19 patients. Although such care was prioritized, a significant proportion of elective operations were canceled for benign and even malignant indications, creating a backlog of surgical cases that remains a burden after more than 2 years since the first peak. A global expert study estimated that during the peak 3-month period of the pandemic, nearly 28.5 million elective surgical cases were canceled worldwide (190 countries), with an overall cancellation rate of 72.3% (81.7% for benign conditions, 37.7% for malignant conditions).[42] The same study estimated that if countries increased surgical volume by 20% following the pandemic, it would take approximately 45 weeks to remedy the backlog created by the pandemic.[42] COVID-19 has also resulted in severe shortages in the supply of several surgical resources hindering the surgical volume of hospitals. In 2022, the American Red Cross, the major supplier of blood products in the United States, declared the most severe blood shortage crisis in more than the prior decade, suggesting that on certain days, hospitals may receive less than 25% of the blood products requested.[39] A significant shortage in contrast media used in computerized tomography imaging disrupted surgical care significantly since May 2022.[43] In response to the significant disruption of elective surgery, The ACS, ASA, Association of Perioperative Registered Nurses (APRN), and American Hospital Association (AHA) issued a joint statement suggesting a roadmap for resuming elective surgery after the COVID-19 pandemic.[44] This roadmap suggested that:

1. The prevalence of COVID-19 cases should be low for at least 14 days before resuming elective operations, and the facility should have the necessary resources (eg, ICU and floor beds, personal protective equipment [PPE], and ventilators) to care for elective surgical patients without the need for crisis-level operations.
2. The hospital should have adequate resources for SARS-CoV-2 laboratory testing and should implement a systematic protocol to test surgical patients and personnel for COVID-19.

3. The hospital should have adequate PPE and other surgical supplies before resuming elective cases.
4. A case prioritization committee should be established with the participation of surgery, anesthesia, and nursing to prioritize elective surgeries to best address the needs of the hospital's patient population.
5. The hospital should develop policies to address the impact of COVID-19 and case cancellations on the five phases of surgical care: preoperative, immediate preoperative, intraoperative, postoperative, and post-discharge care planning.
6. The hospital should collect local data on its COVID-19 and surgical practices and compare these data with regional and national data.
7. The hospital should implement safety and social distancing protocols to mitigate the risk of COVID-19 for patients, personnel, and visitors.

Oncological Surgery

Cancer surgeries are frequently time-sensitive and cannot be safely postponed for 2 to 3 months. These cases are considered "essential" operations and typically not classified as elective.[45] Efforts should be made to maintain cancer surgery despite the challenges posed by the pandemic. Cooperation between health care facilities could help maintain the regional quality of surgical cancer care, despite capacity issues or other problems at individual hospitals. The joint statement by the ACS, ASA, APRN, and AHA for maintaining essential surgery during the pandemic provides a valuable guide for the delivery of essential surgical care.[46]

Anesthesia Considerations

The choice of anesthesia should be primarily dictated by the individual operation and patient characteristics. The use of regional anesthesia (neuraxial anesthesia or nerve blocks) can eliminate the need for endotracheal intubation and decrease aerosol production. If intubation is not required, the patient should wear a surgical mask during the procedure unless contraindicated. Endotracheal intubation and extubation produce high amounts of aerosols and are high-risk procedures for transmission. High-level PPE (respirator, eye/face protection, gown, and gloves) is required for personnel performing these airway procedures. The number of personnel in the operating room during intubation should be minimized. Low volume and low pressure breaths should be delivered during bag-mask ventilation to potentially decrease exposure to aerosol contamination. In patients with difficult airways and no contraindications, rapid sequence intubation is an acceptable strategy to minimize time to intubation and aerosol production.

Postoperative Follow-up

Physicians should anticipate and prepare for challenges in postoperative follow-up during the COVID-19 pandemic. Patients with perioperative SARS-CoV-2 infection have a higher risk of postoperative morbidity and mortality, compared with non-COVID patients undergoing the same operations. Specifically, they have higher rates of postoperative thrombotic and pulmonary complications, and potentially a lower rate of bleeding complications (Argandykov and colleagues 2022, unpublished data). Clinicians should adjust their postoperative protocol and weigh the benefit versus harm of potential interventions (eg, thromboprophylaxis) in light of these data.

Some institutions have implemented telemedicine perioperative appointments to minimize the number of office or ambulatory hospital visits. A single-center retrospective study from the United States concluded that postoperative visits via telemedicine did not increase the risk of readmission compared with in-person visits after oncologic surgery.[47] Health care providers should use telemedicine judiciously as needed, considering patient factors, local COVID-19 prevalence, and institutional resources.

Surgical Research

The clinical burden imposed by the COVID-19 pandemic severely restricted the ability of surgeon-scientists to conduct research studies.[48] The vast majority of research resources were directed toward elucidating the pathogenesis and improving treatment of COVID-19. The impact of the pandemic seems to be more significant on female researchers. A retrospective analysis of submissions to Journal of the American Medical Association Surgery found that a significantly lower percentage of manuscripts with female corresponding authors were submitted in April to May of 2020 versus 2019.[49] After the COVID-19 pandemic, it will be important to address the recession in research areas not related to COVID-19 and the apparent gender disparity in academic publications.

SUMMARY

The ongoing COVID-19 pandemic presents multiple clinical, logistical, and academic challenges for surgery. Surgical providers should adapt to the rapidly evolving pandemic to provide the best possible care to patients, ensure the safety of health care personnel, and advanced surgery through academic research.

DISCLOSURE

The authors have nothing to disclose.

REFERENCES

1. Zhu N, Zhang D, Wang W, et al. A Novel Coronavirus from Patients with Pneumonia in China, 2019. N Engl J Med 2020;382(8):727–33.
2. Albutt K, Luckhurst CM, Alba GA, et al. Design and Impact of a COVID-19 Multidisciplinary Bundled Procedure Team. Ann Surg 2020;272(2):e72–3.
3. Center for Disease Control and Prevention (CDC). Symptoms of COVID-19. Available at: https://www.cdc.gov/coronavirus/2019-ncov/symptoms-testing/symptoms.html. Accessed June 24, 2022.
4. American Society of Anesthesiologists. Anesthesia Patient Safety Foundation. ASA and APSF Joint Statement on Elective Surgery and Anesthesia for Patients after COVID-19 Infection. Available at: https://www.asahq.org/about-asa/newsroom/news-releases/2020/12/asa-and-apsf-joint-statement-on-elective-surgery-and-anesthesia-for-patients-after-covid-19-infection. Accessed June 24, 2022.
5. Gebran A, Gaitanidis A, Argandykov D, et al. Mortality & Pulmonary Complications in Emergency General Surgery Patients with Mortality COVID-19: A Large International Multicenter Study. J Trauma Acute Care Surg 2022;93(1):59–65.
6. Infectious Disease Society of America. COVID-19 Prioritization of Diagnostic Testing. Available at: https://www.idsociety.org/globalassets/idsa/public-health/covid-19-prioritization-of-dx-testing.pdf. Accessed June 23, 2022.
7. Center for Disease Control and Prevention (CDC). Infection Control: Severe acute respiratory syndrome coronavirus 2 (SARS-CoV-2) | CDC. Available at: https://www.cdc.gov/coronavirus/2019-ncov/hcp/infection-control-recommendations.html. Accessed June 23, 2022.

8. World Health Organization (WHO). Infection prevention and control during health care when novel coronavirus (nCoV) infection is suspected. Available at: https://www.who.int/publications/i/item/10665-331495. Accessed June 23, 2022.
9. American Society of Anesthesiologists, Anesthesia Patient Safety Foundation. ASA and APSF Statement on Perioperative Testing for the COVID-19 Virus | American Society of Anesthesiologists (ASA). Available at: https://www.asahq.org/about-asa/newsroom/news-releases/2021/08/asa-and-apsf-statement-on-perioperative-testing-for-the-covid-19-virus. Accessed June 23, 2022.
10. Glasbey JC, Omar O, Nepogodiev D, et al. Preoperative nasopharyngeal swab testing and postoperative pulmonary complications in patients undergoing elective surgery during the SARS-CoV-2 pandemic. Br J Surg 2021;108(1):88–96.
11. Center for Disease Control and Prevention (CDC). Ending Isolation and Precautions for People with COVID-19: Interim Guidance. Available at: https://www.cdc.gov/coronavirus/2019-ncov/hcp/duration-isolation.html. Accessed June 23, 2022.
12. Doglietto F, Vezzoli M, Gheza F, et al. Factors Associated with Surgical Mortality and Complications among Patients with and without Coronavirus Disease 2019 (COVID-19) in Italy. JAMA Surg 2020;155(8):691–702.
13. Knisely A, Zhou ZN, Wu J, et al. Perioperative morbidity and mortality of patients with COVID-19 who undergo urgent and emergent surgical procedures. Ann Surg 2021;273(1):34–40.
14. Bhangu A, Nepogodiev D, Glasbey JC, et al. Mortality and pulmonary complications in patients undergoing surgery with perioperative sars-cov-2 infection: An international cohort study. Lancet 2020;396(10243):27–38.
15. Bertsimas D, Dunn J, Velmahos GC, et al. Surgical Risk Is Not Linear: Derivation and Validation of a Novel, User-friendly, and Machine-learning-based Predictive OpTimal Trees in Emergency Surgery Risk (POTTER) Calculator. Ann Surg 2018;268(4):574–83.
16. Bilimoria KY, Liu Y, Paruch JL, et al. Development and Evaluation of the Universal ACS NSQIP Surgical Risk Calculator: A Decision Aid and Informed Consent Tool for Patients and Surgeons. J Am Coll Surg 2013;217(5):833–42.e3.
17. COVIDSurg Collaborative. Outcomes and Their State-level Variation in Patients Undergoing Surgery With Perioperative SARS-CoV-2 Infection in the USA: A Prospective Multicenter Study. Ann Surg 2022;275(2):247–51.
18. Guadalajara H, Muñoz de Nova JL, Fernandez Gonzalez S, et al. Patterns of acute surgical inflammatory processes presentation of in the COVID-19 outbreak (PIACO Study): Surgery may be the best treatment option. Br J Surg 2020; 107(11):e494–5.
19. González-Calatayud DM, Vargas-Ábrego DB, Gutiérrez-Uvalle DGE, et al. Observational study of the suspected or confirmed cases of sars COV-2 infection needing emergency surgical intervention during the first months of the pandemic in a third level hospital: Case series. Ann Med Surg 2020;60:149–54.
20. Jonker PKC, van der Plas WY, Steinkamp PJ, et al. Perioperative SARS-CoV-2 infections increase mortality, pulmonary complications, and thromboembolic events: A Dutch, multicenter, matched-cohort clinical study. Surgery (United States) 2021;169(2):264–74.
21. Osorio J, Madrazo Z, Videla S, et al. Analysis of outcomes of emergency general and gastrointestinal surgery during the COVID-19 pandemic. Br J Surg 2021; 108(12):1438–47.
22. Timing of surgery following SARS-CoV-2 infection: an international prospective cohort study. Anaesthesia 2021;76(6):748–58.

23. https://www.apsf.org/news-updates/asa-and-apsf-joint-statement-on-elective-surgery-and-anesthesia-for-patients-after-covid-19-infection/. Accessed 23 June 2022.
24. El-Boghdadly K, Cook TM, Goodacre T, et al. Timing of elective surgery and risk assessment after SARS-CoV-2 infection: an update. Anaesthesia 2022;77(5):580–7.
25. Glasbey JC, Nepogodiev D, Simoes JFF, et al. Elective Cancer Surgery in COVID-19-Free Surgical Pathways during the SARS-CoV-2 Pandemic: An International, Multicenter, Comparative Cohort Study. J Clin Oncol 2021;39(1):66–78.
26. Axiotakis LG, Youngerman BE, Casals RK, et al. Risk of Acquiring Perioperative COVID-19 During the Initial Pandemic Peak: A Retrospective Cohort Study. Ann Surg 2020;273(1):41–8.
27. Kaafarani HMA, el Moheb M, Hwabejire JO, et al. Gastrointestinal Complications in Critically Ill Patients With COVID-19. Ann Surg 2020;272(2):e61–2.
28. el Moheb M, Naar L, Christensen MA, et al. Gastrointestinal Complications in Critically Ill Patients with and without COVID-19. JAMA 2020;324(18):1899–901.
29. Winter Beatty J, Clarke JM, Sounderajah V, et al. Impact of the COVID-19 Pandemic on Emergency Adult Surgical Patients and Surgical Services: An International Multi-center Cohort Study and Department Survey. Ann Surg 2021;274(6):904–12.
30. Reichert M, Sartelli M, Weigand MA, et al. Impact of the SARS-CoV-2 pandemic on emergency surgery services—a multi-national survey among WSES members. World J Emerg Surg 2020;15(1). https://doi.org/10.1186/s13017-020-00341-0.
31. Haut ER, Leeds IL, Livingston DH. The Effect on Trauma Care Secondary to the COVID-19 Pandemic: Collateral Damage From Diversion of Resources. Ann Surg 2020;272(3):e204–7.
32. DiFazio LT, Curran T, Bilaniuk JW, et al. The Impact of the COVID-19 Pandemic on Hospital Admissions for Trauma and Acute Care Surgery. Am Surg 2020;86(8):901–3.
33. Manuel Aranda-Narvá ez J, Talló n-Aguilar L, Pareja-Ciuró F, et al. Emergency Surgery and Trauma Care during COVID-19 Pandemic. Recommendations of the Spanish Association of Surgeons §. Cir Esp (Engl Ed 2020;98(8):433–41. Available at: www.elsevier.es/cirugia.
34. Hakkenbrak NAG, Loggers SAI, Lubbers E, et al. Trauma care during the COVID-19 pandemic in the Netherlands: a level 1 trauma multicenter cohort study. Scand J Trauma Resuscitation Emerg Med 2021;29(1). https://doi.org/10.1186/s13049-021-00942-x.
35. Berg GM, Wyse RJ, Morse JL, et al. Decreased adult trauma admission volumes and changing injury patterns during the COVID-19 pandemic at 85 trauma centers in a multistate healthcare system. Trauma Surg Acute Care Open 2021;6(1). https://doi.org/10.1136/tsaco-2020-000642.
36. Hatchimonji JS, Swendiman RA, Seamon MJ, et al. Trauma Does not Quarantine: Violence During the COVID-19 Pandemic. Ann Surg 2020;272(2):e53–4.
37. Holcomb JB, Jenkins D, Rhee P, et al. Damage control resuscitation: Directly addressing the early coagulopathy of trauma. J Trauma 2007;62(2):307–10.
38. Vanderbilt University Medical Center. Blood Conservation Strategies During COVID-19. Published 2020.
39. American Red Cross. Red Cross Declares First-ever Blood Crisis amid Omicron Surge. Available at: https://www.redcross.org/about-us/news-and-events/press-release/2022/blood-donors-needed-now-as-omicron-intensifies.html. Accessed June 23, 2022.

40. Hakiki B, Grippo A, Scarpino M, et al. Effects of COVID-19 pandemic on intensive rehabilitation after severe acquired brain injuries. Neurol Sci 2021;43(2):791–8.
41. Kaufman EJ, Ong AW, Cipolle MD, et al. The impact of COVID-19 infection on outcomes after injury in a state trauma system. J Trauma Acute Care Surg 2021; 91(3):559–65.
42. Nepogodiev D, Omar OM, Glasbey JC, et al. Elective surgery cancellations due to the COVID-19 pandemic: global predictive modelling to inform surgical recovery plans. Br J Surg 2020;107(11):1440–9.
43. American Hospital Association. Shortage of Contrast Media for CT Imaging Affecting Hospitals and Health Systems | AHA. Available at: https://www.aha.org/advisory/2022-05-12-shortage-contrast-media-ct-imaging-affecting-hospitals-and-health-systems. Accessed June 23, 2022.
44. American College of Surgeons, American Society of Anesthesiologists. Association of Perioperative Registered Nurses, American Hospital Association. Joint Statement: Roadmap for Resuming Elective Surgery after COVID-19 Pandemic. Available at: https://www.facs.org/for-medical-professionals/covid-19/clinical-guidance/roadmap-elective-surgery/. Accessed June 23, 2022.
45. Laura A, Thomas B, Jeffrey D, et al. Cancer Surgery and COVID19. Ann Surg Oncol 2020;27(6):1713–6.
46. American College of Surgeons. American Society of Anesthesiologists, Association of Perioperative Registered Nurses, American Hospital Association. Joint Statement: Roadmap for Maintaining Essential Surgery during COVID-19 Pandemic. Available at: https://www.facs.org/for-medical-professionals/covid-19/clinical-guidance/roadmap-maintain-essential-surgery/. Accessed June 23, 2022.
47. Uppal A, Kothari AN, Scally CP, et al. Adoption of Telemedicine for Postoperative Follow-Up After Inpatient Cancer-Related Surgery. JCO Oncol Pract 2022;18(7): e1091–9.
48. Tuttle KR. Impact of the COVID-19 pandemic on clinical research. Nat Rev Nephrol 2020;16(10):562–4.
49. Kibbe MR. Consequences of the COVID-19 Pandemic on Manuscript Submissions by Women. Arch Surg (Chicago 1960) 2020;155(9):803–4.

Diagnostic and Therapeutic Radiology of the GI Tract, Liver, and Pancreas in Patients with COVID

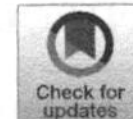

Piero Boraschi, MD[a,*], Francescamaria Donati, MD[a], Ilaria Ambrosini, MD[b], Luciana Bruni, MD[b], Maria Letizia Mazzeo, MD[b], Rachele Tintori, MD[a], Michele Tonerini, MD[c], Emanuele Neri, MD[b]

KEYWORDS

• Gastrointestinal findings • Hepatobiliary findings • Pancreatic findings • COVID-19 • SARS-CoV-2 • Computed tomography • Ultrasound • Interventional radiology

KEY POINTS

- Imaging findings have been recently investigated regarding gastrointestinal, hepatobiliary, and pancreatic involvement with coronavirus disease 2019 (COVID-19) infection.
- Radiological findings of gastrointestinal, hepatic, and pancreatic involvement in patients with COVID-19 are generally nonspecific.
- Ultrasound and particularly computed tomography with multiphasic acquisition are the primary diagnostic methods used in COVID-19 patients to evaluate the significance of gastrointestinal, hepatobiliary, and pancreatic clinical symptoms and signs.
- Imaging should be performed if abdominal or gastrointestinal disease is suspected in COVID-19 patients.
- Diagnostic imaging modalities, particularly computed tomography, are helpful to evaluate and manage COVID-19 patients with gastrointestinal, hepatic, and pancreatic involvement.

[a] 2nd Unit of Radiology, Department of Diagnostic and Interventional Radiology, and Nuclear Medicine, Pisa University Hospital, Via Paradisa 2, Pisa 56124, Italy; [b] Academic Radiology, Department of Translational Research, University of Pisa, Via Roma 67, Pisa 56126, Italy; [c] Unit of Emergency Radiology, Department of Surgical, Medical, Molecular and Critical Area Pathology, Pisa University Hospital, Via Paradisa 2, Pisa 56124, Italy

* Corresponding author. 2nd Unit of Radiology, Department of Diagnostic and Interventional Radiology, and Nuclear Medicine - Pisa University Hospital, Via Paradisa 2, 56124 Pisa, Italy.

E-mail addresses: p.boraschi@gmail.com; p.boraschi@do.med.unipi.it

Twitter: @PBoraschi (P.B.)

Gastroenterol Clin N Am 52 (2023) 185–200

https://doi.org/10.1016/j.gtc.2022.10.006

INTRODUCTION

The lungs are the primarily involved organs in coronavirus disease 2019 (COVID-19), but COVID-19 infection is a systemic disease, with tropism for the vascular system, which can cause variable and widespread clinical manifestations that frequently involve the gastrointestinal tract and hepatobiliary system and infrequently involve the pancreas.[1,2] Accordingly, imaging modalities play a pivotal role in patients with abdominal and gastrointestinal symptoms and signs to investigate possible abdominal features of SARS-CoV-2 infection.[3] Abdominal ultrasound (US) is frequently the first imaging examination that clinicians request to evaluate patients with abdominal discomfort, especially in intensive care unit (ICU) patients.[4] However, US has a limited role in evaluating gastrointestinal involvement, and it is primarily requested to evaluate the hepatobiliary system and portal vein patency.[4,5] In a study of 30 ICU COVID-19 patients, the most frequent findings on abdominal US included hepatomegaly in 23/41 (56%) which is often associated with elevated liver function tests and a bright echo pattern of the liver parenchyma and biliary system disease in 17/41 (41.5%) such as gallbladder distention, biliary sludge, gallbladder wall thickening, and common bile duct dilatation. Nephropathy was the third most common US abnormality which occurred in 7/41 (17%).[4] Nonetheless, US can show life-threatening conditions. For example, Bhayana and colleagues reported on an ICU patient who had portal venous gas incidentally detected at abdominal US and subsequently confirmed by computed tomography (CT).[1]

Abdominal magnetic resonance (MR) is rarely performed in patients with COVID-19 infection because it is time-consuming and difficult to perform in patients with respiratory disease.[6] Moreover, MR rarely leads to a change in diagnosis or management related to COVID-19,[7] as demonstrated by Anderson and colleagues in a study of 1107 COVID-19 patients. Main MRI indications were unrelated to SARS-CoV-2 infection in 75%, and MRI was performed for workup of acute liver dysfunction in 25%.[7]

Abdominal CT plays a crucial role in identifying abdominal involvement due to COVID-19 infection, particularly for the gastrointestinal tract. CT should routinely include the baseline and post-contrast acquisitions in the arterial, portal venous, and delayed phases.

Radiology also plays an important role in the management of COVID-19-related complications using interventional radiology (IR) procedures. Lee and colleagues[8] described the most common interventional procedures in a series of 724 COVID-19 patients: central venous catheter placement for hemodialysis in 31.5% in patients with renal failure; inferior vena cava filter placement in 9.7% in selected patient with venous thromboembolism; angiography/embolization in 4.8% in patients with bleeding complications; gastrostomy tube placement in 9.7%; image-guided biopsy in 10.5%; abscess drainage in 9.7%; and cholecystostomy tube placement in 6.5%.

Gastrointestinal Tract

The gastrointestinal tract is a well-known route of COVID-19 infection as demonstrated by the finding of the SARS-CoV-2 viral ribonucleic acid in stool.[3] The gastrointestinal tract is the most common site of extrapulmonary involvement of COVID-19 disease (11.4%–61.1%),[9] with manifestations of variable severity. As summarized by Zhang and colleagues, subgroups of COVID-19 patients can be identified by (1) the presence of gastrointestinal symptoms without respiratory symptoms; (2) the concurrent presence of gastrointestinal and respiratory symptoms; and (3) gastrointestinal involvement before the occurrence of respiratory symptoms.[3] Gastrointestinal symptoms during SARS-CoV-2 infection are generally nonspecific and usually mild and self-limiting (diarrhea, vomiting, abdominal distension). However, patients can occasionally present with acute abdominal pain due to intestinal obstruction, bowel ischemia, acute appendicitis, hemoperitoneum, or disorders involving other abdominal organs.[9]

As gastrointestinal signs are frequently observed in COVID-19 patients, a correct abdominal diagnosis and correlation with SARS-CoV-2 infections has become more important. Various studies report that abdominal symptoms at the onset of the infection may not be appreciated promptly as related to COVID-19, thus delaying the diagnosis and therapy with a consequent higher risk of complications.[10] Moreover, gastrointestinal involvement in COVID-19 has been associated with a worse disease outcome, expressed by longer hospital stay, and the need for mechanical ventilation.[9,11]

Bhayana and colleagues reported that COVID-19 patients in the ICU are more likely to have gastrointestinal involvement than other in-patients (65% vs 23%, $P = .04$).[1] Horvat and colleagues, in a multicenter study of 81 COVID-19 patients, correlated the abdominal radiological features with clinical outcome; they reported that abnormal abdominal imaging findings were associated with an increased risk of bad outcomes (death/invasive mechanical ventilation; RR = 2.6, $P = .04$), invasive mechanical ventilation (RR = 6.2, $P = .05$), longer hospital stay (adjusted difference: +6.2 days, $P = .1$), and longer ICU stay (adjusted difference: +7.1, $P = .07$).[12]

Abdominal CT is the main imaging modality in the diagnosis of COVID-19 patients with nonspecific abdominal symptoms (including abdominal pain, diarrhea, nausea, and vomiting) and suspicion of complications (intestinal ischemia and sporadic gastrointestinal bleeding).[5,6,12] Abdominal CT may also be useful in suggesting the diagnosis of SARS-CoV-2 infection in patients with abdominal features and ground-glass opacities at lung bases.[6] The most common CT findings in symptomatic and asymptomatic patients are bowel wall abnormalities, bowel wall inflammation (gastritis, enterocolitis), and bowel wall ischemia.[12] Thrombosis of great abdominal vessels can be detected as a filling defect on CT angiography.[1,5,6] However, abdominal imaging findings can be absent in some patients complaining of abdominal symptoms due to the complex pathogenesis of enterocyte damage which is still not clear, with possible factors causing direct viral mucosal injury, increased intraluminal pressure, gut microbiota impairment, lymphoid atrophy, and vessel thrombosis (arterial macro/micro-thrombosis and venous occlusion).[13] The most common CT features of gastritis and enterocolitis are fluid-filled and distended bowel lumen (43%) and mural thickening of large and small intestine due to submucosal edema and mucosal hyperenhancement (**Fig. 1**). Enterocolitis can be segmental in early stages and worsen to become pancolitis.[2] Perivisceral fat stranding, abdominal free fluid, and isolated mesenteric nodal enlargement are common associated findings because of COVID-19-induced inflammatory responses.[2,5] Moreover, thrombosis of the arterioles can cause mesenteric congestion, as demonstrated by autopsy studies.[12]

COVID-19-related bowel ischemia is a life-threatening emergency.[10] CT findings range from a contracted gasless bowel loop appearance (early stage) to dilated gas-filled bowel loops with a paper-thin bowel wall (intermediate stage) and to a late ischemic stage characterized by intestinal wall pneumatosis with or without portomesenteric gas, lack of mucosal enhancement, and luminal dilatation which could cause intestinal perforation (**Fig. 2**). Pneumatosis intestinalis with intramural bowel gas is a rare sign of intestinal ischemia (**Fig. 3**), but it is nonspecific as this finding can also occur with other conditions such as mechanical ventilation or pneumomediastinum.[14] Bowel perforation is not always visible on CT, but may be suspected when associated features such as fat stranding, perivisceral fluid/abscess, or pneumoperitoneum are present.

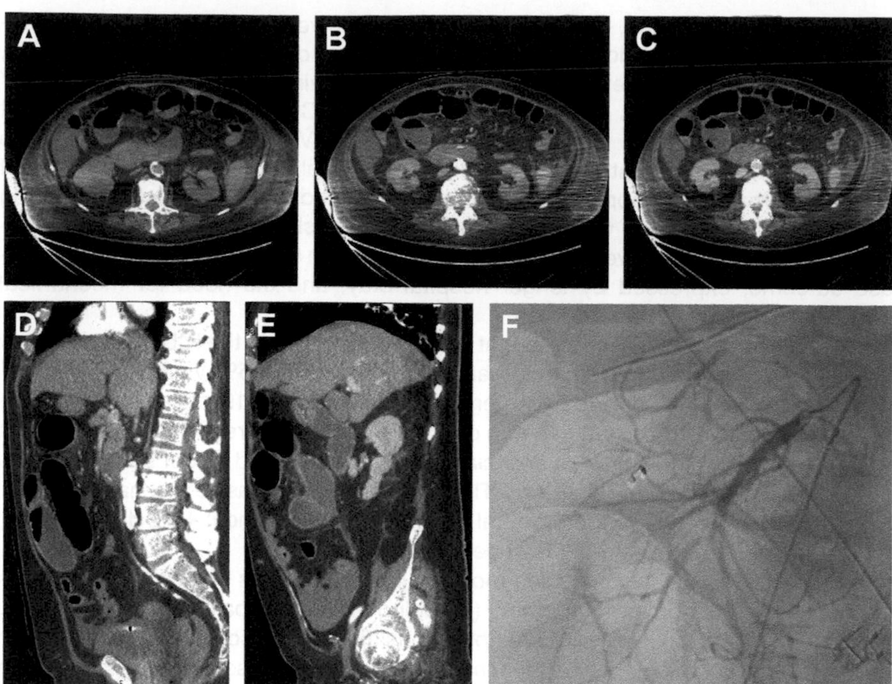

Fig. 1. A 72-year-old man with COVID-19-infection was referred for abdominal CT after presentation with abdominal pain and tenderness and a haemoglobin decline. (*A*) An axial non-contrast CT image showed distended duodenum from hyperdense hematic content in the lumen. (*B*) Arterial phase of contrast-enhanced CT shows a contrast blush in the lumen of the horizontal duodenum that persists in the venous phase (*C*), indicating active arterial bleeding. Peritoneal free-fluid (peri-splenic in the image) was present as an associated finding. (*D*) Sagittal reconstruction shows an active arterial blush into the lumen of the horizontal duodenum. Active bleeding from a duodenal ulcer was stopped by endoscopic therapy. Owing to worsening anemia, an abdominal CT was performed (*D–F*). Non-enhanced sagittal reconstruction (*E*) shows persistence of duodenal distension due to high-density content, extending to the proximal jejunal loop, and increased density of diffuse peritoneal fluid, suggesting hemoperitoneum. Note distension of other bowel loops and peritoneal fluid as signs of gastrointestinal involvement (*E*). Post-contrast CT image did not show signs of active bleeding; however, angiography was still performed. Angiographic study showed arterial blush coming from tiny branches in the duodenum. Super-selective embolization of gastroduodenal branches was performed using coils. Angiographic study of the SMA (Superior Mesenteric Artery) and IMA (Inferior Mesenteric Artery)(*E*) showed no other bleeding source.

Gastrointestinal bleeding is rare and occurs in about 3% of COVID-19 patients.[1,2] It presents as a hyperdense fluid within gastric or bowel lumen detected on CT images (see **Fig. 1**; **Fig. 4**). Martin and colleagues[15] in a matched (1:2) case-control study of 41 cases of COVID-19-related gastrointestinal bleeding (31 upper and 10 lower) found that the most common aetiologies of gastrointestinal bleeding were gastric or duodenal peptic ulcers (80%) in upper gastrointestinal bleeding and rectal ulceration (50%) in lower gastrointestinal bleeding. However, etiology is multifactorial and still not completely known[15]; it could be secondary to factors related to treatment (anticoagulation) and critical illness, more than direct viral damage on enterocytes.[15] GI bleeding in COVID-19-infected patients is reviewed in an accompanying chapter in this

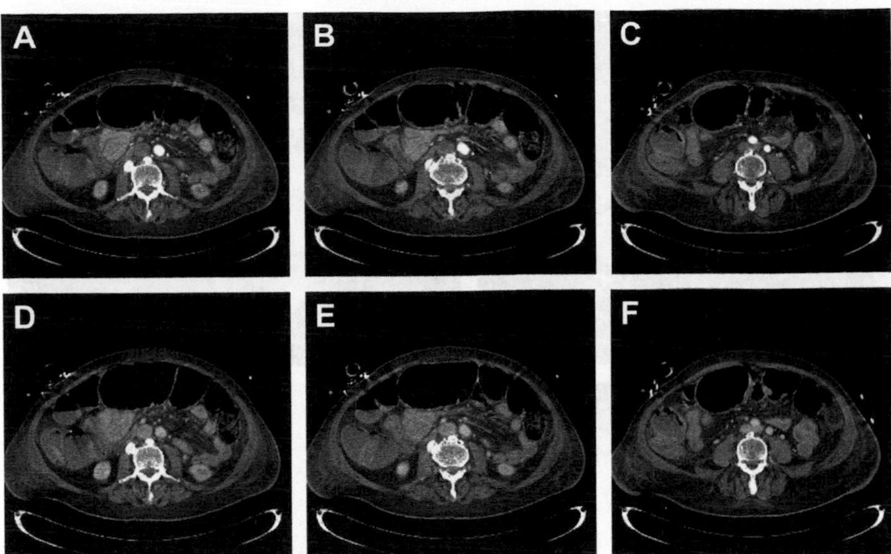

Fig. 2. A 75-year-old man was admitted from the emergency department because of abdominal pain. Despite an absence of respiratory symptoms or signs, a COVID-19Polymerase Chain Reaction (PCR)test was positive. Abdominal CT was performed. Post-contrast acquisitions (*A–C* arterial phase; *D–F* venous phase) show a distended and atonic caecum, reduced enhancement of the bowel wall, and signs of pneumatosis, suggesting intestinal ischemia. A distended, air-filled, and atonic transverse colon was also present.

monograph by Cappell and Friedel.[16] Endoscopy is the standard for the diagnosis and treatment of gastrointestinal bleeding.[17]

Trans-arterial endovascular embolization (TAE) is a viable alternative treatment in patients with COVID-19. In a multicenter retrospective observational study, TAE had a minor risk of aerosol COVID-19 transmission to angiography staff and of respiratory exacerbation in patients undergoing the angiography.[15] TAE is a safe and effective alternative in this patient population with technical and clinical success rates of embolization of 88.2% and 94.1%, respectively.[15] Moreover, another international multicenter retrospective observational study[18] showed that TAE had technical and clinical success in 100% and 90.9% of patients, respectively.[18] Rebleeding occurred in one patient (9%) who then needed a complementary therapeutic endoscopy. Mortality within 30 days after embolization was 0%. Minor complications occurred in 18.2%, including a groin hematoma and an ischemic rectal ulcer, both of which were managed conservatively.[18]

Liver and Biliary Tract

Liver involvement occurs in up to 45% of patients with COVID-19, particularly in patients with severe viral infection.[19,20] Several mechanisms contribute to the liver injury: systemic inflammatory process, drugs, hypoxia, and the direct effect of SARS-CoV-2. The virus directly enters and injures cholangiocytes, which contain the angiotensin-converting enzyme-2 receptor in the same proportion as the alveolar cells of the lungs,[10,21] whereas this receptor is less represented in hepatocytes.[21] The simultaneous presence of multiple pathogenic factors causes a generalized coagulopathy with consequent micro-thrombosis within the sinusoids and consequent necrosis, lymphocytic infiltration of the sinusoids, and hepatic fibrosis or crrhosis.[10,21]

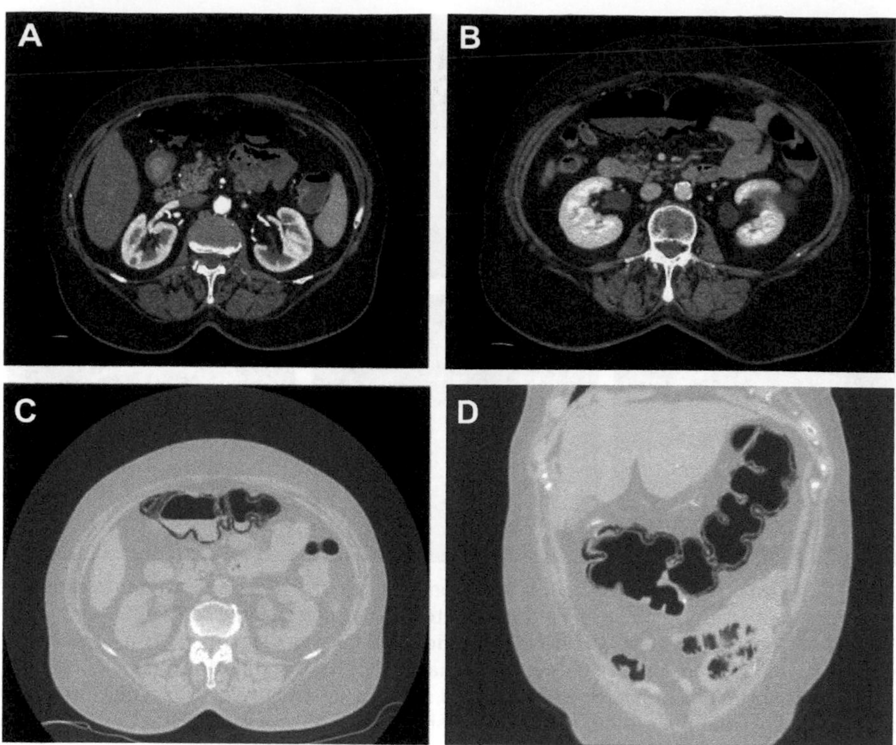

Fig. 3. A 76-year-old woman with COVID-19 infection underwent a thorax CT scan for suspicion of interstitial pneumonia. CT scan was extended to the abdomen due to findings on the transverse colon. CT post-contrast acquisitions (*A, B*) confirmed transverse colon distention with wall thickening, air-fluid levels, and lack of wall enhancement in the arterial phase (*A*). Windowing showed the presence of pneumatosis intestinalis through the wall layers, indicating intestinal ischemia (*C, D*). No obstruction of the major vessels was seen. The patient underwent laparoscopic surgery and resection of the necrotic colon with ileostomy.

The most frequent radiological features are hepatic steatosis, and the formation of gallbladder sludge and gallstones often complicated by cholecystitis and sometimes complicated by secondary sclerosing cholangitis (SSC).[22] There is an increased frequency of hepatic steatosis on CT scans in COVID-19 patients compared with uninfected controls, although some patients may have had abnormal liver function before SARS-CoV-2 infection, from disorders such as nonalcoholic fatty liver disease or chronic hepatitis B.[23] Moreover, the higher prevalence of hepatic steatosis is probably due to the known association between COVID-19 infection and obesity[23] and the known association between pre-existing liver disease and COVID-19 infection. Steatosis is common in COVID-19 patients. It occurs because the virus affects mitochondrial activity, inhibits autophagy, and promotes lipogenesis.[24] The classic signs of steatosis on US are a luminous hepatic pattern (the presence of numerous fine, intense and dense parenchymal echoes, which give the hepatic parenchyma an echogenicity higher than that of the cortex of the right kidney) and the sign of attenuation (deep attenuation of ultrasonic echoes, associated with poor visibility of the diaphragm and echogenic portal, and suprahepatic vascular walls).[25,26] The evaluation

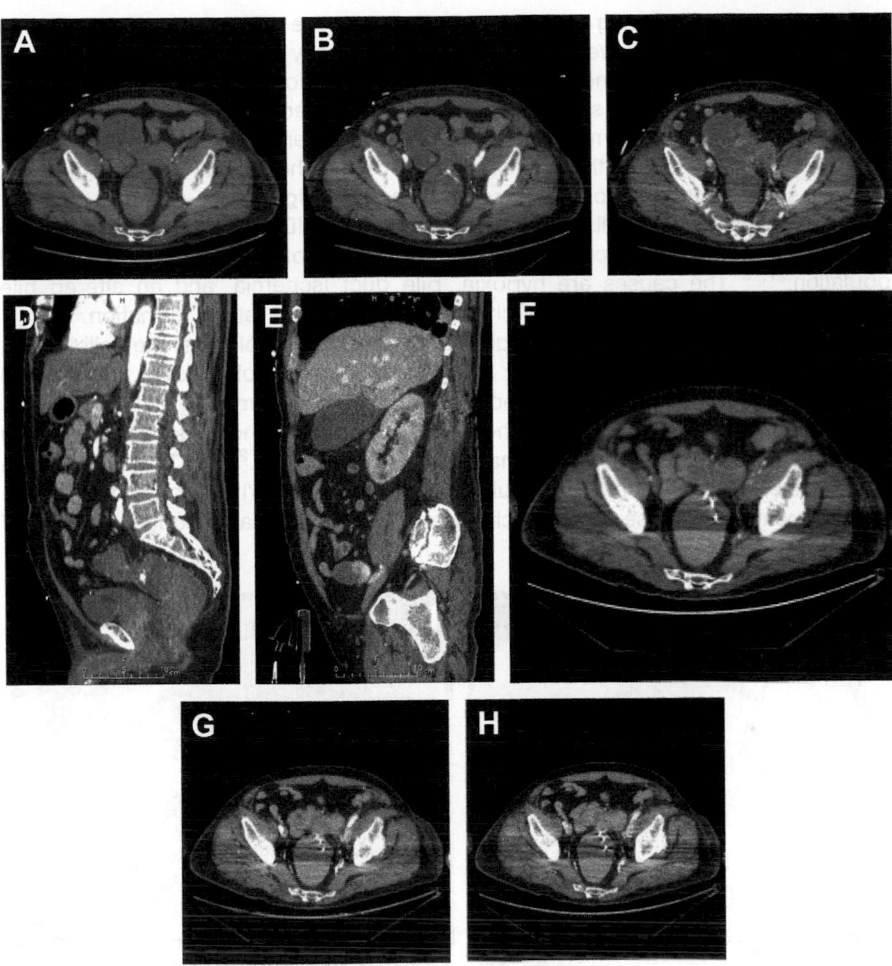

Fig. 4. A 66-year old patient with COVID-19-infection and slight pulmonary symptoms was admitted from the emergency department because of rectal bleeding. Laboratory tests showed lowered haemoglobin; rectal examination seemed to exclude hemorrhoidal bleeding. An abdominal CT scan was performed. (*A*) Axial non-contrast CT image shows distention of sigmoid colon and rectum due to hyperdense intraluminal fluid, suspicious for hematic content. (*B*) Arterial phase of contrast-enhanced CT shows medium contrast blush at left side of rectal-sigmoid junction that persists in the venous phase (*C*), indicating active arterial bleeding. Moreover, in the venous phase a bleeding focus is better appreciated in the proximal sigmoid colon. Patient underwent an endoscopic procedure to stop the bleeding and 5 days later another CT scan was performed. (*D, E*) Sagittal reconstruction shows active arterial blush of medium contrast at rectosigmoid junction (*D*) and proximal sigmoid colon (*E*). (*F–H*) Unenhanced CT images show persistence of hyperdense fluid in rectal ampulla (*D*) without signs of active bleeding in sigmoid colon or rectum, on the arterial (*E*) and venous phases (*F*).

of hepatic steatosis with CT is performed by calculating hepatic hypoattenuation; if the liver density is less than 10 Hounsfield units (HU) compared with the spleen density, the steatosis is mild, whereas if the density is greater than 40 HU, the steatosis is moderate/severe.[26]

MRI is the primary imaging modality for both qualitative and quantitative evaluation of hepatic steatosis. Fatty liver has a high signal intensity on T1-weighted images; in addition, several MRI sequences, including fat suppression sequences and chemical shift imaging with dual-echo sequences, facilitate fat detection. Specifically, chemical displacement imaging determines whether lipid and water protons are present within the same small voxel space (three-dimensional pixel). In the case of fatty liver disease, there is a signal drop in opposed-phase sequences[26] (**Fig. 5**).

Gallbladder sludge and gallstones are common in COVID-19 patients. They develop in 54% of infected patients compared with the incidence of 10% to 20% in the general population.[27,28] The causes are hypoxia, bile duct ischemia, and an altered bile composition, resulting in necrosis of cholangiocytes and gallstone formation.[28]

US is currently the reference technique for evaluating pathology of the gallbladder, macro- and microlithiasis, gallbladder sludge, and cholesterol deposits. Cholesterol deposition appears as hyperechoic spots with the typical "comet sign," biliary sludge as sediment in the sloping portion of the gallbladder lumen, and gallstones appearing as hyperechogenic with a posterior shadow cone, if calcified.[29,30] CT usually plays a marginal role, although it can be helpful in uncooperative COVID-19 patients; calcium stones appear hyperdense, whereas cholesterol stones appear hypodense.[10] Even if

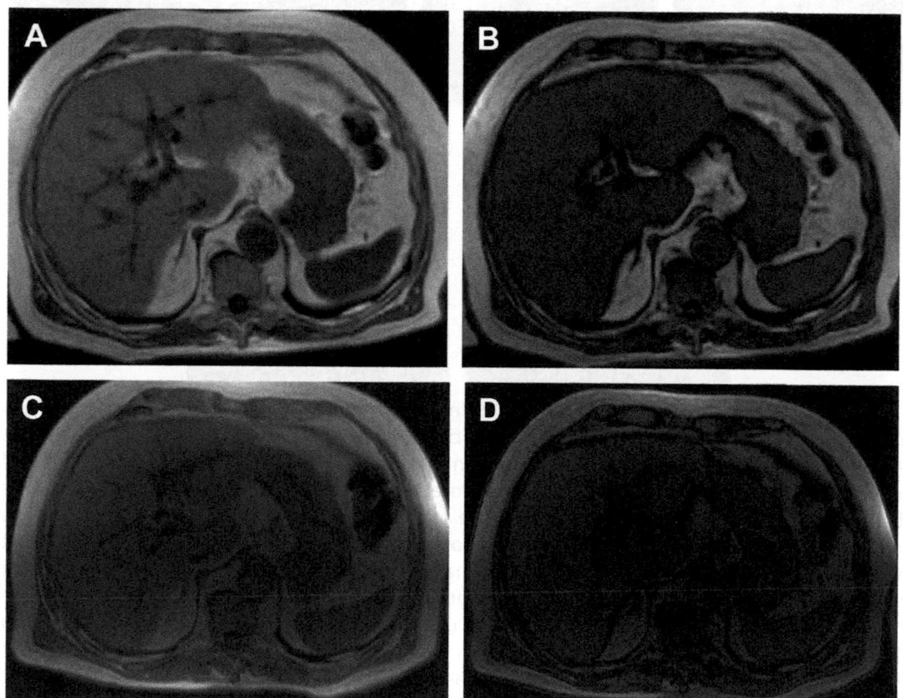

Fig. 5. A 64-year-old man, 3 months after COVID-19 infection, underwent routine MRI for follow-up of pancreatic intraductal papillary mucinous neoplasm (IPMN). Axial T1-weighted "in phase" image (*A*) shows a diffuse liver hyperintensity while axial T1-weighted "opposite phase" and (*B*) demonstrates a loss of signal in the hepatic parenchyma, suggesting hepatic steatosis. On the previous MRI, performed about 6 months earlier, no appreciable differences were found in signal intensity between the axial T1-weighted image "in phase" (*C*) and "opposite phase" (*D*) images at the level of the liver parenchyma, strongly suggesting that the hepatic steatosis increased after the COVID-19 infection.

MRI is the method of choice to detect choledochal stones, it is rarely used in COVID-19 patients as aforementioned. However, gallbladder sludge and biliary sediments are hyperintense on T1-weighted images and iso-hypointense on T2-weighted sequences.[31] Furthermore, gallstones are usually represented on MRI by the characteristic signal void as opposed to the elevated signal intensity of surrounding bile.[32] Biliary stasis and the formation of gallstones can lead to cholecystitis and cholangitis. Some investigators[33] have hypothesized that the cytotoxic effect of the virus can cause ischemia with consequent necrosis of the biliary tract. Furthermore, the virus aggravates cholestasis, by altering the cholangiocyte barrier, and the transport of bile acids.[33]

US is the imaging of choice, but CT can be used to evaluate patients with acute abdominal pain or inconclusive US. Findings indicative of acute cholecystitis include gallbladder over distension, gallbladder wall thickening (>3 mm), mural edematous stratification and hypervascularization, and pericholecystic and perihepatic fluid[34,35](**Fig. 6**).

A small proportion of patients affected by COVID-19 in critical conditions may develop progressive cholestatic damage from consequent SSC. In a series of 34 COVID-19 ICU patients, 9 of them developed severe cholestasis and 4 of them exhibited signs of SSC on MR cholangiopancreatography (MRCP).[36] The MR appearance of SSC is usually similar to that of primary sclerosing cholangitis (**Fig. 7**). The main characteristics of SSC on MRCP are narrowing of the intrahepatic biliary tract with monolobar, bilobar, or segmental distribution, possibly associated with dilation, assuming the appearance of "beads" or a "pruned tree." Involvement of the extrahepatic biliary tree is rare because the intrahepatic bile ducts are vascularized via the

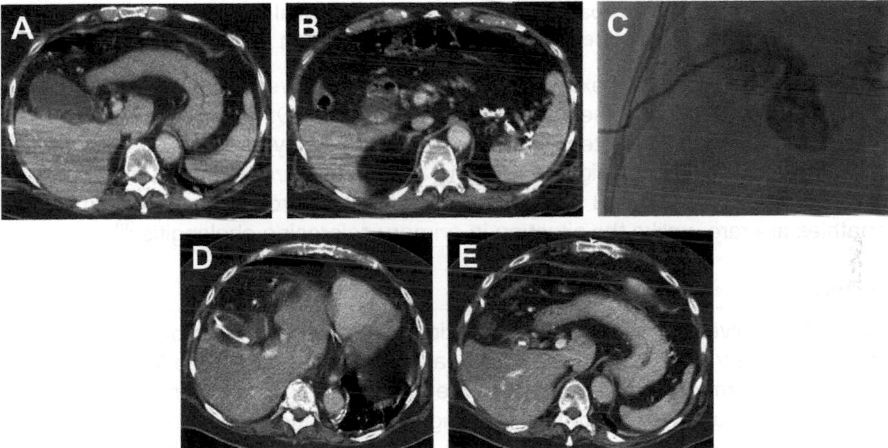

Fig. 6. A 72-year-old man who presented to the emergency department for cholecystitis 2 weeks after severe COVID-19 infection. (*A, B*) Axial CT with contrast on portal venous phase imaging shows an enlarged gallbladder with mural thickening and hypervascularization, with hyperdense calcium stones in the infundibular region, with no biliary tree dilatation. The patient underwent placement of a percutaneous cholecystostomy tube for gallbladder drainage. The procedure was performed with the combined ultrasonography and fluoroscopy. The gallbladder fundus was punctured under ultrasound guidance. (*C*) A pigtail catheter was inserted under fluoroscopic guidance to aspirate purulent bile from the gallbladder. The gallbladder was decompressed at the end of the procedure. (*D, E*) Axial contrast-enhanced CT scans at the portal venous phase show the gallbladder size was reduced after drainage.

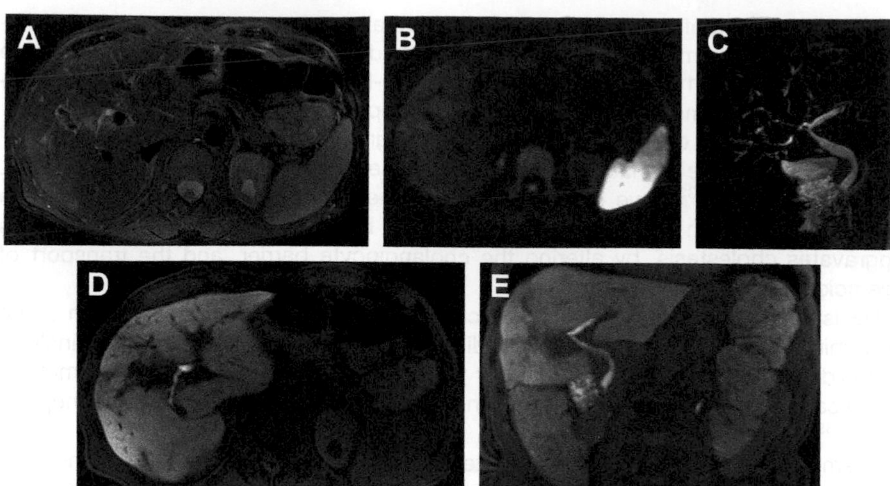

Fig. 7. A 69-year-old male patient with COVID-19 associated SSC after severe COVID-19 infection. (*A*) Axial fat-suppressed propeller T2-weighted MR image shows hepatic contours are rounded, caudate lobe is enlarged, hyperintense signal changes in the liver parenchyma, particularly along the periportal biliary spaces, and slight dilatation of the biliary tree. (*B*) High *b*-value diffusion-weighted image also demonstrates subcapsular and central-hepatic areas of signal changes with mild diffusion restriction. (*C*) Maximum intensity projection MRCP image shows irregularities of the intrahepatic bile ducts with multifocal strictures and dilatations, whereas the extrahepatic biliary tree appears dilated due to stenosis of the hypertrophied papilla. (*D*) Axial and (*E*) coronal post-contrast T1-weighted images in the hepatobiliary phase show patchy hypointense parenchymal areas of decreased contrast enhancement with lack of excretion within the corresponding bile ducts.

hepatic artery, whereas the extrahepatic biliary tree receives a double arterial supply via the hepatic artery and the gastroduodenal artery.[37] Other abnormalities can be represented by high signal intensity of the hepatic parenchyma in the T2-weighted sequences and in diffusion-weighted imaging and by impaired contrast enhancement due to reduced bile flow and areas of cholangitis and fibrosis. Periportal lymphadenopathies are rare, unlike the situation in primary sclerosing cholangitis.[38]

Pancreas

Pancreatic involvement in COVID-19 infection is less frequent compared with bowel and hepatobiliary involvement, but more cases are emerging in the literature, albeit mostly in the form of case reports or single-center studies. Furthermore, only a few studies have focused on abdominal imaging of pancreatic involvement in COVID-19 patients. The first case-series exploring pancreatic pathology in patients with COVID-19 pneumonia reported an incidence of 17% of pancreatic injury,[39] although the radiological findings or the abdominal pain were not described.[40]

The predominant pancreatic gland abnormality is represented by acute pancreatitis (AP), especially in the form of edematous-interstitial pancreatitis referred as pancreatic enlargement, peripancreatic inflammatory changes, and peripancreatic fluid collection.[41,42] According to the revised Atlanta classification, AP is diagnosed if at least two of the following three criteria are present: (1) abdominal pain, (2) elevation of pancreatic enzymes (>three times the upper limit of normal), and (3) typical radiological findings.[43] Nevertheless, COVID-19-related AP requires exclusion of other etiologies for the diagnosis, including gallstones, alcoholism, medications, and other infections.[41] If clinical and biochemical data are inconsistent, contrast-enhanced CT (CECT) should be performed. CECT should include a baseline scan of the abdomen and pelvis followed by arterial and portal venous phases after administration of an iodinated contrast medium at 40 and 65 to 70 seconds, respectively.[44] On CECT, the most typical pattern is either a diffusely enlarged pancreas with homogeneous/slightly heterogeneous enhancement and blurred margins or a combination of an enlarged pancreas with signs of inflammatory changes in peripancreatic fat represented by haziness and mild stranding. Nonencapsulated peripancreatic fluid may also be present[45] (**Fig. 8**). Hinojosa and colleagues reported a case of a 72-year-old man who 8 days after hospitalization for COVID-19 pneumonia underwent chest CT scan to exclude pulmonary embolism; the CT scan extended to the upper abdomen and revealed pancreatic pseudocysts at the pancreatic head and tail, findings that were not present at the initial CT performed on admission. No other findings of peripancreatic inflammation or ductal dilatation or pancreatic enzyme alteration were present.[46]

A pancreatic pseudocyst is a late phase collection typically occurring 4 weeks after the onset of AP. It consists of an encapsulated fluid collection with an enhancing wall. The fluid is homogeneous and hypoattenuating at CECT.[47] Schepis and colleagues reported a patient with a pancreatic pseudocyst undergoing percutaneous US-guided transgastric drainage because of partial gastric obstruction. Moreover, analysis of the drained fluid revealed the presence of three genes of SARS-CoV-2.[48]

Pancreatic involvement has also been described in children with COVID-19 infection or multisystem inflammatory syndrome in children (MIS-C).[49] Stevens and colleagues

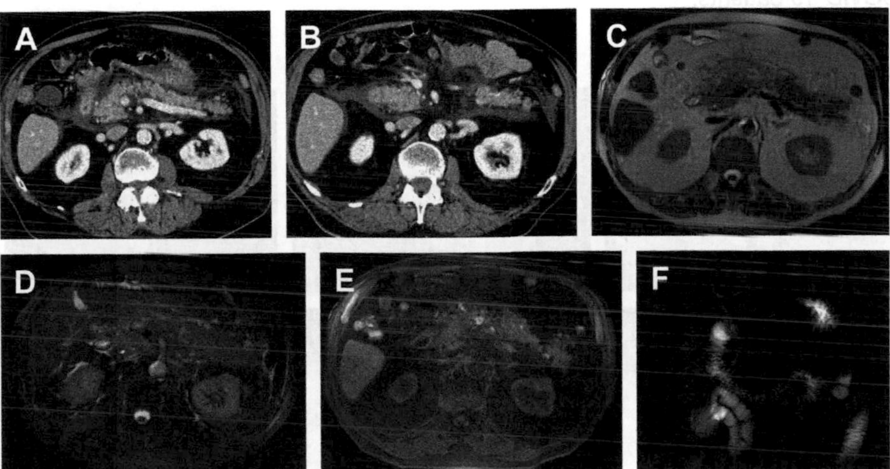

Fig. 8. A 79-year-old man with COVID-19-related slight respiratory symptoms developed acute abdominal pain 10 days later. Patient presented to the emergency department and underwent an abdominal CT scan for a significantly increased serum amylase and lipase. (*A, B*) Axial contrast-enhanced CT images show loss of the normal pancreatic lobulation of the pancreatic head, and fluid collections in the peripancreatic space and in the anterior pararenal spaces. Axial magnetic resonance T2-weighted (*C*) and axial T2-weighted fat-sat-suppression image (*D*), obtained 10 days after the onset of AP, reveal peripancreatic fat stranding and the resolution of fluid collections. (*E*) Axial fat-suppressed T1-weighted image exhibits high signal intensity foci in the pancreas and peripancreatic fat tissue, consistent with necrotic/hemorrhagic components. (*F*) Thick-slab MR cholangiopancreatography (MRCP) demonstrates a normal caliber of the pancreatic and biliary ductal system.

presented the first case of AP in MIS-C; it occurred in a 10-year-old girl with previous COVID-19 infection who presented to the emergency department with abdominal pain, pyrexia, fatigue, and hyperlipasemia; CT scan revealed pancreatomegaly and peripancreatic fatty change, from AP[50] (**Fig. 9**).

A few cases of necrotizing pancreatitis and its complications in COVID-19 infection have also been described. Parenchymal necrosis has to be considered when, in the pancreatic phase, there is low attenuation/no homogeneous enhancement of any part of the gland. Small necrotic areas could be mistaken for heterogeneous parenchyma in interstitial edematous AP.[47] A young man with positive nasal swab for SARS-CoV-2 underwent chest and abdomen CT scans for pulmonary symptoms and abdominal pain; CT-depicted multifocal bilateral ground-glass opacities consistent with COVID-19 infection and revealed non-enhancing head and body of the pancreas with fat stranding.[51] A necrotizing pancreatitis infected by *Clostridium perfringens* has been reported, expressed by gas within the peripancreatic fluid collection.[52] Among complications of necrotizing pancreatitis, hemorrhage has to be appreciated on CT scan. It can result from parietal erosion of peripancreatic arteries and is usually treated via vascular embolization (**Fig. 10**). Although a few patients with necrotizing emphysematous pancreatitis have been described, attention must be paid to this complication in severe COVID-19 infection. AP in COVID-19 patients is rare with a low prevalence of pancreatitis in hospitalized COVID-19 patients, a worse prognosis in patients with COVID-19, and a higher mortality.[41,53] In this setting, imaging plays a crucial role in the early diagnosis, in particular when clinical and biochemical findings are inconclusive, but especially to monitor the patient with complications and to guide clinicians in the workup of AP and to reduce morbidity and mortality in COVID-19 patients.[10]

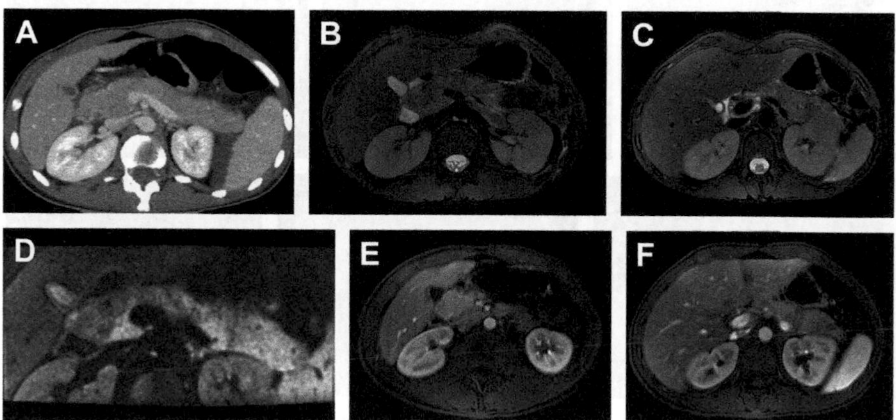

Fig. 9. A 17-year-old woman was hospitalized for the onset of conjunctivitis, joint pain, bilateral palmar erythema, cutaneous manifestations to the lower limb and abdominal pain 1 year after COVID-19 infection. (*A*) CECT scan shows an enlarged pancreas with loss of the normal pancreatic lobulation. Peri-splenic fluid collection is also present. (*B, C*) Axial MR T2-weighted fat-sat-suppression PROPELLER images demonstrate patchy inhomogeneous pancreatic parenchyma with areas of high signal intensity. The main pancreatic duct is not dilated. (*D*) Reduced field-of-view (FOV) diffusion-weighted image with a *b* value of 1000 s/mm^2 well exhibits areas of proton diffusivity restriction in the pancreatic parenchyma. (*E, F*) An inhomogeneous contrast uptake after gadolinium injection was observed on T1-weighted liver acquisition with volume acceleration (LAVA) sequences.

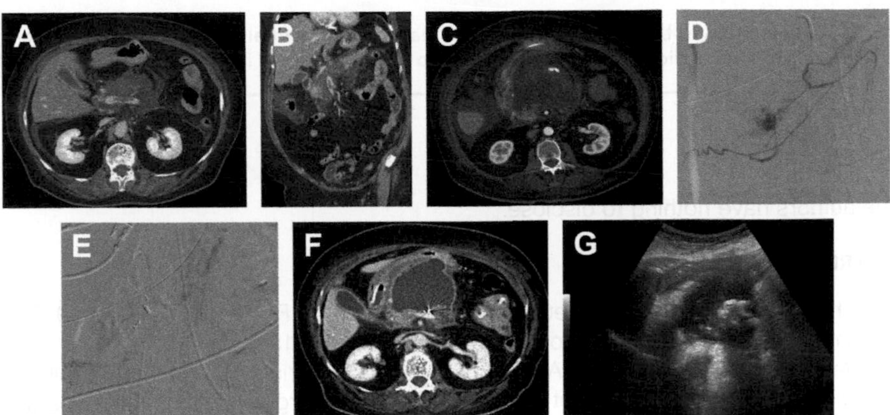

Fig. 10. A 78-year-old woman presented to the emergency room for abdominal pain, nausea, and vomiting. Intestinal obstruction was suspected. (*A*) Axial CECT on portal venous phase shows peripancreatic heterogeneous fluid collections, fat stranding and splenic vein thrombosis. (*B*) Coronal reconstruction of CECT image on portal venous phase demonstrates hypoattenuating region in the head and body of the pancreas (consistent with parenchymal necrosis) along with ill-defined heterogeneous peripancreatic fluid collections and mesenteric vein thrombosis. (*C*) Axial CECT image in the arterial phase, acquired 2 weeks later for worsening abdominal pain, reveals an extravasation of contrast material within the peripancreatic necrotic collection, a finding that is suggestive of hemorrhage. (*D*) Digital subtraction angiography (DSA) obtained after super-selective catheterization of a dorsal pancreatic artery branch confirms active bleeding. (*E*) Angiography post-embolization confirmed adequate vessel occlusion. (*F*) Axial CECT image obtained 5 weeks after the onset of AP demonstrates a well-defined walled-off-necrosis (WON) in the body of the pancreas measuring 9 × 6 cm. Note the naso-jejunal feeding tube in the stomach and jejunum that was inserted to bypass the mass effect determined by the WON. (*G*) Transabdominal US image reveals a well-defined hypoechoic collection with internal echogenic spots consisting of solid necrotic/hemorrhagic debris.

SUMMARY

Gastrointestinal, hepatobiliary, and pancreatic clinical manifestations in COVID-19 patients have been recently investigated using imaging modalities, including US and particularly CT. The radiologist must be familiar with imaging features of potential gastrointestinal, hepatobiliary, and pancreatic COVID-19 involvement to promptly diagnosis and manage these patients.[7] Even if radiological findings of gastrointestinal, hepatic, and pancreatic involvement in patients with COVID-19 are nonspecific, imaging should be performed if abdominal or gastrointestinal disease is suspected in these patients. Furthermore, diagnostic imaging, particularly CT, is helpful to evaluate and manage gastrointestinal, hepatic, and pancreatic disease in COVID-19 patients.

CLINICS CARE POINTS

- Ultrasound and particularly computed tomography should be performed if abdominal or gastrointestinal disease is suspected in COVID-19 patients
- Imaging modalities play a pivotal role in patients with abdominal and gastrointestinal symptoms and signs to investigate possible abdominal features of SARS-CoV-2 infection

- The radiologist must be familiar with imaging features of potential gastrointestinal, hepatobiliary, and pancreatic COVID-19 involvement to promptly report it to the clinicians.

DISCLOSURE

The authors have nothing to disclose.

REFERENCES

1. Bhayana R, Som A, Li MD, et al. Abdominal Imaging Findings in COVID-19: Preliminary Observations. Radiology 2020;297(1):E207–15.
2. Varadarajan V, Shabani M. Ambale Venkatesh B, Lima JAC. Role of Imaging in Diagnosis and Management of COVID-19: A Multiorgan Multimodality Imaging Review. Front Med 2021;8:765975.
3. Zhang J, Garrett S, Sun J. Gastrointestinal symptoms, pathophysiology, and treatment in COVID-19. Genes Dis 2021;8(4):385–400.
4. Abdelmohsen MA, Alkandari BM, Gupta VK, et al. Diagnostic value of abdominal sonography in confirmed COVID-19 intensive care patients. Egypt J Radiol Nucl Med 2020;(1):51. https://doi.org/10.1186/s43055-020-00317-9.
5. Revzin MV, Raza S, Srivastava NC, et al. Multisystem imaging manifestations of COVID-19, part 2: From cardiac complications to pediatric manifestations. Radiographics 2020;40(7):1866–92.
6. Balaban DV, Baston OM, Jinga M. Abdominal imaging in COVID-19. World J Radiol 2021;13(7):227–32.
7. Anderson MA, Goiffon RJ, Lennartz S, et al. Abdominal Imaging Utilization during the First COVID-19 Surge and Utility of Abdominal MRI. Tomography 2021;7(4):972–9.
8. Lee KS, Talenfeld AD, Browne WF, et al. Role of interventional radiology in the treatment of COVID-19 patients: Early experience from an epicenter. Clin Imaging 2021;71:143–6.
9. Kariyawasam JC, Jayarajah U, Riza R, et al. Gastrointestinal manifestations in COVID-19. Trans R Soc Trop Med Hyg 2021;115(12):1362–88.
10. Boraschi P, Giugliano L, Mercogliano G, et al. Abdominal and gastrointestinal manifestations in COVID-19 patients: Is imaging useful? World J Gastroenterol 2021;27(26):4143–59.
11. Pan L, Mu M, Yang P, et al. Clinical Characteristics of COVID-19 Patients With Digestive Symptoms in Hubei, China: A Descriptive, Cross-Sectional, Multicenter Study. Am J Gastroenterol 2020;115(5):766–73.
12. Horvat N, Pinto PVA, Araujo-Filho J de AB, et al. Abdominal gastrointestinal imaging findings on computed tomography in patients with COVID-19 and correlation with clinical outcomes. Eur J Radiol Open 2021;8:100326.
13. Keshavarz P, Rafiee F, Kavandi H, et al. Ischemic gastrointestinal complications of COVID-19: a systematic review on imaging presentation. Clin Imaging 2021; 73:86–95.
14. Caruso D, Zerunian M, Pucciarelli F, et al. Imaging of abdominal complications of COVID-19 infection. BJR Open 2021;2(1):20200052.
15. Ierardi AM, Coppola A, Tortora S, et al. Gastrointestinal Bleeding in Patients with SARS-CoV-2 Infection Managed by Interventional Radiology. J Clin Med Res 2021;(20):10. https://doi.org/10.3390/jcm10204758.
16. Cappell MS, Friedel DM. Gastrointestinal bleeding in COVID-19-infected patients. Gastroenterol Clin North Am 2022. In press.

17. Martin TA, Wan DW, Hajifathalian K, et al. Gastrointestinal Bleeding in Patients With Coronavirus Disease 2019: A Matched Case-Control Study. Am J Gastroenterol 2020;115(10):1609–16.
18. Ierardi AM, Del Giudice C, Coppola A, et al. Gastrointestinal Hemorrhages in Patients With COVID-19 Managed With Transarterial Embolization. Am J Gastroenterol 2021;116(4):838–40.
19. Xu L, Liu J, Lu M, et al. Liver injury during highly pathogenic human coronavirus infections. Liver Int 2020;40(5):998–1004.
20. Garrido I, Liberal R, Macedo G. Review article: COVID-19 and liver disease-what we know on 1st May 2020. Aliment Pharmacol Ther 2020;52(2):267–75.
21. Chai X, Hu L, Zhang Y, et al. Specific ACE2 Expression in Cholangiocytes May Cause Liver Damage After 2019-nCoV Infection. Biorxiv 2020. https://doi.org/10.1101/2020.02.03.931766. 2020.02.03.931766.
22. Tafreshi S, Whiteside I, Levine I, et al. A case of secondary sclerosing cholangitis due to COVID-19. Clin Imaging 2021;80:239–42.
23. Medeiros AK, Barbisan CC, Cruz IR, et al. Higher frequency of hepatic steatosis at CT among COVID-19-positive patients. Abdom Radiol (Ny) 2020;45(9):2748–54.
24. Nardo AD, Schneeweiss-Gleixner M, Bakail M, et al. Pathophysiological mechanisms of liver injury in COVID-19. Liver Int 2021;41(1):20–32.
25. Lee SS, Park SH. Radiologic evaluation of nonalcoholic fatty liver disease. World J Gastroenterol 2014;20(23):7392–402.
26. Zhang YN, Fowler KJ, Hamilton G, et al. Liver fat imaging-a clinical overview of ultrasound, CT, and MR imaging. Br J Radiol 2018;91(1089):20170959.
27. Revzin MV, Scoutt L, Smitaman E, et al. The gallbladder: uncommon gallbladder conditions and unusual presentations of the common gallbladder pathological processes. Abdom Imaging 2015;40(2):385–99.
28. Tian S, Xiong Y, Liu H, et al. Pathological study of the 2019 novel coronavirus disease (COVID-19) through postmortem core biopsies. Mod Pathol 2020;33(6):1007–14.
29. Yu MH, Kim YJ, Park HS, et al. Benign gallbladder diseases: Imaging techniques and tips for differentiating with malignant gallbladder diseases. World J Gastroenterol 2020;26(22):2967–86.
30. Oh SH, Han HY, Kim HJ. Comet tail artifact on ultrasonography: is it a reliable finding of benign gallbladder diseases? Ultrasonography 2019;38(3):221–30.
31. Seong M, Kang TW, Kim M, et al. Tumefactive gallbladder sludge: the MRI findings. Clin Radiol 2016;71(4):402, e9-e402.e15.
32. Tsai HM, Lin XZ, Chen CY, et al. MRI of gallstones with different compositions. AJR Am J Roentgenol 2004;182(6):1513–9.
33. Leonhardt S, Veltzke-Schlieker W, Adler A, et al. Trigger mechanisms of secondary sclerosing cholangitis in critically ill patients. Crit Care 2015;19:131.
34. Chawla A, Bosco JI, Lim TC, et al. Imaging of acute cholecystitis and cholecystitis-associated complications in the emergency setting. Singapore Med J 2015;56(8):438–43, quiz 444.
35. Tonolini M, Ravelli A, Villa C, et al. Urgent MRI with MR cholangiopancreatography (MRCP) of acute cholecystitis and related complications: diagnostic role and spectrum of imaging findings. Emerg Radiol 2012;19(4):341–8.
36. Bütikofer S, Lenggenhager D, Wendel Garcia PD, et al. Secondary sclerosing cholangitis as cause of persistent jaundice in patients with severe COVID-19. Liver Int 2021;41(10):2404–17.

37. Ramesh Babu CS, Sharma M. Biliary tract anatomy and its relationship with venous drainage. J Clin Exp Hepatol 2014;4(Suppl 1):S18–26.
38. Ghafoor S, Germann M, Jüngst C, et al. Imaging features of COVID-19-associated secondary sclerosing cholangitis on magnetic resonance cholangiopancreatography: a retrospective analysis. Insights Imaging 2022;13(1):128.
39. Wang F, Wang H, Fan J, et al. Pancreatic Injury Patterns in Patients With Coronavirus Disease 19 Pneumonia. Gastroenterology 2020;159(1):367–70.
40. Bulthuis MC, Boxhoorn L, Beudel M, et al. Acute pancreatitis in COVID-19 patients: true risk? Scand J Gastroenterol 2021;56(5):585–7.
41. Onoyama T, Koda H, Hamamoto W, et al. Review on acute pancreatitis attributed to COVID-19 infection. World J Gastroenterol 2022;28(19):2034–56.
42. Vaidya T, Nanivadekar A, Patel R. Imaging spectrum of abdominal manifestations of COVID-19. World J Radiol 2021;13(6):157–70.
43. Banks PA, Bollen TL, Dervenis C, et al. Classification of acute pancreatitis–2012: revision of the Atlanta classification and definitions by international consensus. Gut 2013;62(1):102–11.
44. UK Guidelines for the Management of Acute Pancreatitis. 2005.
45. Mazrouei SSA, Saeed GA. Al Helali AA. COVID-19-associated acute pancreatitis: a rare cause of acute abdomen. Radiol Case Rep 2020;15(9):1601–3.
46. Hinojosa V, Gamboa E, Varon J. Pancreatic Pseudocysts as a Late Manifestation of COVID-19. Cureus 2022;14(2):e22181.
47. Shyu JY, Sainani NI, Sahni VA, et al. Necrotizing pancreatitis: diagnosis, imaging, and intervention. Radiographics 2014;34(5):1218–39.
48. Schepis T, Larghi A, Papa A, et al. SARS-CoV2 RNA detection in a pancreatic pseudocyst sample. Pancreatology 2020;20(5):1011–2.
49. Pegoraro F, Trapani S, Indolfi G. Gastrointestinal, hepatic and pancreatic manifestations of COVID-19 in children. Clin Res Hepatol Gastroenterol 2022;46(4):101818.
50. Stevens JP, Brownell JN, Freeman AJ, et al. COVID-19-associated Multisystem Inflammatory Syndrome in Children Presenting as Acute Pancreatitis. J Pediatr Gastroenterol Nutr 2020;71(5). 669–671.
51. Mohammadi Arbati M, Molseghi MH. COVID-19 Presenting as Acute Necrotizing Pancreatitis. J Investig Med High Impact Case Rep 2021;9. 23247096211009393.
52. Sánchez-Gollarte A, Jiménez-Álvarez L, Pérez-González M, et al. necrotizing pancreatitis: an unusual pathogen in pancreatic necrosis infection. Access Microbiol 2021;(9):3, 000261.
53. Goyal H, Kopel J, Ristić B, et al. The pancreas and COVID-19: a clinical conundrum. Am J Transl Res 2021;13(10):11004–13.

Pathologic Characteristics of Digestive Tract and Liver in Patients with Coronavirus Disease 2019

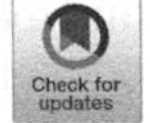

Chunxiu Yang, PhD[a,1], Lijun Cai, MD[b,1], Shu-Yuan Xiao, MD[c,*]

KEYWORDS

• COVID-19 • Pathologic characteristics • SARS-CoV-2 • Lymphocytic infiltration

KEY POINTS

- The common digestive manifestations associated with coronavirus disease-2019 (COVID-19) include anorexia, nausea, vomiting, and diarrhea; the clearance of the viruses in COVID-19 patients with digestive symptoms is usually delayed.
- COVID-19-associated gastrointestinal histopathology is characterized by mucosal damage and lymphocytic infiltration.
- The most common hepatic changes are steatosis, mild lobular and portal inflammation, congestion/sinusoidal dilatation, lobular necrosis, and cholestasis.

INTRODUCTION

With the high prevalence of coronavirus disease-2019 (COVID-19), there has been increasing understanding of the pathologic changes associated with the severe acute respiratory syndrome coronavirus 2 (SARS-CoV-2). The virus can infect multiple organs and cause multiorgan symptoms, causing a wide range of clinical manifestations,[1] including respiratory, cardiovascular, gastrointestinal (GI), and neurologic symptoms (including loss of smell and taste),[2,3] as well as skin manifestations[4] (erythema and papules). A meta-analysis has shown that 17.6% of patients with COVID-19 have GI symptoms, and that viral RNA is detected in stool samples in 48.1% of patients.[5] Neglecting GI symptoms may sometimes delay a timely diagnosis

[a] Department of Pathology, Union Hospital, Tongji Medical College, Huazhong University of Science and Technology, Wuhan, China; [b] Department of Pathology, Zhongnan Hospital of Wuhan University, Wuhan, China; [c] Department of Pathology, University of Chicago Medicine, University of Chicago Medicine, MC6101, Anatomic Pathology, 5841 South Maryland Avenue, Chicago, IL 60637, USA
[1] Co-first authors.
* Corresponding author.
E-mail address: Shu-Yuan.Xiao@uchospitals.edu

Gastroenterol Clin N Am 52 (2023) 201–214
https://doi.org/10.1016/j.gtc.2022.09.003

and may permit the unchecked fecal-oral transmission of the virus. Ulcerative lesions occur in the GI tract in some patients, but only a few studies have described the histopathology of these lesions.[6] In addition, hepatic injury is a frequent complication of COVID-19 and is associated with the severity of the disease. Studies in patients with COVID-19 have shown the incidence of liver injury ranges from 14.8% to 62%, usually indicated by abnormal alanine aminotransferase (ALT) and aspartate aminotransferase (AST) levels accompanied by slightly elevated bilirubin levels.[7–10] In fatal cases, the incidence of liver injury may reach up to 58% to 78%.[7] Pathologic findings in the GI tract and liver come mostly from autopsies or postmortem biopsies but may include pathologic examination of GI biopsies obtained premortem by GI endoscopy. This review summarizes the pathologic changes in the digestive system and liver associated with COVID-19, including the injuries induced by SARS-CoV2 infection of GI epithelial cells and the systemic immune responses.

Esophageal Pathology

Although the clinical manifestations of COVID-19 are usually dominated by respiratory symptoms, some patients may lack symptoms and imaging features of COVID-19 pneumonia but only show GI symptoms.[11] SARS-CoV-2 infection may lead to esophageal mucosal injury, with acute esophagus necrosis (AEN) occurring in critically ill patients.[12] Two case reports have shown esophageal bleeding and multiple round herpetic-like erosions and ulcers by endoscopy in patients with GI symptoms, and SARS-CoV-2 RNA was detected in these esophageal lesions.[12,13] At the autopsy, two necrotic ulcers were detected at the hypopharynx (**Fig. 1**A, B). Histopathology showed full-thickness inflammatory cell infiltration with thinning of the pharyngeal wall at the level of the ulcer center (**Fig. 1**C, D).[6] Meanwhile, in the presence of cells positive for SARS-CoV-2 spike protein subunit 1, histologic examination showed moderate lymphocytic infiltration in the esophageal mucosa (**Fig. 1**E–H),[6] consistent with the histopathological features of viral esophagitis.

Gastric and Intestinal Pathology

The incidence of GI symptoms in patients with COVID-19 is shown in **Table 1**.

The appearance of GI symptoms in patients with COVID-19 seems to indicate disease progression, as GI symptoms are more common in severe and critically ill patients, and are associated with an increased risk of adverse outcomes.[14–16] Interestingly, other case-control studies had previously shown that the presence of GI symptoms was associated with longer illness duration, a trend toward lower ICU admissions, and lower mortality,[17] and the presence of GI symptoms could predict reduced disease severity and mortality.[18] The presence of SARS-CoV-2 RNA in feces is related to GI symptoms. Fecal shedding of viral RNA suggests prolonged GI infection.[19] In addition, the virus may persist in the GI tract after it was cleared from the respiratory tract.[19]

A multicenter study showed that ulcers were the most common lesions observed in upper GI endoscopy in patients with COVID-19, with the lesions sometimes accompanied by active bleeding.[20] Bhayana and colleagues[21] retrospectively analyzed the abdominal imaging findings of 412 patients with COVID-19, and a variety of abnormalities were observed. Bowel-wall abnormalities were found on 13 computed tomography (CT) images (31%), which were associated with intensive care unit (ICU) admission. Pneumatosis or portal venous gas was observed in four abdominal CT images obtained in patients in the ICU. Unusual yellow discoloration of the bowel was observed in three cases and bowel infraction in two cases. Pathologic examinations revealed ischemic enteritis, with patchy necrosis and fibrin thrombi in arterioles.

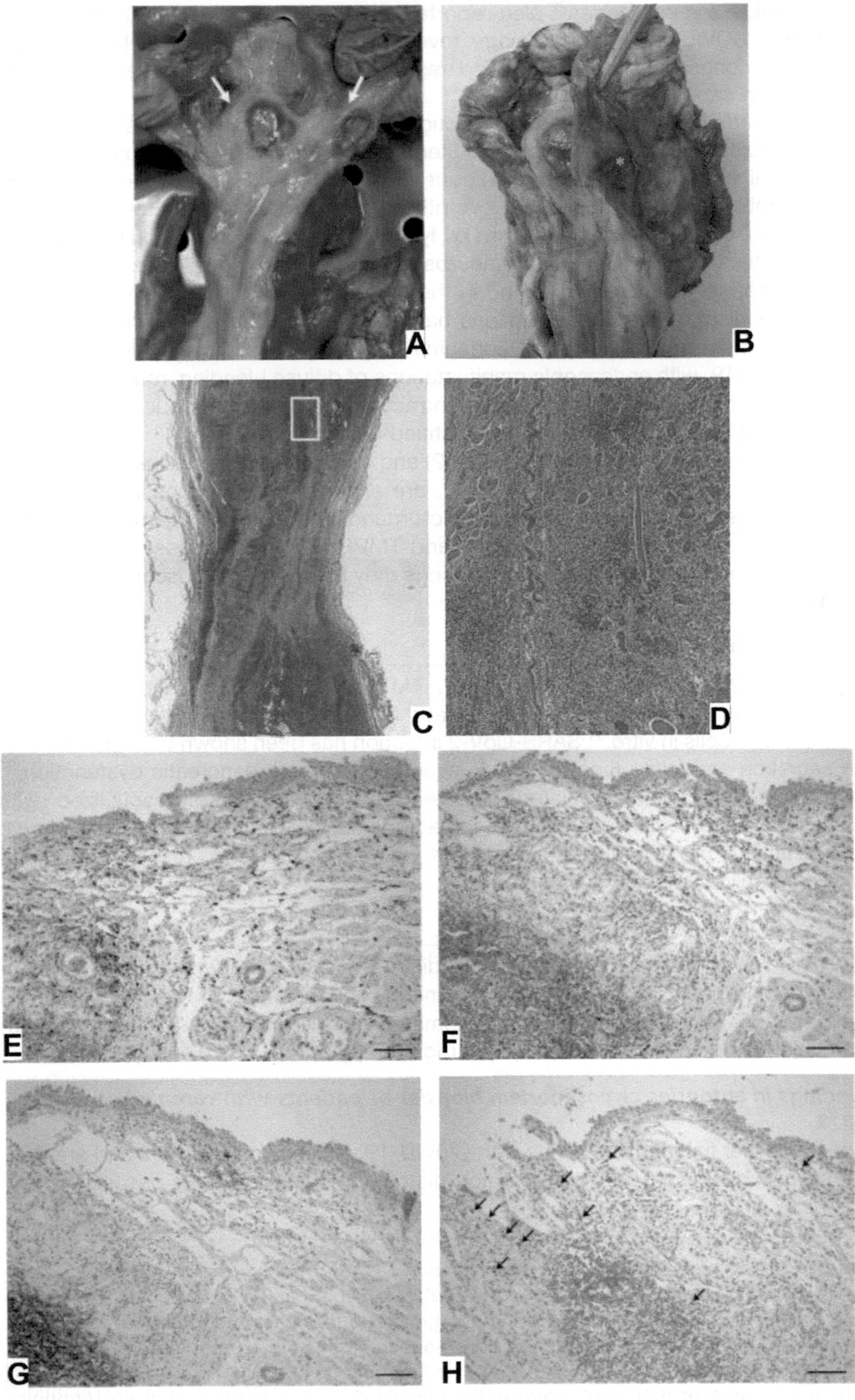
A
B
C
D
E
F
G
H

Amarapurkar and colleagues[22] also reported a case of hemorrhagic enteritis associated with COVID-19. Histopathology revealed extensive transmural hemorrhages with many congested and dilated blood vessels, and fibrin thrombi were occasionally observed in capillaries.

The GI pathology of SARS-CoV-2 infection had been verified in autopsy and biopsy studies. Liu and colleagues[23] observed alternating segmental dilatations and stenoses of the small bowel at the autopsy of a patient with COVID-19, associated with SARS-CoV-2 replication in GI mucosa.[19,20] Another report described GI alterations in patients with COVID-19 as characterized by lymphoplasmacytic infiltration in the lamina propria of the GI tract.[19] Coagulative necrosis, micro-hemorrhages, microthrombi, and vascular congestion had been found in the colonic mucosa, suggesting ischemia is one mechanism of injury. Such lesions have been found to be positive for COVID-19 by immunohistochemistry.[20] Duodenitis may also occur in critically ill patients with COVID-19, with endoscopic manifestations of diffuse bleeding, mucosal edema, and severe inflammation with erosions. Intracytoplasmic and intranuclear inclusions consistent with a viral infection were identified in duodenal crypts.[24]

Angiotensin-converting enzyme 2 (ACE2) and transmembrane protease serine type 2 (TMPRSS2) receptors for SARS-CoV-2, are expressed in GI mucosa.[25,26] Experimental studies have shown human gastric organoids are susceptible to SARS-CoV-2 infection.[27] In addition, as both ACE2 and TMPRSS2 are expressed in the enteric nervous system, gut sensory-motor functions may be affected in susceptible patients with COVID-19.[28]

Pancreatic Pathology

SARS-CoV-2 receptors, including ACE2, TMPRSS2, NRP1,[29,30] and TFRC,[29] are expressed at very low levels in pancreatic β-cells; studies showed SARS-CoV-2 tropism for β cells in vitro.[31] SARS-CoV-2 infection has been shown to suppress insulin secretion and injure β cells ex vivo, eventually causing pancreatic dysfunction,[31] which leads to infection-related diabetes.[32] Among patients hospitalized with COVID-19, the prevalence of acute pancreatitis is 0.27%. COVID-19-associated acute pancreatitis is more frequently associated with severe systemic disease and multiorgan complications.[33]

Liver Pathology

SARS-CoV-2 can cause hepatic injury via direct binding to ACE2 receptors in cholangiocytes and hepatocytes, antibody dependent enhancement of infection, systemic inflammatory response syndrome, inflammatory cytokine storms, ischemia/reperfusion injury, and adverse events due to drug therapy.[9,34–37]

Findings in autopsies or postmortem biopsies of patients with coronavirus disease-2019

The main liver findings in patients with COVID-19 are shown in **Table 2** and are illustrated in **Fig. 2**A–E. The most common histopathological changes associated with

Fig. 1. Macroscopic examination of fresh (*A*) and fixed (*B*) hypopharynx, with two necrotic ulcer (*white arrows* in A). (*C*) Histopathology of ulcer in hypopharynx. (*D*) Inflammatory infiltration of the muscle layer with necrosis and degeneration of the skeletal muscle fibers (*E–H*). Moderate lympho-monocytic infiltration in esophageal mucosa (*E*—anti-CD68; *F*—anti-CD3; *G*—anti-CD20; *H*—positive for SARS-CoV-2 spike subunit 1, *black arrows*). (Porzionato A, Stocco E, Emmi A, et al. Hypopharyngeal Ulcers in COVID-19: Histopathological and Virological Analyses - A Case Report. Frontiers in immunology. 2021;12:676828. https://doi.org/10.3389/fimmu.2021.676828)

Table 1
Incidence of gastrointestinal symptoms in patients with coronavirus disease-2019

Studies	Number of Patients, *n*	GI Symptoms, *n* (%)	Anorexia, *n* (%)	Nausea, *n* (%)	Vomiting, *n* (%)	Diarrhea, *n* (%)	Abdominal Pain, *n* (%)	Virus RNA in Stool (+),*n* (%)
Xiao et al,[19] 2020	73	NA	NA	NA	NA	NA	NA	39(53.4)
Nobel et al,[17] 2020	278	97(34.9)	NA	63(64.9)		56(57.7)	NA	NA
Luo et al,[68] 2020	1141	183(16.0)	180(98.4)	134(73.2)	119(65.0)	68(37.2)	45(24.6)	NA
Hunt et al,[33] 2021	206	48(23.3)	NA	NA	NA	67(32.5)	NA	NA
Cheung et al,[5] 2020	59	15(25.4)	NA	NA	1(6.7)	13(86.7)	7(46.7)	9(60.0)
Pan et al,[69] 2020	204	103(50.5)	81(78.6)	NA	4(3.9)	35(34.0)	2(1.9)	NA
Jin et al,[15] 2019	651	74(11.4)	NA	17(23.0)	18(24.3)	56(75.7)	NA	NA
Wang et al,[70] 2020	138	NA	NA	14(10.1)	5(3.6)	14(10.1)	3(2.2)	NA
Ferm et al,[71] 2020	892	219(24.6)	105(11.8)	148(16.6)	91(10.2)	177(19.8)	70(7.8)	NA

Abbreviation: NA, not available.

Table 2
Summary of main hepatic findings in patients with coronavirus disease-2019

Ref.	No. Cases	Specimen Type	Steatosis	Portal Inflammation	Lobular Inflammation	Congestion/ Sinusoidal Dilation	Lobular Necrosis	Cholestasis	Hepatocyte Apoptosis	Vascular Pathology and/or Thrombosis
Greuel et al,[40] 2021	6	Autopsies	2/6 (33.3%)	–	–	–	–	1/6 (16.7%)	–	–
Xu et al,[44] 2020	1	Postmortem biopsy	1/1 (100%)	1/1 (100%)	1/1 (100%)	–	–	–	–	–
Tian et al,[50] 2020	4	Postmortem biopsies	1/4 (25%)	–	1/4 (25%)	3/4 (75%)	1/4 (25%)	–	–	–
Wang et al,[8] 2020	2	Postmortem biopsies	2/2 (100%)	2/2 (100%)	1/2 (50%)	–	–	–	2/2 (100%)	–
Sonzogni et al,[45] 2020	48	Postmortem biopsies	26/48 (54.2%)	32/48 (66.7%)	24/48 (50%)	–	18/48 (37.5%)	–	–	48/48 (100%)
Cai et al,[9] 2020	1	Postmortem biopsy	1/1 (100%)	–	1/1 (100%)	–	–	–	–	–
McConnell et al,[54] 2021	43	Postmortem biopsies	20/43 (46.5%)	10/43 (23.3%)	–	42/43 (97.7%)	–	–	–	–
Beigmohammadi et al,[47] 2021	7	Postmortem biopsies	7/7 (100%)	7/7 (100%)	–	7/7 (100%)	1/7 (14.3%)	2/7 (28.6%)	–	–
Lagana et al,[46] 2020,	40	Autopsies	30/40 (75%)	20/40 (50%)	–	–	20/40 (50%)	15/40 (37.5%)	10/40 (25%)	6/40 (15%)
Yurdaisik et al,[49] 2021	7	Postmortem biopsies	4/7 (57.1%)	2/7 (28.6%)	5/7 (71.4%)	1/7 (14.3%)	6/7 (85.7%)	2/7 (28.6%)	–	1/7 (14.3%)
Ramos-Rincon et al,[52] 2022	5	Postmortem biopsies	1/2 (50%)	–	–	–	1/5 (20%)	1/5 (20%)	–	–
Barton et al,[41] 2020	2	Autopsies	1/2 (50%)	–	–	–	–	–	–	–

Zhao et al,[43] 2021	17	Autopsies	12/17 (70.6%)	8/17 (47.1%)	5/17 (29.4%)	–	2/17 (11.8%)	–	–	–
Bradley et al,[48] 2020	14	Autopsies	9/14 (64.3%)	4/14 (28.6%)	1/14 (7.1%)	11/14 (78.6%)	4/14 (28.6%)	–	–	–
Wang XX et al,[51] 2021	1	Postmortem biopsy	1/1 (100%)	–	1/1 (100%)	–	1/1 (100%)	1/1 (100%)	1/1 (100%)	–
Chornenkyy et al,[55] 2021	8	Autopsies	4/8 (50%)	7/8 (87.5%)	6/8 (75%)	6/8 (75%)	4/8 (50%)	1/8 (12.5%)	–	–
Falasca et al,[58] 2020	22	Autopsies	12/22 (54.5%)	–	11/22 (50%)	10/22 (45.5%)	–	–	–	–
Fassan et al,[56] 2021	25	Autopsies	9/25 (36%)	–	–	21/24 (87.5%)	2/25 (8%)	–	–	3/25 (12%)
	3	Liver biopsies	2/3 (66.7%)	2/3 (66.7%)	1/3 (33.3%)	–	1/3 (33.3%)	–	–	–
Fraga et al,[59] 2020	1	Liver biopsy	–	1/1 (100%)	–	–	–	–	1/1 (100%)	–
Fiel et al,[57] 2021	2	Liver biopsies	–	2/2 (100%)	1/2 (50%)	–	2/2 (100%)	–	1/2 (50%)	–

–, finding was not described or found.

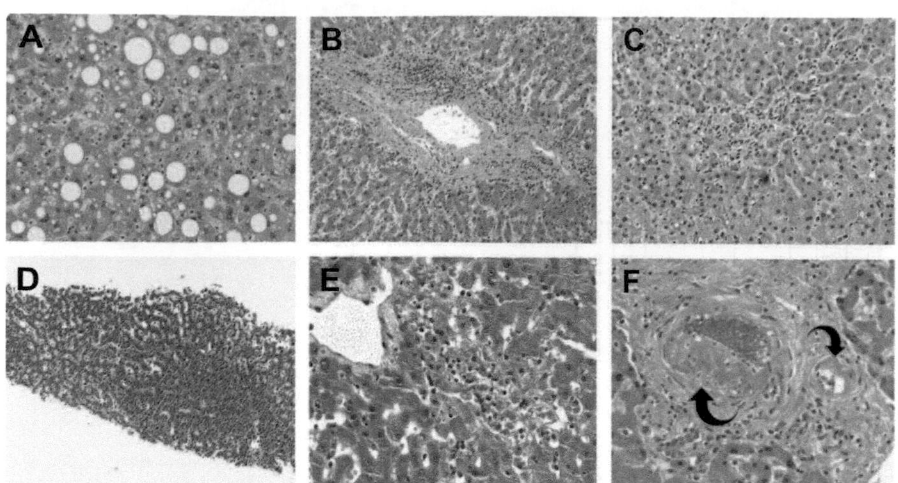

Fig. 2. Histology of liver changes in patients with COVID-19. (*A*) Steatosis. (*B*) Mild portal activity. (*C*) Mild lobular activity. (*D*) Mild sinusoidal dilatation with increased lymphocytic infiltration. (*E*) Focal centrilobular hepatic necrosis. (*F*) Portal arteriolar muscular hyperplasia (*left arrow*) and hyalinosis of a smaller branch of portal arteriole (*right arrow*). ([A] Zhao CL, Rapkiewicz A, Maghsoodi-Deerwester M, et al. Pathological findings in the postmortem liver of patients with coronavirus disease 2019 (COVID-19). Human pathology. Mar 2021;109:59-68. https://doi.org/10.1016/j.humpath.2020.11.015 (Ref. 43); [B, C] Chornenkyy Y, Mejia-Bautista M, Brucal M, et al. Liver Pathology and SARS-CoV-2 Detection in Formalin-Fixed Tissue of Patients With COVID-19. American journal of clinical pathology. May 18 2021;155(6):802-814. https://doi.org/10.1093/ajcp/aqab009 (Ref. 55); [D, E] Tian S, Xiong Y, Liu H, et al. Pathological study of the 2019 novel coronavirus disease (COVID-19) through postmortem core biopsies. Modern pathology : an official journal of the United States and Canadian Academy of Pathology, Inc. Jun 2020;33(6):1007-1014. https://doi.org/10.1038/s41379-020-0536-x (Ref. 50); [F] Lagana SM, Kudose S, Iuga AC, et al. Hepatic pathology in patients dying of COVID-19: a series of 40 cases including clinical, histologic, and virologic data. Modern pathology : an official journal of the United States and Canadian Academy of Pathology, Inc. Nov 2020;33(11):2147-2155. https://doi.org/10.3389/fimmu.2021.676828)

SARS-CoV-2 are hepatic steatosis, mild lobular and portal inflammation, congestion/sinusoidal dilatation, lobular necrosis, and cholestasis.[38,39]

In several autopsy studies, hepatic steatosis of variable severity was the main findings,[40–42] which may be related to high BMI, as well as hypoxia and shock induced by COVID-19-related complications. It is well documented that shock and hypoxia can lead to lipid accumulation in hepatocytes and cause liver injury.[43] Postmortem liver biopsy examination carried out by Xu and colleagues[44] showed moderate microvesicular steatosis and mild lobular and portal activity, indicating the injury could have been caused by either SARS-CoV-2 infection or drug-induced liver injury. In another study of 48 postmortem liver biopsies performed on patients with COVID-19, the histologic assessment also revealed microvesicular and macrovesicular steatosis (54%), mild portal inflammation (66%), and lobular inflammation (50%).[45] The same histologic findings were described in another study of 17 patients.[43] In a study of 40 autopsies, Lagana and colleagues[46] described gross findings of hepatic fibrosis in two patients. Histologically, macrovesicular steatosis was the most common finding, involving 30 patients (75%). Mild lobular necroinflammation and portal inflammation were present in 20 cases (50%) each.

In studies by Beigmohammadi and colleagues[47] and Bradley and colleagues,[48] congestion, steatosis and minimal-to-mild portal inflammation were the most common findings, whereas lobular inflammation was not prominent. Conversely, Yurdaisik and colleagues[49] observed lobular inflammation in most cases. Tian and colleagues[50] reported mild sinusoidal dilatation and focal macrovesicular steatosis in postmortem liver biopsies of four patients. There was mild lobular lymphocytic infiltration, which was insignificant in portal areas; the same findings were reported in another pathologic study.[9,51]

In addition, patchy hepatic necrosis has been described in postmortem liver biopsies and autopsies,[43,48–53] mainly in centrilobular areas (zone 3) and without evident inflammatory cellular infiltration. This pattern is consistent with acute ischemic injury. More severe changes such as confluent necrosis[45,47] and coagulative necrosis[51] were observed in rare cases.

Other histopathological changes frequently described in patients with COVID-19 include the proliferation of the intrahepatic bile ducts and the presence of intracanalicular bile plugs, consistent with cholestasis.[40,49,51–53] In fact, 38% of patients were shown to have lobular cholestasis among 40 autopsied cases, which were generally mild and focal.[46] Four (10%) of these patients had ductular cholestasis.[46] However, bile duct injury has not been observed.[43]

In postmortem wedge liver biopsies of 48 patients, Sonzogni and colleagues[45] noted alterations of vascular structures, both acute (thrombosis of portal and sinusoidal vessels, luminal ectasia) and chronic (fibrous thickening of vascular wall or phlebosclerosis, and abnormalities of the portal intrahepatic vasculature). Lagana and colleagues[46] reported similar changes, such as phlebosclerosis and sinusoidal microthrombi in six cases (15%).[43] Portal arterioles were abnormal (**Fig. 2**F) in nine cases (22.5%), including arteriolar muscular hyperplasia, hyalinosis of the vessel wall, and fibrinoid necrosis with endothelial apoptosis. These findings strongly suggest marked derangement of the intrahepatic blood vessel network secondary to systemic changes induced by the viral infection.

Other uncommon histologic changes include histiocytic hyperplasia in the portal tract,[43] platelet-fibrin microthrombi in the hepatic sinusoids, central vein, or portal vein, and rare megakaryocytes in sinusoids.[43] Minor to massive hepatocytic apoptosis,[8,51] and mild ballooning degeneration[9,40,46,47,54] have been described as well. Presence of SARS- CoV-2 in hepatocytes has been confirmed by in situ hybridization or RT-PCR.[45,46,50,52,55–57]

Liver pathology of patients with coronavirus disease-2019 in controlled studies

To further delineate the role of pre-existing conditions, Falasca and colleagues[58] showed in 22 COVID-19 autopsies (18 with comorbidities and 4 without comorbidities), that the incidence of macroscopic parenchyma congestion, histologic sinusoidal congestion, steatosis, and inflammatory infiltrate were similar between the two groups.[58]

In another postmortem study, patients with COVID-19 ($n = 8$) were compared with controls ($n = 4$). Minimal to focal mild portal tract chronic inflammation ($P < 0.05$) and mild focal lobular activity ($P = 0.06$) were more frequently observed in COVID patients.[46]

McConnell and colleagues[54] compared postmortem liver biopsies between 43 patients with COVID-19 versus normal controls ($n = 12$). Dilated sinusoids with congestion ($P < 0.01$), lobular inflammation ($P < 0.01$), steatosis ($P = 0.02$), and sinusoidal erythrocyte aggregation ($P < 0.01$) were more frequently observed in patients with COVID-19.

Pathology of liver biopsies in living patients with coronavirus disease-2019
Although findings at autopsy are often "contaminated" by terminal iatrogenic changes, liver biopsies performed in patient's premortem likely present more specific pathologic findings. Such findings include mild portal inflammation, scattered hepatocyte apoptosis, ground-glass hepatocytes consistent with cytoplasmic accumulation of fibrinogen,[59] activation of Kupffer cells, and steatosis.[56] In another study of 2 patients without significant lung disease, acute hepatitis, prominent bile duct damage, foci of centrilobular necrosis, and endothelitis were identified, although some of these changes may be due to post-transplant changes in one of the patients.[57]

Liver pathology in patients with underlying chronic liver diseases
Overall, 2% to 11% of patients with COVID-19 had underlying chronic liver disease.[37] Fatty liver disease or non-alcoholic steatohepatitis accounted for 42% of COVID-19 patients with preexisting liver diseases.[60] Hepatic dysfunction was significantly higher in patients with preexisting liver disease, especially in patients with cirrhosis and this was associated with poor outcomes.[60]

In a study of 202 consecutive patients with COVID-19,[61] patients with NAFLD had a higher risk of disease progression ($P < 0.0001$) and longer viral shedding ($P < 0.0001$) than those without NAFLD. Postmortem liver biopsies in one of these patients showed microvesicular steatosis with overactivation of T cells. However, other autopsy and biopsy studies only showed histologic findings consistent with shock liver[62] or the preexisting liver disease.[50]

Liver pathology in patients after vaccination
Hepatitis has been observed in some individuals after vaccination, that share some histologic features with autoimmune liver disease[63,64]; some contain diffusely distributed highly activated T cells.[65] Moreover, among the infiltrating T cells, there is an enrichment of T cells that are reactive to SARS-CoV-2, suggesting that the vaccine-induced cells can contribute to hepatic inflammation. In a cohort of 16 patients who presented with hepatic dysfunction after vaccination, 10 underwent liver biopsy. All showed portal inflammation (60% of which was graded as moderate or severe).[66]

In a case report of an 86-year-old man who died of acute renal and respiratory failure after receiving the first dose of the BNT162b2 mRNA COVID-19 vaccine, the autopsy showed stenosis and sinus dilatation in the liver.[67]

In summary, the most common histologic changes associated with SARS-CoV-2 in the liver are steatosis, mild lobular and portal hepatitis, congestion with sinusoidal dilatation, lobular necrosis, and cholestasis. Hepatocyte apoptosis, vascular pathology with or without thrombosis, histiocytic hyperplasia, and Kupffer cells hyperplasia may also occur.

CLINICS CARE POINTS

- GI symtoms due to involvement by COVID-19 are non-specific. Diagnosis may be facilitated by exclusion of other etiology and positive COVID test.
- Pathologically GI involvement is mainly characterized by lymphocytic infiltration of the mucosa.
- In patients with hepatic involvement, non-specific portal and/or lobular lymphocytic infiltration, mild steatosis, and rarely, spotty necrosis may be pathologic findings.

REFERENCES

1. Aiyegbusi OL, Hughes SE, Turner G, et al. Symptoms, complications and management of long COVID: a review. J R Soc Med 2021;114(9):428–42.
2. Mullol J, Alobid I, Marino-Sanchez F, et al. The Loss of Smell and Taste in the COVID-19 Outbreak: a Tale of Many Countries. Curr Allergy asthma Rep 2020; 20(10):61.
3. Glezer I, Bruni-Cardoso A, Schechtman D, et al. Viral infection and smell loss: The case of COVID-19. J Neurochem 2021;157(4):930–43.
4. Daneshgaran G, Dubin DP, Gould DJ. Cutaneous Manifestations of COVID-19: An Evidence-Based Review. Am J Clin Dermatol 2020;21(5):627–39.
5. Cheung KS, Hung IFN, Chan PPY, et al. Gastrointestinal Manifestations of SARS-CoV-2 Infection and Virus Load in Fecal Samples From a Hong Kong Cohort: Systematic Review and Meta-analysis. Gastroenterology 2020;159(1):81–95.
6. Porzionato A, Stocco E, Emmi A, et al. Hypopharyngeal Ulcers in COVID-19: Histopathological and Virological Analyses - A Case Report. Front Immunol 2021;12: 676828.
7. Xu L, Liu J, Lu M, et al. Liver injury during highly pathogenic human coronavirus infections. Liver Int 2020;40(5):998–1004.
8. Wang Y, Liu S, Liu H, et al. SARS-CoV-2 infection of the liver directly contributes to hepatic impairment in patients with COVID-19. J Hepatol 2020;73(4):807–16.
9. Cai Q, Huang D, Yu H, et al. COVID-19: Abnormal liver function tests. J Hepatol 2020;73(3):566–74.
10. Hajifathalian K, Krisko T, Mehta A, et al. Gastrointestinal and Hepatic Manifestations of 2019 Novel Coronavirus Disease in a Large Cohort of Infected Patients From New York: Clinical Implications. Gastroenterology 2020;159(3): 1137–1140 e2.
11. Lin L, Jiang X, Zhang Z, et al. Gastrointestinal symptoms of 95 cases with SARS-CoV-2 infection. Gut 2020;69(6):997–1001.
12. Deliwala SS, Gurvits GE. Acute Esophageal Necrosis in a Patient With COVID-19. Am J Gastroenterol 2021;116(10):1977.
13. Rahim F, Kapliyil Subramanian S, Larson S. Case Report of Acute Esophageal Necrosis (Gurvits Syndrome) in Vaccinated, COVID-19-Infected Patient. Cureus 2022;14(2):e22241.
14. Zhang SY, Lian JS, Hu JH, et al. Clinical characteristics of different subtypes and risk factors for the severity of illness in patients with COVID-19 in Zhejiang, China. Infect Dis poverty 2020;9(1):85.
15. Jin X, Lian JS, Hu JH, et al. Epidemiological, clinical and virological characteristics of 74 cases of coronavirus-infected disease 2019 (COVID-19) with gastrointestinal symptoms. Gut 2020;69(6):1002–9.
16. Zhang MM, Chen LN, Qian JM. Gastrointestinal manifestations and possible mechanisms of COVID-19 in different periods. J Dig Dis 2021;22(12):683–94.
17. Nobel YR, Phipps M, Zucker J, et al. Gastrointestinal Symptoms and Coronavirus Disease 2019: A Case-Control Study From the United States. Gastroenterology 2020;159(1):373–375 e2.
18. Livanos AE, Jha D, Cossarini F, et al. Intestinal Host Response to SARS-CoV-2 Infection and COVID-19 Outcomes in Patients With Gastrointestinal Symptoms. Gastroenterology 2021;160(7):2435–2450 e34.
19. Xiao F, Tang M, Zheng X, et al. Evidence for Gastrointestinal Infection of SARS-CoV-2. Gastroenterology 2020;158(6):1831–1833 e3.

20. Vanella G, Capurso G, Burti C, et al. Gastrointestinal mucosal damage in patients with COVID-19 undergoing endoscopy: an international multicentre study. BMJ open Gastroenterol 2021;8(1).
21. Bhayana R, Som A, Li MD, et al. Abdominal Imaging Findings in COVID-19: Preliminary Observations. Radiology 2020;297(1):E207–15.
22. Amarapurkar AD, Vichare P, Pandya N, et al. Haemorrhagic enteritis and COVID-19: causality or coincidence. J Clin Pathol 2020;73(10):686.
23. Liu Q, Wang RS, Qu GQ, et al. Gross examination report of a COVID-19 death autopsy. Fa yi xue za zhi 2020;36(1):21–3.
24. Neuberger M, Jungbluth A, Irlbeck M, et al. Duodenal tropism of SARS-CoV-2 and clinical findings in critically ill COVID-19 patients. Infection 2022. https://doi.org/10.1007/s15010-022-01769-z.
25. Yang C, Xiao SY. COVID-19 and inflammatory bowel disease: A pathophysiological assessment. Biomed Pharmacother 2021;135:111233.
26. Trougakos IP, Stamatelopoulos K, Terpos E, et al. Insights to SARS-CoV-2 life cycle, pathophysiology, and rationalized treatments that target COVID-19 clinical complications. J Biomed Sci 2021;28(1):9.
27. Giobbe GG, Bonfante F, Jones BC, et al. SARS-CoV-2 infection and replication in human gastric organoids. Nat Commun 2021;12(1):6610.
28. Marasco G, Lenti MV, Cremon C, et al. Implications of SARS-CoV-2 infection for neurogastroenterology. Neurogastroenterol Motil 2021;33(3):e14104.
29. Cantuti-Castelvetri L, Ojha R, Pedro LD, et al. Neuropilin-1 facilitates SARS-CoV-2 cell entry and infectivity. Science 2020;370(6518):856–60.
30. Daly JL, Simonetti B, Klein K, et al. Neuropilin-1 is a host factor for SARS-CoV-2 infection. Science 2020;370(6518):861–5.
31. Wu CT, Lidsky PV, Xiao Y, et al. SARS-CoV-2 infects human pancreatic beta cells and elicits beta cell impairment. Cell Metab 2021;33(8):1565–1576 e5.
32. Muller JA, Gross R, Conzelmann C, et al. SARS-CoV-2 infects and replicates in cells of the human endocrine and exocrine pancreas. Nat Metab 2021;3(2):149–65.
33. Hunt RH, East JE, Lanas A, et al. COVID-19 and Gastrointestinal Disease: Implications for the Gastroenterologist. Dig Dis 2021;39(2):119–39.
34. Mohamed DZ, Ghoneim ME, Abu-Risha SE, et al. Gastrointestinal and hepatic diseases during the COVID-19 pandemic: Manifestations, mechanism and management. World J Of Gastroenterol 2021;27(28):4504–35.
35. Lei HY, Ding YH, Nie K, et al. Potential effects of SARS-CoV-2 on the gastrointestinal tract and liver. Biomed Pharmacother 2021;133:111064.
36. Li Y, Xiao SY. Hepatic involvement in COVID-19 patients: Pathology, pathogenesis, and clinical implications. J Med Virol 2020;92(9):1491–4.
37. Jothimani D, Venugopal R, Abedin MF, et al. COVID-19 and the liver. J Hepatol 2020;73(5):1231–40.
38. Zghal M, Bouhamed M, Mellouli M, et al. Liver injury in COVID-19: pathological findings. Pan Afr Med J 2022;41:56.
39. Moreira JLS, Barbosa SMB, Vieira JG, et al. Liver histopathological changes and COVID-19: What does literature have to tell us? Dig Liver Dis 2022;54(3):296–8.
40. Greuel S, Ihlow J, Dragomir MP, et al. COVID-19: Autopsy findings in six patients between 26 and 46 years of age. Int J Infect Dis : IJID 2021;108:274–81.
41. Barton LM, Duval EJ, Stroberg E, et al. COVID-19 Autopsies, Oklahoma, USA. Am J Clin Pathol 2020;153(6):725–33.

42. Mikhaleva LM, Cherniaev AL, Samsonova MV, et al. Pathological Features in 100 Deceased Patients With COVID-19 in Correlation With Clinical and Laboratory Data. Pathol Oncol Res : POR 2021;27:1609900.
43. Zhao CL, Rapkiewicz A, Maghsoodi-Deerwester M, et al. Pathological findings in the postmortem liver of patients with coronavirus disease 2019 (COVID-19). Hum Pathol 2021;109:59–68.
44. Xu Z, Shi L, Wang Y, et al. Pathological findings of COVID-19 associated with acute respiratory distress syndrome. Lancet Respir Med 2020;8(4):420–2.
45. Sonzogni A, Previtali G, Seghezzi M, et al. Liver histopathology in severe COVID 19 respiratory failure is suggestive of vascular alterations. Liver Int 2020;40(9): 2110–6.
46. Lagana SM, Kudose S, Iuga AC, et al. Hepatic pathology in patients dying of COVID-19: a series of 40 cases including clinical, histologic, and virologic data. Mod Pathol 2020;33(11):2147–55.
47. Beigmohammadi MT, Jahanbin B, Safaei M, et al. Pathological Findings of Post-mortem Biopsies From Lung, Heart, and Liver of 7 Deceased COVID-19 Patients. Int J Surg Pathol 2021;29(2):135–45.
48. Bradley BT, Maioli H, Johnston R, et al. Histopathology and ultrastructural findings of fatal COVID-19 infections in Washington State: a case series. Lancet 2020;396(10247):320–32.
49. Yurdaisik I, Demiroz AS, Oz AB, et al. Postmortem Biopsies of the Lung, Heart, Liver, and Spleen of COVID-19 Patients. Cureus 2021;13(12):e20734.
50. Tian S, Xiong Y, Liu H, et al. Pathological study of the 2019 novel coronavirus disease (COVID-19) through postmortem core biopsies. Mod Pathol 2020;33(6): 1007–14.
51. Wang XX, Shao C, Huang XJ, et al. Histopathological features of multiorgan percutaneous tissue core biopsy in patients with COVID-19. J Clin Pathol 2021; 74(8):522–7.
52. Ramos-Rincon JM, Alenda C, Garcia-Sevila R, et al. Histopathological and virological features of lung, heart and liver percutaneous tissue core biopsy in patients with COVID-19: A clinicopathological case series. Malays J Pathol 2022; 44(1):83–92.
53. Yao XH, Li TY, He ZC, et al. [A pathological report of three COVID-19 cases by minimal Invasive autopsies]. Chin J Pathol 2020;49(5):411–7.
54. McConnell MJ, Kawaguchi N, Kondo R, et al. Liver injury in COVID-19 and IL-6 trans-signaling-induced endotheliopathy. J Hepatol 2021;75(3):647–58.
55. Chornenkyy Y, Mejia-Bautista M, Brucal M, et al. Liver Pathology and SARS-CoV-2 Detection in Formalin-Fixed Tissue of Patients With COVID-19. Am J Clin Pathol 2021;155(6):802–14.
56. Fassan M, Mescoli C, Sbaraglia M, et al. Liver histopathology in COVID-19 patients: A mono-Institutional series of liver biopsies and autopsy specimens. Pathol Res Pract 2021;221:153451.
57. Fiel MI, El Jamal SM, Paniz-Mondolfi A, et al. Findings of Hepatic Severe Acute Respiratory Syndrome Coronavirus-2 Infection. Cell Mol Gastroenterol Hepatol 2021;11(3):763–70.
58. Falasca L, Nardacci R, Colombo D, et al. Postmortem Findings in Italian Patients With COVID-19: A Descriptive Full Autopsy Study of Cases With and Without Comorbidities. J Infect Dis 2020;222(11):1807–15.
59. Fraga M, Moradpour D, Artru F, et al. Hepatocellular type II fibrinogen inclusions in a patient with severe COVID-19 and hepatitis. J Hepatol 2020;73(4):967–70.

60. Singh S, Khan A. Clinical Characteristics and Outcomes of Coronavirus Disease 2019 Among Patients With Preexisting Liver Disease in the United States: A Multicenter Research Network Study. Gastroenterology 2020;159(2):768–771 e3.
61. Ji D, Qin E, Xu J, et al. Non-alcoholic fatty liver diseases in patients with COVID-19: A retrospective study. J Hepatol 2020;73(2):451–3.
62. Wichmann D, Sperhake JP, Lutgehetmann M, et al. Autopsy Findings and Venous Thromboembolism in Patients With COVID-19: A Prospective Cohort Study. Ann Intern Med 2020;173(4):268–77.
63. Bril F, Al Diffalha S, Dean M, et al. Autoimmune hepatitis developing after coronavirus disease 2019 (COVID-19) vaccine: Causality or casualty? J Hepatol 2021;75(1):222–4.
64. Tan CK, Wong YJ, Wang LM, et al. Autoimmune hepatitis following COVID-19 vaccination: True causality or mere association? J Hepatol 2021;75(5):1250–2.
65. Boettler T, Csernalabics B, Salie H, et al. SARS-CoV-2 vaccination can elicit a CD8 T-cell dominant hepatitis. J Hepatol 2022;77(3):653–9.
66. Shroff H, Satapathy SK, Crawford JM, et al. Liver injury following SARS-CoV-2 vaccination: A multicenter case series. J Hepatol 2022;76(1):211–4.
67. Hansen T, Titze U, Kulamadayil-Heidenreich NSA, et al. First case of postmortem study in a patient vaccinated against SARS-CoV-2. Int J Infect Dis 2021;107:172–5.
68. Luo S, Zhang X, Xu H. Don't Overlook Digestive Symptoms in Patients With 2019 Novel Coronavirus Disease (COVID-19). Clin Gastroenterol Hepatol 2020;18(7):1636–7.
69. Pan L, Mu M, Yang P, et al. Clinical Characteristics of COVID-19 Patients With Digestive Symptoms in Hubei, China: A Descriptive, Cross-Sectional, Multicenter Study. Am J Gastroenterol 2020;115(5):766–73.
70. Wang D, Hu B, Hu C, et al. Clinical Characteristics of 138 Hospitalized Patients With 2019 Novel Coronavirus-Infected Pneumonia in Wuhan, China. JAMA 2020;323(11):1061–9.
71. Ferm S, Fisher C, Pakala T, et al. Analysis of Gastrointestinal and Hepatic Manifestations of SARS-CoV-2 Infection in 892 Patients in Queens, NY. Clin Gastroenterol Hepatol 2020;18(10):2378–2379 e1.

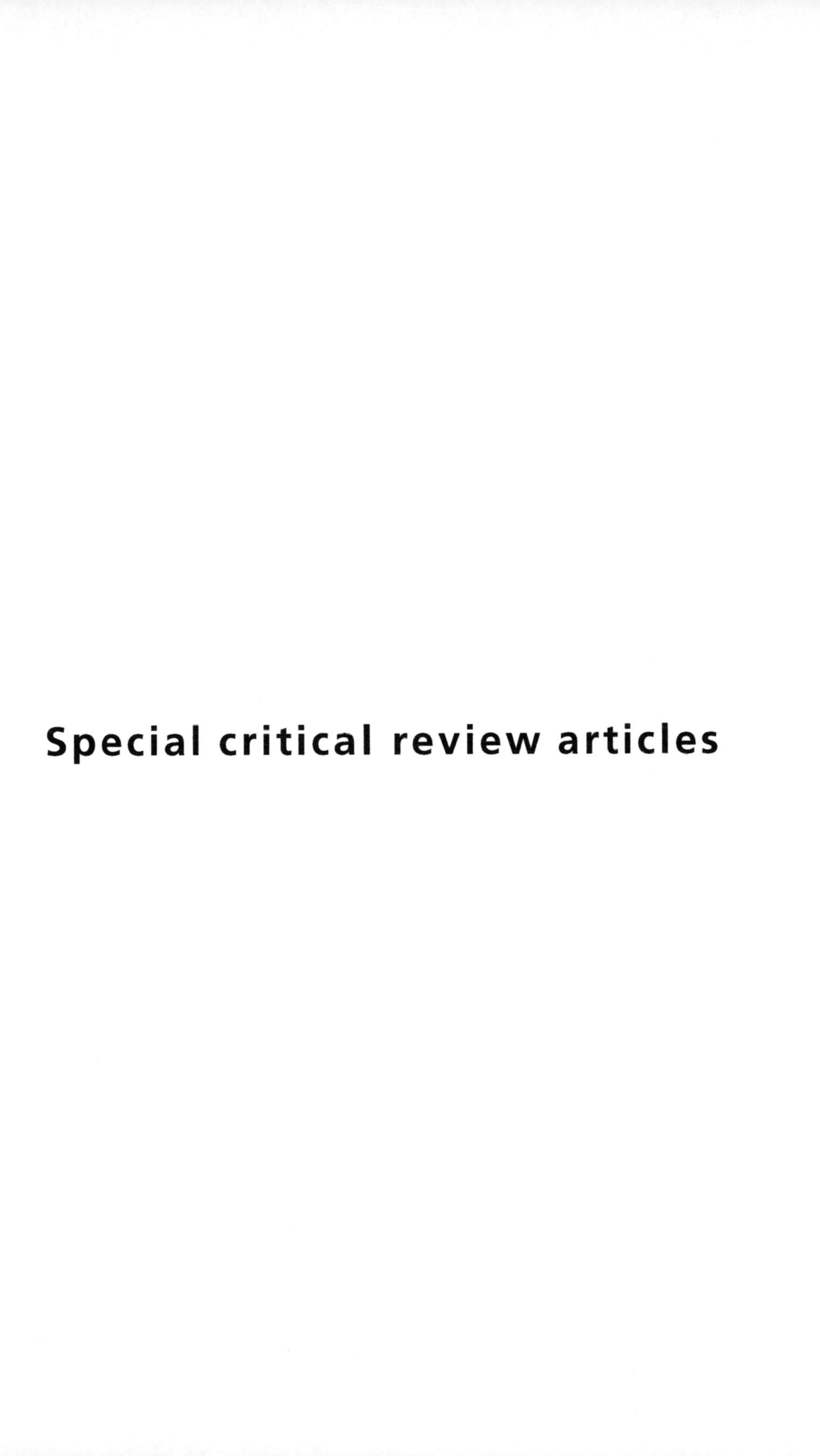

Special critical review articles

Critical Review Two-Years Thereafter of the Effectiveness of the Revolutionary Changes in a Gastroenterology Division at A Medical School Teaching Hospital in Response to the COVID-19 Pandemic

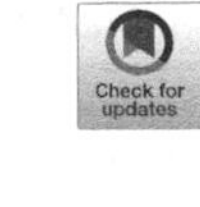

Medical School, Residency, and Gastrointestinal Fellowship Education and Clinical Practice of Gastroenterology Attendings and Gastrointestinal Endoscopy

Mitchell S. Cappell, MD, PhD

KEYWORDS

• COVID-19 • Coronavirus • SARS • Pandemic • Gastroenterology fellowship • Academic gastroenterology • Gastroenterology clinical service

KEY POINTS

- The effectiveness of the revolutionary changes during the COVID-19 pandemic in an academic gastroenterology division (William Beaumont Hospital at Royal Oak, the primary teaching hospital of Oakland University Medical School) were critically reviewed, from the perspective of two years thereafter, in two special articles. This article focuses on changes in GI physician clinical practice, physician emotional stress, GI graduate medical education, GI professional societies, and pandemic control. Most pandemic-induced revolutionary changes were advantageous, while some were not.

Continued

Funding: None.
Gastroenterology Service, Department of Medicine, Aleda E. Lutz VA Medical Center at Saginaw, Building 1, Room 3212, 1500 Weiss Street, Saginaw, MI 48602, USA
E-mail address: Mitchell.cappell@va.gov

Gastroenterol Clin N Am 52 (2023) 215–234
https://doi.org/10.1016/j.gtc.2022.12.003
0889-8553/23/Published by Elsevier Inc.

Continued

- Beneficial changes during severe pandemic included: temporarily pulling GI fellows to supervise exclusively COVID-19 patient wards; endoscopies reduced to perform only emergent/urgent cases; change from "live" to "virtual" lectures and meetings; fellows promoted/graduated on time despite missing minor requirements due to pandemic; GI clinic reduced by 50%; GI fellowship program director contacted GI fellows biweekly to monitor their psychological stress; and ACGME cancelled annual fellowship survey in 2020.
- These profound, beneficial GI-Divisional changes maximized clinical resources devoted to pandemic and minimized risk of infection transmission.
- Disadvantageous changes: Huge, hospital revenue shortfall during pandemic exacerbated by Hospital's paying $84.5 million-fine to government for Stark-Law/anti-kickback violations; hospital employee terminations during pandemic; and reduced GI fellowship support staff. Replacement of long-term academic anesthesiology group by low-cost anesthesiology group and many resignations of GI nurses (after hospital prevented nursing unionization) caused severe personnel shortages causing about 50% reduction in GI endoscopies and severe endoscopy delays. Numerous highly respected, elderly, senior leaders (e.g, chief medical officer, department chairs) terminated without cause.
- Disadvantageous, massive, cost-cutting degraded this academic institution while offering hospital for sale to about 100 hospital suiters, until eventually "selling" hospital to Spectrum Health, without faculty input.

Abbreviations	
COVID-19	Coronavirus disease 2019
PMC	PubMed Central
US	United States
mRNA	messenger ribonucleic acid
GI	gastrointestinal or gastroenterology
GME	Graduate Medical Education
FDA	Food and Drug Administration
ACGME	Accreditation Council for Graduate Medical Education
RRC	Residency Review Committee
ICU	intensive care unit
IRB	Institutional Review Board
VA	Veterans Administration

INTRODUCTION

The reader is hereby notified that there are two special critical review articles by the same author, Mitchell S. Cappell, MD, PhD, in this issue that have similar titles but discuss different topics that are related in that they both deal with the effectiveness of the revolutionary changes due to the pandemic at Oakland University William Beaumont School of Medicine and the affiliated teaching hospital, Beaumont Hospital at Royal Oak. The reader may want to review both articles together since they are closely related to each other.

The medical system throughout the world was "shocked" by an abrupt and unanticipated looming medical catastrophe, the coronavirus disease 2019 (COVID-19) pandemic in late 2019 to early 2020, unprecedented in modern medical history, that raised the specter of a medical catastrophe ranging from the medieval Black Death

(Bubonic Plague) that annihilated about one-third of the then-European population[1] to the "Spanish" flu 100 years ago that killed an estimated 50 million Americans and Europeans.[2] The COVID-19 pandemic proved to cause approximately 6 million documented deaths and several million more suspected but unproven deaths worldwide, including more than 1 million deaths in the United States during its first 2 years.[3] The magnitude of the resultant COVID-19 pandemic locally at Beaumont Hospital, a local pandemic epicenter in metropolitan Detroit, was an unprecedentedly abrupt and prolonged surge of COVID-19 infections starting from 0 inpatients on March 9, 2020,[4] to more than 300 inpatients (>25% of total inpatient census) in April 2020, and to more than 200 inpatients in April 2021,[5] with a cumulative total of approximately 13,000 distinct patients admitted to this one Hospital with COVID-19 infection from March 2020 to April 2021.

Confronted by this exceedingly dangerous, potentially highly lethal, and unprecedented challenge in March 2020, the medical and scientific community mobilized explosively and en masse, such as an overwhelming immunologic cytokine storm combating an invading viral infection such as COVID-19. The enormous reaction is demonstrated by 309,558 published articles listed in Pub Med and 434,877 published articles listed in PMC on the pandemic from January 2020 to November 3, 2022,[6] and by the astronomic total cumulative spending of US$4,600,000,000,000.00 by the United States Government (!),[7] excluding spending by the private sector in America and by the private and public sectors of other Western democratic economies.

This extraordinary investment led to 5 outstanding achievements in combating the pandemic: (1) diagnostic tests, (2) relatively effective vaccines using novel mRNA technologies to both prevent and mitigate the pandemic, (3) improved general therapy to reduce mortality (eg, improved management of respiratory decompensation), (4) reduced contagiousness by instituting effective infection control measures (eg, N95 face masks), and (5) moderately effective therapy to improve infection prognosis (eg, Plaxovid).

- Other notable achievements included elucidating its infectious pathophysiology, clinical presentation, and natural history. These summative achievements gloss over interim fitful and incremental advancements, typical of scientific progress, that even included some interim mishaps. Nonetheless, the cumulative progress has remarkably saved many millions of lives during the pandemic, such as the development of vaccines, which saved an estimated 14,600,000 lives from January 2020 to December 2021, excluding lives saved in the vast Chinese population. The cost of this benefit is crudely calculated by dividing US government expenditures per life saved as US$328,571.43,[8] or by a more precise mathematical model, using different costs and lives saved estimates, of a mean US$40, 800 (range: US$7,400– $81,500) per life saved.[9] These cost estimates of US$328,571 or US$40,800 are comparable to that of lives saved from numerous universally accepted medical interventions, such as triaging critically ill patients to intensive care units.[10] Moreover, the cost per life saved is reduced by factoring in the benefits of increasing worker productivity due to mitigation of workers' COVID-19 infections. I salute these accomplishments by the American government, National Institutes of Health, American pharma and academia, in partnership with other Western democracies, international organizations, and institutions.

I personally modestly contributed to this plethora of research by contributing 10 articles on the effects of COVID-19 on clinical gastroenterology (GI) and by editing the current issue of the Gastroenterology Clinics of North America devoted to GI and hepatic manifestations of COVID-19 infection. In March 2020, at the pandemic onset, I resolved to suddenly cease all my previous research and revolutionarily devote all my new research to the GI effects of this pandemic, like Abraham the patriarch who suddenly abandoned his birthplace to travel on a mission to the promised land. I began my crusade . by publishing a report in early April 2020 about a COVID-19-infected-patient expiring from acute renal failure consequent to severe dehydration from moderately severe diarrhea.[11] This report published in the Am J Gastroenterol was one of the first 40 publications in the world on the pandemic; I believe this paper was notable in demonstrating that diarrhea from COVID-19 infection can contribute to patient mortality by causing acute renal failure from dehydration and electrolyte imbalances.

The pandemic dramatically changed the practice and work schedule of GIs, including me. The rate of performing GI endoscopy plummeted to less than 10% of baseline in 11 New York City hospitals[12] and to about 4% of baseline (!) at William Beaumont Hospital in suburban Detroit[13] just after the pandemic onset. I witnessed, experienced, actively participated, and prospectively reported on the clinical, administrative, research, and financial responses of the Division at William Beaumont Hospital at Royal Oak, a very large (1200 bed), tertiary university hospital in my position as a full-time clinician in the Division, clinical educator as codirector of the preclinical GI course in the affiliated medical school, director of the GI fellowship, and as the former chief of GI. My clinical practice became significantly focused on COVID-19 infection with the inundation of COVID-19 infected patients at the Hospital. I wrote a comprehensive and detailed analysis of the changes brought about by the pandemic that was published nearly 2 years ago in Dig Dis Sci.[14] The previous study was envisioned as a microcosm of the reorganization throughout academic and clinical GI and was proposed as a representative model for academic GI divisions in America. However, study of this flagship Hospital of the Beaumont Hospital network may magnify the pandemic effects because Beaumont Hospital is a tertiary referral center for very sick COVID-19-infected patients with complicated disease, in an intense metropolitan pandemic epicenter.

This earlier study may have benefited clinical and academic GIs, hospital administrators, governmental health-care regulators, medical ethicists, and medical historians in reporting the profound and pervasive effects of the pandemic on GI. Literature review revealed little, but still important, data published elsewhere on the pandemic impact on the clinical and academic missions of GI divisions.[15–20] My previous study was distinguished by its depth and comprehensiveness, including new, previously unreported data concerning the reorganization, some of which might otherwise have never been reported.

The current companion study critically analyzes the effectives of the previously published revolutionary changes of the GI division mostly enacted from March to September 2020, from the perspective of some 2 years later. This critical analysis is divided into two related but different works that critically analyze different aspects of the previously published revolutionary changes. The reader is referred to the companion work on the critical study of different aspects of the revolutionary changes in the Hospital and the Medical School in response to the pandemic (also published in this monograph in Gastrointest Clin of N Am. While the changes are mostly effective, some changes are questionably effective, and occasionally changes are ineffective.

METHODS

The previous work published in Dig Dis Sci[14] continuously collected prospective data from March 2020 to May 2021 (mostly March-September 2020) that reported the revolutionary changes in GI at this clinical and academic institution, the primary teaching hospital of Oakland-University-William-Beaumont-School-of-Medicine since the medical school was founded 12 years ago. The hospital employs more than 400 house officers in-training annually for more than 25 years and has continuously maintained an accredited GI fellowship since 1973. This study reported direct changes in the Division, and indirect effects on the Division from changes in the Department of Medicine, institutional Graduate Medical Education (GME) Department, Hospital administration, affiliated medical school, Accreditation Council for Graduate Medical Education (ACGME), professional GI/hepatology organizations, and governmental regulators.

This work is claimed as expert opinion based on the investigator's expertise in hospital administration from serving as Chief of GI at the Hospital, November 2006 to September 2019, just before the pandemic onset; as GI fellowship program director at various institutions for more than 21 years including GI fellowship program director at William Beaumont Hospital from 2006 to 2021; as medical school GI preclinical course codirector at Oakland University William Beaumont Hospital School of Medicine for more than 11 years; as a member of the Hospital GME Committee for more than 15 years, as a member of the Hospital Endoscopy Committee for more than 15 years, and as a member of the medical school Curriculum Committee for more than 11 years. The author also has considerable experience in academic GI research as a member of the Food and Drug Administration (FDA) Advisory Committee for GI drugs for 5 years[21]; and as author of more than peer-reviewed professional publications in GI, including several publications on academic GI divisions or fellowships., I can claim expertise on GI manifestations of COVID-19 infection, as author of 5 previously published articles on COVID-19 infection[11,14,22–24] and 5 currently published articles in the present monograph.

The medical school and Hospital are nonprofit, private, institutions, unaffiliated with municipal or state governments. Medical students normally spend most of their preclinical years attending required courses on major bodily organ systems, such as cardiology or GI, aside from attending several basic science courses, such as biochemistry. Faculty delivering clinical lectures in bodily organ system courses are mostly physicians employed full-time at the Hospital but some physicians are in private practice affiliated with the Hospital, whereas the basic science faculty for these courses are full-time employees of the Graduate School of Medical Sciences at Oakland University.

The Division has a current complement of 6 GI fellows in total (2020–2021) and was fully accredited by ACGME without warnings or citations. The Division maintains a liver transplant service for more than 10 years accredited by United Network Organ Sharing. The Division maintains a large GI consultative and endoscopic clinical service, encompassing about 36 GIs in private practice primarily affiliated with the Hospital in 2020 to 2021, with a recent drastic decline to about 28 clinical faculty due to a large private GI group and another faculty member quitting the Hospital, and 3 full-time hospital-employed GIs; has a busy endoscopy suite performing more than 23,000 GI endoscopies annually before the pandemic with a large, recent, drastic, and sustained plunge by about 50% or more due to the pandemic and about 22% of the GI staff leaving the Hospital. The reader is directed to a closely related special article on the same subject in this monograph, but covering a set of different topics.

Review

The following critically reviews the effectiveness of the previously reported changes/reorganization of the clinical, teaching, research, and financial functions of this Division due to the pandemic from March 2020 to May 2021, from the perspective of two years afterward, as follows:

Changes in preclinical and clinical medical school education due to pandemic
Background: The medical school at Oakland University enrolls 125 medical students per year, for a full complement of 500 medical students for all 4 medical school years. The first 2 (preclinical) years were taught almost entirely at the Oakland University campus in Rochester, Michigan with basic science faculty supplied by the Graduate School of Oakland University and nearly all clinical faculty supplied by the William Beaumont Hospital at Royal Oak, an equal partner of the medical school. The last 2 (clinical) years are taught almost entirely at William Beaumont Hospital at Royal Oak, which is one of the 8 hospitals in the Beaumont Hospital system that are all located in the Greater metropolitan Detroit area. Occasional clinical rotations were held at William Beaumont Hospital at Troy, and rarely at other Beaumont network hospitals. Medical students rarely take clinical electives at other medical schools, outside the Hospital network, with approval required from medical school administration. Oakland University is in Rochester, MI, about 20 miles away, or 30 to 45 minutes by car, from Beaumont Hospital in Royal Oak.

1. In mid-March 2020, the medical school abruptly, emergently, and completely ceased operations due to the raging pandemic onset in the Detroit epicenter. After 96 hours of intense deliberations, the medical school reopened with medical school lectures for the first 2 years all changed in format from live lectures, presented in classrooms crowded with medical students exposing them to COVID-19 infection, to lectures presented virtually by tapes rebroadcast remotely by Internet through a private, secure, audiovisual connection.[25] These lectures had been originally audiovisually taped when delivered live during the prior academic year 2019 to 2020. Colleges and universities, similarly, used videotaped course lectures that were retransmitted in the same manner for the same reasons.

Opinion: As course codirector for the GI course, I was not invited to participate in these deliberations or decisions about the medical school. I was first officially notified on April 24, 2020, that the second-year medical school course in GI would start on schedule in September 2020 but use audiovisually taped lectures. The memo did not, at the time, specify whether the course lectures would be recycled lectures, that were taped from the prior year, as was occurring in the earlier courses running March to June 2020, or would use newly created audiovisually taped lectures. I, therefore, suspended preparation for the GI course from March to July 2020 including postponing the scheduling of lecture dates and times, recruiting clinical lecturers, revising the course curriculum, and meeting the course codirector for basic science until the medical school administration resolved this issue. First-year and second-year medical school Curriculum Committee meetings, with clinical and basic science course codirectors, medical school administrators, and student representatives, were held as usual monthly in April to July 2020 but were severely curtailed by partial medical school closure, by frequent sudden committee meeting cancelations without advance notice, and by holding them virtually by telephone or audiovisual conference through the Internet rather than live and face-to-face, to prevent exposure of committee members to COVID-19 infection by physically meeting in crowded classrooms.

2. As course codirector, I was first, and belatedly, informed in July 2020, just 1 month before the GI course was to begin, that the GI course, like all future medical school courses, would change from the recycled, previously taped, lectures, derived from the academic year 2019 to 2020 to newly created audiovisual lectures taped just before the upcoming 2020 to 2021 courses to avoid presenting 1-year-old lectures. Unfortunately, the course codirectors were provided little time to recruit faculty for

the upcoming course and for the recruited faculty to prepare new lectures. Lecture formats were changed to comply with new curriculum guidelines recommended in Spring 2020 by the Curriculum Committee. Taped questions posed by medical students attending the live lectures in 2019 to 2020 were eliminated; the newly taped audiovisual 2020 lectures were not videotaped before a live audience and, therefore, lacked questions asked by medical students.

Benefits: The 30 “live” clinical lectures for the 5-week-long GI course presented during September to October 2019 were replaced by newly created audiovisual tapes of lectures for September to October 2020, thereby eliminating the canned questions asked by medical students as recorded in the prior year’s lecture. This change was beneficial because the canned questions from the prior year came across as awkward and lame because the questions were not spontaneous. The new course format prevented medical students from being exposed to COVID-19 from previously sitting 1.3 m from each other in fixed chairs during physical lectures held face-to-face in traditional classrooms and theoretically thereby eliminated the risks of medical students contracting COVID-19 from each other. Moreover, canceling the previous format of live lectures freed-up lecturers from a nearly 2-hour round-trip commute from the Hospital to the medical school, with the travel time then becoming available for patient care. The newly created lectures were only about 1-month-old compared with the previously used lectures that were 1-year-old.

Opinion: Unfortunately, senior administrators rendered decisions on medical school courses without soliciting advice from course codirectors, including me, who could have offered sage advice based on direct teaching experience and should have been consulted if only as a courtesy. Course codirectors were ordered to recruit new lecturers abruptly and hastily and create a new course schedule on short notice. The medical school administration temporarily used WebEx and then another commercially available, remote access, Internet system to broadcast videotaped lectures but both formats proved cumbersome and impractical, and the administration then settled on audiovisual tapes using Microsoft Teams, which functioned excellently.

These changes answered well the prior criticisms but did not permit medical students to ask questions during the lectures. This perforce lacked a critical part of the classic Socratic method of teaching, which had evolved during 2.5 millennia, of students spontaneously asking questions during the lecture and relegated students to purely passive learning without being able to ask questions or interact with the lecturer whatsoever.

3. Three clinical lectures scheduled for the renal and urology course running in August 2020, just before the GI course, were abruptly canceled on the day of their lectures, without warning, because the lecturers made technical mistakes using the Internet lecture system due to their lack of training by information technologist (IT) personnel because IT personnel were cut by 20% and unavailable to supply routine technical support just when these personnel were needed most to set up virtual computerized technology during the pandemic onset. These cancellations left 125 medical students in the lurch because of waiting for a scheduled medical school lecture that did not occur. These lectures were then successfully taped audiovisually and rebroadcast several days later. Planning for the September to October 2020 GI course encountered similar setbacks because audiovisual taping was supervised by academicians, from the medical school, rather than IT personnel, with IT personnel only available for assistance remotely by telephone by special request due to the shortage of IT personnel. This arrangement caused

confusion and errors due to inadequately trained academicians supervising the taping of lectures. Only pretaped lectures were used because “live” broadcasting of virtual lectures through the Internet had caused many lecture cancelations due to computer glitches. Ironically, 3 lectures presented by computer-savvy GI attendings who thought they did not need IT technical support for taping their lectures had to cancel their lectures on the day of their scheduled broadcast because of computer glitches, whereas I, a rank IT amateur, delivered my 8 lectures without computer glitches because I arranged for and relied on IT assistance in advance.

4. *Modifications:* By January 2021, audiovisual recording of lectures improved with simplified, automated audiovisual Internet connections, rather than teleconferences made by the lecturer, and computer glitches became rare. Lectures were delivered “live” but virtually using Zoom or Microsoft Teams without audiovisual taping of lectures. In early 2021, Microsoft Teams became the official commercial channel for audiovisual conferences and lectures for the Medical School and Hospital.

Opinion: Such technology allowed students to ask questions virtually in “real” time. Microsoft Teams significantly improved interactions between teachers and students but still prevented face-to-face interactions that might have exposed students to contracting COVID-19 infection. Students and lecturers were unable to interact through gestures or other nonverbal cues due to the virtual connection. These lost interactions haves undetermined the value of virtual lectures. Yet, Microsoft Teams and Zoom offer the best possible verisimilitude of physical lectures in the virtual world despite these minor quibbles.

5. The 6 laboratory sessions for the GI second-year medical school course, each lasting from 1.5 to 2 hours, covered upper GI anatomy and histology, lower GI anatomy and histology, and hepatobiliary and pancreatic anatomy and histology. These sessions were changed in 2020 from physical, “traditional” laboratories delivered face-to-face by proctors in classrooms using actual anatomic, pathologic, and histologic specimens to virtual sessions presented in real time by a preceptor using photographic images of specimens accompanied by oral explanations of the illustrated slides. Students could ask preceptors virtual questions in real time (March 2000–current). After presenting a slide, the preceptor asked students questions about the slide, which each student answered out loud. Students’ answers were followed by the preceptor presenting and explaining the correct answer virtually. Laboratory sessions ended with questions by medical students answered live and virtually by the laboratory preceptor.

Opinion: Laboratory sessions pose a special challenge for virtual reality. For example, how does a medical student virtually appreciate the nodularity and fibrosis of a cirrhotic liver? Verisimilitude for virtual laboratory sessions will require further technological breakthroughs.

6. Elective clinical rotations for fourth-year medical students in medical subspecialties, including GI, were canceled (March–December 2020), and resumed (January 2021–current). Clinical rotations at other institutions for third or fourth-year medical students were suspended (March 2020–February 2021) and resumed (March 2021–current). Similarly, clinical clerkships or rotations from medical students visiting from other medical schools were suspended (March 2020–February 2021), and resumed (March 2021–current). Elective clinical GI rotations for third-year or fourth-year medical students were canceled during the early pandemic

(March 2020–February 2021).[25] Substantial medical school closure for subspecialty clinical rotations freed-up subspecialty attendings from teaching responsibilities to medical students and permitted these clinicians to devote more time to the clinical care of COVID-19-infected patients.

Opinion: With decreasing threats to the health of patients or medical students after the first 9 months of the pandemic, clinical rotations of medical students did not need to be cancelled. The medical students were then allowed to do elective rotations in medical subspecialties. The absence of medical students earlier rotating in GI detracted from their medical education and harmed the GI consultative service because the very busy service depended on the medical students to help in performing GI consults.

7. All eligible fourth-year medical students graduated on time, as scheduled, and were awarded their diplomas in both May 2020 and May 2021, despite missing small parts of scheduled clinical rotations or electives due to the pandemic.[26]
8. Medical students were exempted from evaluating and treating hospitalized patients with active COVID-19 infection but could waive this exemption (March 2020–current). These policies reduced risks of medical students contracting COVID-19 infection.
9. Clinical clerkships substantially modified (March–June 2020) by employing objective structured clinical examinations, which were disseminated virtually using commercial platforms such as WebEx. Substantial parts of the third-year clinical clerkships and fourth-year clinical electives used remote (virtual) teaching. For example, teaching sessions on performing phlebotomy were canceled.

Opinion: Graduation of medical students on time was essential. This graduation prevented unwarranted delays in their medical career. They missed small parts of the usually mandatory medical curriculum because of the pandemic.

10. The medical school granted all medical students (years I–IV), a US$1,000.00 discount on tuition for the academic year 2020–2021 due to cost savings from substituting virtual for physical lectures and in recognition of the hardships endured by the medical students in attending classes during the pandemic.

Opinion: The medical students appreciated this nice gesture. Although it was likely only symbolic, it was likely all that the medical school could afford during the pandemic.

Changes in teaching and clinical supervision of medical residents and gastroenterology fellows in gastroenterology division due to the pandemic

1. The Division standardly had 5 face-to-face divisional lectures or conferences per week before the pandemic, which were uniformly canceled during the early pandemic to reduce pandemic transmission and to conserve physician manpower for clinical duties (March–August 2020). Lectures were resumed (September 2020–current) with audiovisual conferencing by Microsoft Teams with the speaker located remotely. To compensate for canceled divisional lectures, the Division periodically offered GI fellows and rotating medical residents complementary lectures delivered by national GI experts through the Internet, sponsored by the American College of Gastroenterology.
2. GI and medical grand rounds were canceled (March–August 2020) thereby freeing up 1 hour per lecture for each of the many voluntary GI and other clinical faculty and reduced their risks of contracting COVID-19 infection from attending these lectures

in crowded classrooms. GI and medical conferences were reinstituted September 2020, with conferences held remotely (virtually) by Microsoft Teams, without live attendance by lecturers or attendees.

3. Medical resident rotations on GI electives (2 residents per month) were suspended, and these residents were pulled from the GI service to work on general medicine wards devoted exclusively to COVID-19-infected patients (March–July 2020). Residents reverted to their prepandemic GI clinical schedule in August 2020. Medical resident research rotations in GI electives were suspended (March–December 2020) to accommodate the heavy clinical burden to treat COVID-19-infected patients.

Opinion: Starting January 2021 medical residents were permitted to have GI research electives but were discouraged by the Hospital from doing so because of the heavy clinical burden of the pandemic.

4. Four GI fellows were deployed from GI service to act as medical attendings to supervise medical residents and physicians assistants in newly created medical wards exclusively for COVID-19-infected patients (April and May 2020). Before the pandemic, 3 GI teams manned 3 general GI teaching service teams per month performing GI consults, patient follow-ups, and GI endoscopies, with each team containing 1 GI fellow supervised by 1 GI attending; 1 further GI fellow was assigned to advanced endoscopy including diagnostic and therapeutic endoscopic retrograde cholangiopancreatography (ERCP) and endoscopic ultrasound (EUS) supervised by a GI attending certified in advanced and therapeutic endoscopy; 1 GI fellow was assigned to hepatology/liver transplant service supervised by an attending hepatologist; and 1 GI fellow was assigned to GI electives in GI research or special clinical rotations (such as, inflammatory bowel disease or GI motility). This reassignment as medical attendings supervising COVID-19 wards was legally permissible because all GI fellows were licensed to (independently) practice internal medicine as medical attendings after completing 3 years of medical residency before starting GI fellowship. One GI fellow covered the hepatology/liver transplant service under supervision by an attending hepatologist, and 1 GI fellow covered GI consults, follow-ups, and endoscopies exclusively for staff and private patients with COVID-19 infection under supervision by a GI attending. In summary, 4 GI fellows were reassigned in April to May 2020 from covering exclusively GI consults as GI fellows to supervise general medical wards as medical attendings for exclusively COVID-19 infected patients, and the 2 other GI fellows were assigned to cover the GI or hepatology consultative services treating mostly COVID-19-infected patients. The rotation of GI fellows on medical wards exclusively treating COVID-19 patients was rescinded June 1, 2020, at which time all GI fellows reverted to the prepandemic schedule of covering only GI wards. This change became possible because of the decreasing daily census of COVID-19-infected patients. A new wave of COVID-19 infection peaked in April 2021 with the census of COVID-19-infected hospitalized patients again reaching more than 200/d.[5] Four GI fellows were transferred from GI service to serve as medical attendings to supervise medical residents and physician's assistants exclusively treating COVID-19-infected patients (April–May 2020). Resumed regular GI schedules (June 2020–current).

5. GI fellows excused from performing GI endoscopies on their patients (March–April 2020) forcing GI attendings to perform endoscopies alone on patients on the GI teaching service. This policy was rescinded (May 2020–June 2021) allowing GI fellows to assist in GI endoscopies performed on their patients.

Opinion: The original policy exempting GI fellows from GI endoscopies was ill conceived because it harmed their endoscopic training and exposed GI attendings, some of whom were relatively elderly and had risk factors for severe COVID-19 complications, to be exposed to COVID-19 infection during GI endoscopy. Nearly half of GI attendings are elderly.

6. Due to the reduction of endoscopies assigned to GI fellows (March–May 2020), the Division proportionally reduced the minimum threshold of specialized GI endoscopies (ERCP and EUS) required during the 3-year fellowship for certification for specialized endoscopies.
7. Before the pandemic, medical attendings and residents could schedule patients for GI clinic without GI fellow approval but with the pandemic onset, the GI service instituted in March 2020 prescreening of patients for upcoming GI clinics. GI fellows reviewed patients' medical records and briefly contacted patients by telephone to determine whether a patient should be seen in GI clinic. Patients with relatively urgent indications were scheduled for occuring relatively soon in GI clinics, whereas patients for elective indications had their GI clinic visits postponed for more than 8 weeks. Prescreening reduced the total number of GI clinic visits from about 36 to 18 patients per week to reduce the stress on the GI service from the overload of COVID-19-infected patients. Before the pandemic, GI patients were uniformly seen in person in GI clinic in private examining rooms. GI fellows had interviewed patients face-to-face, performed physical examinations on their patients, and returned with their supervisory GI attending to review the patients' GI condition and discuss their recommendations with patients. During the early COVID-19 surge (March– June 2020), all GI clinic visits became virtual via telemedicine: patients were contacted, interviewed, received recommendations, ordered to undergo tests, and prescribed medicines by videoconference or telephone. In person (live) GI clinic visits were reinstituted starting July 2020 but GI telemedicine clinic visits were also continued. Currently, about half of GI clinic visits are live and in-person, and about half are virtual by telemedicine. Patients who are sicker and have more urgent indications for clinic visits are seen "live," whereas other patients are seen by telemedicine. Due to the pandemic, patients seen in person at clinic could not be accompanied by a companion unless medically necessary (eg, patient with dementia).

Opinion: GI clinic appointments were triaged according to severity of disease. This is a reasonable solution for allocating scarce medical resources. It is frequently done to determine the priority of seeing patients in busy emergency rooms.

8. National Board of Medical Examiners tests in certain medical specialties (eg, emergency medicine) postponed during the pandemic peak and offered later using remote proctoring.
9. GI fellowship applicant interviews changed in 2020 from physical interviews to virtual interviews via Internet to reduce applicants' exposure to COVID-19 infection during the pandemic. The virtual interview process closely simulated the physical interview process before the pandemic, by having individual interviews conducted virtually by Internet, by supplying a taped audiovisual tour of hospital facilities, by providing applicants a detailed list of the monthly GI fellowship schedules and listing employment conditions via the Internet, and by arranging for applicants to confidentially meet current GI fellows virtually via Microsoft Teams, with GI attendings excluded to ensure meeting confidentiality.[22] The Alliance for Academic Internal Medicine recommended that the fellowship interview process should be entirely virtual in 2021.

Opinion: The Hospital received a record number of 400 applications for GI fellowship positions in 2020, possibly because of instituting virtual interviews attributed to the greatly reduced investment in time and money by interviewees for virtual interviews due to eliminating the time and cost involved in physical interviews, including airplane travel and overnight stay at a hotel for physical visits. This virtual interview process was set-up to closely resemble the previous physical face-to-face interview process.

Changes in clinical practice of gastroenterology attendings due to pandemic

1. One GI attending reassigned from general GI consultative services to GI services for exclusively COVID-19-infected patients due to clinical demand (April–May 2020). As aforementioned, in April–May 2020, the normal 3 GI consultative teams for general GI patients, each consisting of 1 GI fellow and 1 supervising GI attending per team, were disbanded and replaced by 1 GI consultative service designated exclusively for COVID-19-infected patients covered by 1 GI fellow and supervised by 1 GI attending. One additional GI consultative team for overflow staff GI patients, previously manned by a physician's assistant and supervised by a GI attending was maintained but also became substantially devoted to COVID-19-infected patients due to the pandemic surge. The hepatology consultative service was maintained with 1 GI fellow and 1 hepatology attending but also substantially became a consultative service for COVID-19-infected patients due to the pandemic. The GI schedule reverted to the prepandemic format for GI attendings in June 2020 as the volume of COVID-19-infected patients decreased.
2. Hospital Physician-in-Chief directed GI and other subspecialty consultants to obtain patient histories and advise patients after consultation through telemedicine (April 2020–May 2021) to maintain greater than 2 meters distance from patients with confirmed or suspected COVID-19 infection to minimize consultant risks. GI consultants could avoid physical examinations altogether by relying on physical examinations performed earlier on the same day by emergency room or medical ward attendings to avoid exposure to COVID-19-infected patients (starting April 2020).
3. The Centers for Medicare and Medicaid Services (CMS) established a new billing code in April 2020 to reimburse physicians for telemedicine.[27]

Opinion: E-consults through telemedicine represented a significant advance in medical care in selected circumstances. E-consults are more convenient and less costly to patients, but e-consults have inherent limitations due to lack of physical examinations, and less forceful recommendations offered to patients when presented virtually. Physical faceto-face visits should still be offered to sicker and more complicated patients.

4. Due to a critical shortage of staff physicians during the pandemic surge, the Hospital requested full-time employed physicians to voluntarily relinquish planned vacations during April 2020.

   Opinion: In response to this Hospital request, I voluntarily relinquished a 1-week vacation during the Spring holidays (April 2020), during which I had already planned to visit my family in Florida.

Changes in gastrointestinal endoscopy practice due to pandemic

1. All elective and semielective GI endoscopies, whether outpatient or inpatient, and regardless of patient COVID-19 status, were cancelled late March to June

1, 2020, and then postponed (June 2020–May 2021) due to insufficient hospital supplies of personal protective equipment, especially N95 masks, shortages of endoscopy nurses and anesthesiologists, and to reduce risks to endoscopy staff of contracting COVID-19 infection from infected patients during GI endoscopy. Patients with urgent or emergent indications still underwent GI endoscopy. Patients underwent mandatory prophylactic endotracheal intubation, and mechanical ventilation for EGD from mid-March until April 17, 2020 to reduce the risks to endoscopy personnel of contracting COVID-19 infection.[28] An association of COVID-19 infection with diarrhea and finding of infectious COVID-19 viral mRNA in stool[29] raised the possibility of transmitting COVID-19 infection to endoscopy personnel during colonoscopy and concern about whether prophylactic endotracheal intubation and artificial mechanical ventilation was warranted for COVID-19-infected patients undergoing colonoscopy. Mandatory intubation for EGD performed on inpatients was rescinded (April 2020)[28] and made voluntary after 4 national/international GI and hepatology professional societies declared in a joint statement that endotracheal intubation and mechanical ventilation in such situations should not be mandatory. GI endoscopies performed on COVID-19-infected patients were, if possible, scheduled as the last procedure of the day in an endoscopy room to minimize risks of viral contamination of endoscopy rooms, just as was practiced for many years for HIV-seropositive patients undergoing GI endoscopy.

Opinion: Change for all patients undergoing EGD from mandatory endotracheal intubation to elective intubation in selected patients was reasonable. Mandatory intubation exposed patients to risks of subsequentextubation failure after EGD, which could prove dangerous to patients with COVID-19 pneumonia. Subsequent data seem to show that the risk of contracting COVID-19 infection during GI endoscopy is manageable (but not nil) during the pandemic.

2. Endoscopy suite did not routinely screen patients for COVID-19 infection before performing endoscopy until July 2020, although patients undergoing elective surgery were screened for this infection beginning several months earlier.

Opinion: Screening patients scheduled for GI endoscopy was important to prevent COVID-19 exposure of endoscopy staff.

3. Hundreds of outpatient GI endoscopies (including both EGDs and colonoscopies) for GI clinic patients faced long delays (often amounting to many months) because of less inpatient endoscopy slots available due to a large decrease in number of endoscopy nurses, attending anesthesiologists, and nurse-anesthetists and longer turnaround times for disinfecting rooms between endoscopies due to the pandemic. The Hospital has encouraged private and hospitalemployed GI attendings to perform extra GI endoscopy sessions to decrease the extremely long waiting times for ambulatory endoscopies of GI clinic patients. GI clinic patients now have a half-day endoscopy block per week in the hospital endoscopy suite to shorten the endoscopy waiting list for clinic endoscopies but this action has still left substantial delays.

Opinion: I thought delays in outpatient GI endoscopic procedures were primarily due to shortages in endoscopy nurses and anesthesiology attendings attributed to the hospital discouraging unionization of the nurses and the hospital replacing its affiliated anesthesiology group. The change of staff was foolishly timed to occur during the near pandemic peak.

US$84.5 million settlement by Beaumont Hospital for claims against it by the United States Department of Justice for improper payments by the hospital to physicians in apparent violation of the antikickback or Stark Law

1. Beaumont Hospital in 2018 voluntarily agreed to pay US$84.5 million to the Department of Justice (and to regulatory authorities of the State of Michigan) to settle allegations of violation of the antikickback statue (Stark Law) under the False Claims Act. The Hospital allegedly improperly paid 8 cardiologists and others in 2004 to 2012 to refer patients to the Hospital.[30]

Opinion: The Hospital agreement to pay the United States Department of Justice US$84.5 million in 2018 to settle alleged violations of the antikickback statue (Stark Law) in paying physicians affiliated with Beaumont for patient referrals does not formally constitute an admission of guilt. However, the settlement and payment of US$84.5 million by the Hospital speaks for itself. In my opinion, this settlement has severely tarnished the Hospital's reputation and played a large role in the Hospital's reaction to the pandemic that began less than 2 years after the settlement 30 discussion (See Discussion).

DISCUSSION

The COVID-19 pandemic proved to be a cataclysmic threat to public health throughout the world. This threat was substantially mitigated by outstanding efforts by medical researchers, Pharma, clinical institutions, medical schools, research institutes, and regulatory authorities in America, Europe, and the rest of the world. Yet the pandemic still caused more than six million known deaths worldwide and likely caused several million more undocumented deaths despite all this mitigation. Perhaps the most important pandemic mitigation was the development of vaccines based on novel mRNA technology, as implemented for the Pfizer-BioNTech and other COVID-19 vaccines. This achievement has been a triumph of Pharma, especially of Pfizer, under the supervision of the Food and Drug Administration (FDA), the National Institutes of Health, and European regulatory institutions. This achievement has been widely documented. However, the overwhelming response by the medical community included numerous other scientific and clinical achievements, as enumerated in the Introduction, that also helped mitigate the pandemic and probably also saved many more millions of lives.

Another landmark achievement has been the flourishing of novel virtual technology that has so ubiquitously replaced physical meetings with virtual meetings throughout healthcare and society. This transformation is inexorably linked to the pandemic. Although this transformation would likely have evolved slowly over time, regardless of the pandemic, to render time management of meetings more efficient and less costly, this transformation occurred revolutionarily in terms of its speed and scope due to the pandemic. The primary driver for this transformation was the pandemic: physical meetings, which entail close physical contact and introduce significant risks of transmission of COVID-19 infection, are replaced by virtual meetings, which entail remote contact, with virtually no risks of transmitting COVID- 19 infection. Virtual meetings have greatly reduced contagiousness by reducing the frequency and duration of interpersonal contacts at physical meetings during the pandemic. This effect has been pervasive throughout clinical medicine, including hospital visits, hospital admissions, outpatient clinic visits, and ambulatory office visits. Virtual teaching has also been adopted for medical education in medical schools, graduate school medical programs, postgraduate medical education, and medical research. The occurrence of virtual teaching and virtual GI care has been thoroughly documented in this and the accompanying article, as illustrated for residency and fellowship lectures, hospital lectures, research symposia, and other functions. Virtual meetings have also revolutionized teaching in general at colleges, universities, high schools, and even primary schools. Virtual hearings have become ubiquitous in legal proceedings such as depositions and trials. Professional medical conventions, such as that of the American Gastroenterology Association or the American College of Gastroenterology changed from physical meetings planned in physical convention halls to virtual meetings during the height of the pandemic. Virtual meetings have also transformed the corporate workplace by allowing many employees to work from home. For example, a close family member of mine works mostly from home via virtual technology as a physician's assistant while performing medical research under contract at a prestigious United States Hospital. This allows her to work full-time while also raising five children.

This work documents the growing pains in developing and establishing virtual meetings. Despite the intense clinical need to quickly adapt virtual technology during the pandemic, this process evolved over many months during the early pandemic. For example, the first attempts at holding virtual meetings by the medical school curriculum committee involved conference calls which have since become obsolete for managing large committee meetings. The technology was far inferior to that available just one year later when Microsoft Teams and Zoom became commonplace and popular. Conference calls were also plagued by intermittent loss of communication, poor connectivity, variable sound volume and quality in a large conference room depending upon proximity to the speaker microphone, and people speaking up simultaneously on top of each other because of the lack of visual contact and cues. Moreover, large conference calls only partly eliminate the risk of contagiousness during the pandemic because many people are still present in a large conference room with some residual physical contact while listening to the conference call. The next iteration of virtual technology involved WebEx which also entailed problems.

Medical school lectures were initially transmitted via audiovisual tapes saved from videotapes of the previous year's lectures which had been standardly videotaped live during the presentation. This initial strategy was implemented easily because the previous year's lectures were standardly available.

The medical school then planned to improve the virtual technology to help mitigate the pandemic after a brief review process. This medical school badly planned and implemented this review process, as it was plagued by mistakes and bungling in its implementation and long delays. The medical school administration kept to themselves their planned modifications for too long. I checked biweekly in April through June with the medical school administration regarding revised plans for virtual transmission of the GI course which was scheduled to start at the end of August 2020 but was provided no information except that the administration was still working on its plans. Belatedly, in July 2020, just one month before the second-year medical school GI lectures which I codirected was set to begin, the medical school administration informed me that the schedule of course lectures would have to be created anew and a new roster of course lecturers would have to be recruited for the 2020 GI course. I as a GI course co-director, despite my many years of teaching experience at the medical school, was not consulted on how to arrange the new annual course, even if only as a courtesy. Course codirectors were abruptly ordered to hastily recruit new lecturers and create a new course schedule on exceedingly short notice. The course codirectors were provided little time to recruit faculty and the recruited faculty in turn were provided little time to prepare their new lectures. This caused great stress on the GI clinical faculty as if the clinical faculty were not under enough psychological pressure from the COVID-19 pandemic.

The Medical School made a serious mistake in cutting back across the board the number of information technologist (It) personnel by 20% to save money during the early pandemic rather than preserving or even increasing the number of IT personnel that were essential to create the transition to virtual technology during the early pandemic. IT cutbacks directly led to cancelling six lectures, three lectures for the renal and urology course, and three lectures for the GI course with disastrous consequences. Each lecture cancellation caused 125 medical students to attend a one-hour scheduled lecture for naught. Cancellation of one lecture ended costing about $15,000 in tuition money estimated at about $125 per lecture per student multiplied by 125 medical students. Three clinical lectures scheduled for the renal and urology course running in August 2020, just before the GI course, were abruptly canceled on the day of their lectures, without warning, because the lecturers made technical mistakes using the Internet lecture system due to their inexperience with the virtual technology and the lack of supervision by IT personnel because of the IT personnel cutbacks. Planning for the September–October 2020 GI course encountered three cancelled lectures at the last minute because audiovisual taping was supervised by academicians, from the medical school, rather than IT personnel, with IT personnel only available remotely for assistance by telephone and only if arranged in advance by special request due to the shortage of IT personnel. IT was unavailable to supply routine technical support for the lecturers just when IT were needed most to set up and guide academicians about virtual computerized technology during the pandemic onset. These failed lectures were successfully retaped audio-visually and rebroadcast several days later. Only pretaped lectures were used because "live" broadcasting of virtual lectures via the Internet had caused many lecture cancelations due to computer glitches. The lectures delivered in September 2020 used hybrid technology with the talk delivered by audiovisual tapes awkwardly controlled by computer. The newly created lectures thankfully eliminated the canned questions posed by medical students attending the live lectures previously in 2019–2020; the newly taped audiovisual 2020 lectures were not videotaped before a live audience and, therefore, lacked questions asked by medical students.

Four iterations during the next approximately eight months of the pandemic using various virtual technologies finally produced a practical, and efficient virtual technology. In early 2021, Microsoft Teams became the official commercial Website for audiovisual conferences and lectures for the Medical School and Hospital. Microsoft Teams was named as the official virtual technology website. Microsoft Teams functioned nearly flawlessly! Zoom is an equally capable alternative technology. Capitalism, I believe, stimulated the rapid progress to develop highly efficient virtual technology, just as capitalism stimulated Pharma to develop relatively effective modern vaccines that saved many millions of lives from the pandemic.

By January 2021, audiovisual recording of lectures improved with simplified, automated audiovisual Internet connections, rather than teleconferences made by the lecturer, and computer glitches became exceedingly rare. Lectures were delivered "live" but virtually using Microsoft Teams without the need to audio-visually tape the lectures. Such technology allowed students to ask questions virtually in "real" time. Microsoft Teams significantly improved interactions between teachers and students but still prevented face-to-face interactions that might have exposed students to contracting COVID-19 infection. However, Microsoft Teams still had limited interactions between students and lecturers due to their interacting virtually without gestures or other nonverbal cues. These lost interactions slightly undetermined the value of virtual lectures.

With gradually decreasing threats to the health of patients or medical students after the first nine months of the pandemic, clinical rotations of medical students did not need to be cancelled. Medical students were then allowed to do elective rotations in medical subspecialties. The absence of medical students in earlier GI rotations, due to the pandemic, detracted from their medical education and harmed the GI service because the very busy consultative service depended upon medical students to help in performing GI consults.

E-consults via telemedicine represent a significant advance in medical care in selected circumstances. It offers a convenient alternative to face-to-face medical care that are less costly, but e-consults have inherent limitations due to lack of physical examinations, and less forceful recommendations offered to patients when presented virtually rather than physically and in person. The convenience of e-consults is illustrated by a patient cancelling a scheduled physical consult with me because of the need to travel a long distance in a snowstorm to make the scheduled appointment. The patient was accommodated at the same time slot by converting his scheduled physical consult to an e-consult at the same time. E-consults were approved and adapted by the Centers for Medicare and Medicaid Services in response to the pandemic just after the pandemic onset. It represents an innovation in health care which was accelerated because of the dire need for it due to the pandemic. After using somewhat clumsy interim virtual technologies, the Hospital formally adopted Microsoft Teams about eight months thereafter as the standard for e-consults.

Notable mistakes on performing EGD early in the pandemic were excusing GI fellows form performing endoscopy and mandating endotracheal intubation for all patients undergoing EGD with suspected COVID-19 infection. The use of mandatory endotracheal intubation was unwarranted because of the significant risk of failure to extubate patients with severe COVID-19 associated pneumonia. Delays in outpatient GI endoscopic procedures were primarily due to shortages in endoscopy nurses and anesthesiology attendings attributed to the hospital discouraging unionization of the nurses and the Hospital abruptly dismissing its long-term affiliated, academic anesthesiology group.

Hospital payment to the United States Department of Justice of 84.5 million dollars in 2018 to settle alleged violations of the antikickback statue (Stark Law) played a critical role in the hospital's subpar response to the pandemic. The hospital was buffeted by severe economic losses early in 2020 from the COVID-19 pandemic just after paying this huge "penalty".[30] This huge penalty severely tarnished the Hospital's reputation and the Hospital lost potential patients due to its tarnished reputation. I felt the loss of the reputation of the Hospital every day after the settlement was announced. I think this monetary loss played a role in the disastrous termination of the 20-year-long affiliation with the academic anesthesiology group which proved disastrous to the Hospital being able to staff an adequate number of endoscopy rooms. The announced settlement greatly affected the morale of Beaumont Hospital's employed and voluntary physicians. The diminished Hospital finances and reputation inexorably led the Hospital to being offered to more than 100 other health institutions, two failed acquisitions or mergers, and finally its sale, or merger, to Spectrum Health in 2021-2022.[33] Dr. David Felten, the former Vice President of Research at the Hospital, was the main whistleblower against the Hospital in its settlement with the Department of Justice, is set to shortly receive his whistleblower award for reporting against the Hospital.[31] Eric Starkman has written a series of exposes about the chaos in the GI endoscopy suite at Beaumont Hospital during the pandemic focusing on the acute shortage of endoscopy nurses.[32]

ACKNOWLEDGMENTS

Dr M.S. Cappell initiated this article and wrote the entire article. The Hospital Institutional Review Board (IRB) approved the previous published study on April 14, 2020.[14] The current study does not require IRB approval because it is solely a review article with no report of original patient data and provides expert opinion based only on previously published data. Dr M.S. Cappell is employed as a gastroenterologist at the Aleda E. Lutz Veterans Affairs Hospital at Saginaw in Michigan. The Veteran's Administration Hospital System and the federal government of the United States have no position or opinion on this publication written by Dr Cappell.

CONFLICTS OF INTEREST

The author declares no conflict of interest. In particular, Dr M.S. Cappell, as a member of the United States FDA Advisory Committee for Gastrointestinal Drugs, 2013 to 2018,[21] affirms that this article does not discuss any proprietary, confidential, pharmaceutical data submitted to the FDA and reviewed by Dr M.S. Cappell. Dr M.S. Cappell was more than 3 years ago a member of the speaker's bureau for AstraZeneca and Daiichi Sankyo, comarketers of Movantik. Dr M.S. Cappell had one-time consultancies for Mallinckrodt and Shire more than 3 years ago. This study does not discuss any drug manufactured or marketed by AstraZeneca, Daiichi Sankyo, Shire, or Mallinckrodt.

Dr. M. S. Cappell dedicates these two related special critical review articles in this issue to Dr. Anthony Fauci, the Head of Infectious Diseases at the National Institutes of Health, who has served selflessly in this capacity or other positions as a public servant at the National Institutes of Health over a long career, and who despite this dedicated service was the subject of vitriol because of advocating vaccination for the pandemic that has been proven to have saved millions of lives throughout the world.

DISCLAIMER

Dr. M. S. Cappell is employed as a gastroenterologist at the Aleda E. Lutz Veterans Administration Hospital in Saginaw, MI and by the United States Government. These institutions do not have an opinion on the views expressed by Dr. Cappell herein.

REFERENCES

1. Black Death. Editors. At: History.com. Original: September 17, 2010. Updated July 6, 2020. Available at: www.history.com/topics/middle-ages/black-death Accessed November 14, 2022.
2. Spanish Flu. Editors. At History.com. Editors updated: May 19,2020. Original: October 12, 2010. 2020. Available at: www.history.com/topics/world-war-i/1918-flu-pandemic. Accessed November 14, 2022.
3. Mathieu E, Ritchie H. Rodés-Guirao, et al., (2020–2022) "coronavirus pandemic (COVID-19), Our World in Data, 2023. Available at: https://ourworldindata.org/coronavirus. Accessed January 26, 2023.
4. WXYZ (ABC Television News). First cases of coronavirus confirmed in Michigan. One each in Oakland and Wayne counties. Available at: www.web.archive.org/web/20200311025008/https://www.wxyz.com/news/coronavirus/first-cases-ofcoronavirus-confirmed-in-michigan-one-each-in-oakland-and-wayne-counties. Accessed April 14, 2020.
5. Smith M. and Mervosh S., Michigan's Covid wards are filling up with younger patients. New York Time April 25, 2021, Available at: www.nytimes.com/2021/04/25/

us/michigan-covid-younger-people-hospitalized.html. Accessed November 3, 2022.

6. NCBI SARS-CoV-2 resources. National Institute of Health, Library of Medicine, National Center for Biotechnology Information. SARS-CoV-2 Data. Available at: www.ncbi.nlm.nih.gov/sars-cov-2/. Accessed November 3, 2022.
7. Federal response to COVID-19. This is how much was spent so far in response to COVID. Available at: www.usaspending.gov/disaster/covid-19?publicLaw=all. Accessed November 3, 2022.
8. Watson OJ, Barnsley G, Toor J, et al. Global impact of the first year of COVID-19 vaccination: a mathematical modelling study. Lancet Infect Dis 2022;22(9): 1293–302.
9. Savinkina A, Bilinski A, Fitzpatrick M, et al. Estimating deaths averted and cost per life saved by scaling up mRNA COVID-19 vaccination in low-income and lower-middle-income countries in the COVID-19 Omicron variant era: a modelling study. BMJ Open 2022;12(9):e061752.
10. Edbrooke DL, Minelli C, Mills GH, et al. Implications of ICU triage decisions on patient mortality: a cost-effectiveness analysis. Crit Care 2011;15(1):R56.
11. Cappell MS. Moderately severe diarrhea and impaired renal function with COVID-19 infection. Am J Gastroenterol 2020;115:947–8.
12. Mahadev S, Aroniadis OC, Barraza LH, et al. Gastrointestinal endoscopy during the coronavirus pandemic in the New York area: results from a multi-institutional survey. Endosc Int Open 2020;8(12):E1865–71.
13. Data obtained from William Beaumont Hospital endoscopy suite, 3601 West 13 Mile Road, Royal Oak, Michigan, 48073.
14. Cappell MS. Local COVID-19 epicenter in Detroit metropolitan area causing profound and pervasive reorganization of clinical, educational, research, and financial programs of a large academic gastroenterology division with a GI fellowship and primary medical school affiliation. Dig Dis Sci 2021;66(11): 3635–58.
15. Papaefthymiou A, Koffas A, Kountouras J, et al. The impact of COVID-19 pandemic on gastrointestinal diseases: a single-center cross-sectional study in central Greece. Ann Gastroenterol 2021;34:323–30.
16. Koo CS, Siah KTH, Koh CJ. Endoscopy training in COVID 19: Challenges and hope for a better age. J Gastroenterol Hepatol 2021. https://doi.org/10.1111/jgh.15524.
17. Li J, Li C, Wang X, et al. Considerations and perspectives on digestive diseases during the COVID-19 pandemic: a narrative review. Ann Palliat Med 2021;10: 4858–67.
18. Tepper DL, Burger AP, Weissman MA. Hands down, COVID-19 will change medical practice. Am J Manag Care 2020;26:e274–5.
19. Crespo J, Fernández-Carrillo C, Iruzubieta CP, et al. Massive impact of coronavirus disease 2019 pandemic on gastroenterology and hepatology departments and doctors in Spain. J Gastroenterol Hepatol 2021;36(6):1627–33.
20. Gross SA, Robbins DH, Greenwald DA, et al. Preparation in the Big Apple: New York City, A new epicenter of the COVID-19 pandemic. Am J Gastroenterol 2020; 115:801–4. Accessed May 4, 2021.
21. Ambulatory Surgery Centers: Gastroenterologist Dr. Mitchell Cappell Appointed to FDA GI Advisory Committee, Becker's Hospital Review. Thursday, September 20, 2012.Available at: https://www.beckershospitalreview.com/asc/gastroenterologist-dr-mitchell-cappell-appointed-to-fda-gi-advisory-committee.html. Accessed December 8, 2022.

22. Cappell MS. Novel modifications for a virtual interview visit to simulate the traditional, live, site visit for GI fellowship applicants for an academic GI fellowship program due to the COVID-19 pandemic. Dig Dis Sci 2021;66:1370–1.
23. Gill I, Shaheen AA, Edhi AI, Amin M, Rana K, Cappell MS. Novel case report: A previously reported, but pathophysiologically unexplained, association between collagenous colitis and protein-losing enteropathy may be explained by an undetected link with collagenous duodenitis. Dig Dis Sci. 4557–4564.
24. Cappell MS. Problems for gastrointestinal patients with diarrheal disorders: Limited access to public bathrooms because previously open public bathrooms have closed due to COVID-19 pandemic and inadequate number of bathrooms in some endoscopy suites. Am J Gastroenterol 2021;116:1355–6.
25. Coronavirus outbreak forces OUWB medical students to embrace 'new normal' in learning. Oakland University William Beaumont School of Medicine, Mar 24, 2020. Available at: https://oakland.edu/medicine/news/auto-list-news/2020/Coronavirus-outbreak-forces-OUWB-medical-students-to. Accessed December 8,2022.
26. Oakland University William Beaumont School of Medicine. Getting across the finish line: How OUWB keeps next-gen physicians on track during pandemic. Friday, May 01, 2020. Available at: https://www.oakland.edu/medicine/news/auto-list-news/2020/Getting-across-the-finishline-How-OUWB-keeps-next-gen-physicians-on-track-during-pandemic. Accessed May 4, 2021.
27. Centers for Medicare & Medicaid Services. President Trump Expands Telehealth Benefits for Medicare Beneficiaries During COVID-19 Outbreak. CMS.gov, Mar 17, 2020. Available at: www.cms.gov/newsroom/press-releases/president-trump-expands-telehealth-benefits-medicare-beneficiaries-duringcovid-19-outbreak. Accessed April 14, 2020.
28. AASLD, ACG, AGA, and ASGE. Gastroenterology professional society guidance on endoscopic procedures during the COVID-19 pandemic. Available at: https://webfiles.gi.org/links/media/Joint_GI_Society_Guidance_on_Endoscopic_Procedure_During_COVID19_FINAL_impending_3312020.pdf. Accessed May 4, 2021.
29. Gu J, Han B, Wang J. COVID-19: Gastrointestinal manifestations and potential fecal-oral transmission. Gastroenterology 2020. https://doi.org/10.1053/j.gastro. pii: S0016-5085(20)30281-X. [Epub ahead of print] No abstract available. PMID:32142785 Accessed March 27, 2020.
30. The United States Department of Justice, Office of Public Affairs. Detroit area hospital system to pay $84.5 million to settle false claims act allegations arising from improper payments to referring Physicians, Available at: www.justice.gov/opa/pr/detroit-area-hospital-system-pay-845-million-settle-false-claims-act-allegations-arising, 2018. Accessed January 27, 2023.
31. 8 physicians identified in Beaumont Hospital $84.5M illegal kickback FCA settlement, Whistleblower News Review December, 24, 2022. Accessed December 24, 2022.
32. Starkman E. Sh** Show at Beaumont – Endoscopy suite In chaos amid nursing shortage. August 27, 2021. Deadline Detroit. https://business.deadlinedetroit.com/articles/28695/starkman_sh_show_at_beaumont_endoscopy_suite_in_chaos_amid_nursing_shortage. Accessed December 24, 2022.
33. Starkman: Beaumont's Woes Prove CEO Tina Freese Decker Unfit To Run Michigan's Biggest Hospital System. Deadline Detroit. August 19, 2022. https://www.deadlinedetroit.com/articles/31125/starkman_beaumont_s_woes_prove_ceo_tina_freese_decker_unfit_to_run_michigan_s_biggest_hospital_system. Accessed August 19, 2022.

A Critical Review from the Perspective of 2 Years Thereafter of the Effectiveness of Revolutionary Changes in a Gastroenterology Division at a Medical School Teaching Hospital due to the Coronavirus Disease-2019 Pandemic

Gastrointestinal Physician Clinical Practice and Emotional Stresses, Gastrointestinal Graduate Medical Education, Gastrointestinal Professional Societies, and Pandemic Control

Mitchell S. Cappell, MD, PhD

KEYWORDS

• COVID-19 • Coronavirus • SARS • Pandemic • Gastroenterology fellowship
• Academic gastroenterology • Gastroenterology clinical service

KEY POINTS

- The effectiveness of the revolutionary changes during the COVID-19 pandemic in an academic gastroenterology division (William Beaumont Hospital at Royal Oak, the primary teaching hospital of Oakland University Medical School) were critically reviewed, from the perspective of two years thereafter, in two special articles. This article focuses on changes in GI physician clinical practice, physician emotional stress, GI graduate medical education, GI professional societies, and pandemic control.

Continued

Funding: None.
Gastroenterology Service, Department of Medicine, Aleda E. Lutz VA Medical Center at Saginaw, Building 1, Room 3212, 1500 Weiss Street, Saginaw, MI 48602, USA
E-mail address: mitchell.cappell@va.gov

Gastroenterol Clin N Am 52 (2023) 235–259
https://doi.org/10.1016/j.gtc.2022.12.004
0889-8553/23/Published by Elsevier Inc.

Continued

- Most of the pandemic-induced revolutionary changes were beneficial, while some were disadvantageous.
- Beneficial changes during severe pandemic included: temporarily pulling GI fellows to supervise exclusively COVID-19 patient wards; endoscopies reduced to perform only emergent/urgent cases; change from "live" to "virtual" lectures and meetings; fellows promoted/graduated on time despite missing minor requirements due to pandemic; GI clinic reduced by 50%; GI fellowship program director contacted GI fellows biweekly to monitor their psychological stress; and ACGME cancelled annual fellowship survey in 2020. These profound, beneficial GI-Divisional changes maximized clinical resources devoted to pandemic and minimized risk of infection transmission.
- Disadvantageous changes: Huge, hospital revenue shortfall during pandemicexacerbated by Hospital's paying $84.5 million-fine to government for Stark-Law/anti-kickback violations; hospital employee terminations during pandemic; and reduced GI fellowship support staff. Replacement of long-term academic anesthesiology group by low-cost anesthesiology group and many resignations of GI nurses (after hospital prevented nursing unionization) caused severe personnel shortages causing about 50% reduction in GI endoscopies and severe endoscopy delays. Numerous highly respected, elderly, senior leaders (e.g., chief medical officer, department chairs) terminated without cause.
- Disadvantageous, massive, cost-cutting degraded this academic institution while offering hospital for sale to about 100 hospital suiters, until eventually "selling" hospital to Spectrum Health, without faculty input.

Abbreviations	
COVID-19	Coronavirus disease 2019
PMC	PubMed Central
US	United States
mRNA	messenger ribonucleic acid
GI	gastrointestinal
GME	Graduate Medical Education
FDA	Food and Drug Administration
ACGME	Accreditation Council for Graduate Medical Education
RRC	Residency Review Committee
ICU	intensive care unit
IRB	Institutional Review Board
VA	Veterans Administration

INTRODUCTION

The spending by America and Western Europe and to a lesser extent but still importantly other countries and international organizations, especially the World Health Organization, have been enormous encompassing an astronomical total cumulative spending of 4,600,000,000,000.00 dollars just by the US Government (!)[1] alone. Likewise, the basic and clinical research expended by academia, pharma, and organizations including the Centers for Disease Control, National Institutes of Health (NIH), and World Health Organization have, likewise, been enormous encompassing 309,558 (!) published articles listed in PubMed and 434,877 published articles listed in PMC on the pandemic from January 2020 to November 3, 2022.[2] Indeed, I liken this worldwide response to a cytokine storm that represents an overwhelming immunologic defensive response against an invading virus, such as coronavirus disease-2019 (COVID-19). What have Western societies and the entirety of civilization obtained from their extraordinary investment in the capitol, resources, scientific research, and clinical investigation?

Extraordinary achievements, including in just 2 years combating the pandemic by developing: (1) diagnostic tests; (2) relatively effective vaccines using novel mRNA technologies to both prevent and mitigate infection; (3) improved general therapy to reduce mortality (eg, improved management of respiratory decompensation); (4) reduced contagiousness by instituting effective infection control measures (eg, N95 face masks); and (5) moderately effective therapy to improve infection prognosis (eg, Plaxovid). Other notable achievements include elucidating its infectious pathophysiology, clinical presentation, and natural history. These summative achievements gloss over interim fitful and incremental advancements, typical of scientific progress, which even included some interim mishaps.

None the less, the cumulative progress is remarkable. Just the development of relatively effective vaccines, using novel mRNA technology, has saved an estimated 14,600,000 lives worldwide from January 2020 to December 2021, exclusive of China (which has not been well analyzed in terms of lives saved). This benefit is crudely calculated by dividing US government expenditures per world-wide life saved as $328,571.43,[3] or by a more precise mathematical model, using different costs and lives saved estimates, of a mean US $40,800 (range: US $7400 to $81,500) per life saved.[4] These cost estimates of $328,571 or $40,800 are comparable to that of lives saved from numerous universally accepted medical interventions, such as triaging critically ill patients to intensive care units (ICUs)[37]. Moreover, the cost per life saved is reduced by factoring in the benefits of increasing worker productivity due to the mitigation of workers' COVID-19 infections. I salute these accomplishments by the American government, NIH, American pharma, and academia, in partnership with other Western democracies, international organizations, and institutions.

In the second part of the study, we analyze the nitty-gritty of the advances in the management of the pandemic by focusing on academic and clinical gastroenterology in specific and comprehensive detail. I believe the reported experience in clinical, academic, and professional organizations in gastroenterology by focusing on one tertiary care Hospital and its affiliated medical school can (1) serve as a microcosm of the revolutionary changes to mobilize academia, hospitals, and pharma against this virus to effectively combat it, (2) lay out a road map to combat, I believe, the almost inevitable next pandemic, and (3) use this experience to learn from mistakes done during this pandemic to prepare for the next pandemic.

This work has been divided into two related parts because of its extraordinary length and its covering of two different but related aspects of the Hospital and Medical School responses to the pandemic. For the convenience of the readership and to reduce redundancy from overlapping text in the two parts, the Introduction is much abbreviated in this second part.

METHODS

I wrote a comprehensive and detailed analysis of the changes brought about by the pandemic in Beaumont Hospital and the Medical School that was published nearly two years ago in Dig Dis Sci.[21] The previous work prospectively and continuously collected data from March 2020-May 2021 (mostly March-September 2020) that reported the revolutionary changes in GI at this clinical and academic institution, the primary teaching hospital of Oakland-University-William-Beaumont-School-of-Medicine since the medical school was founded 12 years ago. The previous work was envisioned as a microcosm of the reorganization throughout academic and clinical GI and was proposed as a representative model for academic GI divisions in America. The current companion works critically analyze the effectives of the previously published revolutionary changes of the GI division mostly enacted from March-September 2020, from the perspective of some two years later. The first critical review conveniently proceeds this second one.[38] While the changes are mostly effective, some changes are questionably effective, and occasionally changes are ineffective. This work consists of two closely related but different works. To avoid redundancy, the Methods section is not repeated in this related article and the reader is referred to the other related article to view the complete Methods section.

Consequences of Pandemic on Income of Hospital and Gastrointestinal Practitioners

1. Pandemic onset caused American unemployment to soar to 14.8%) and a massive and the gross domestic product to sharply decline by 31.4% (April to June 2020), with temporary business closures due to stay-at-home policies of consumers.[39] In response to this economic contraction, the US Federal Reserve Bank drastically lowered interest rates to stimulate the economy, and the federal government passed four large stimulus packages (early 2020 to early 2021) to help revive the economy and relieve economic pressures on families and businesses impacted by the pandemic.[5] These interventions caused a moderate, gradual economic recovery, reflected by improvements in GDP and decreasing unemployment (July 2020 to May 2021).

Opinion: I personally experienced the economic effects of the initial pandemic, by buying a large house at a deeply discounted price because of the absence of buyers at the pandemic onset and I purchased a mortgage at an extremely low fixed-interest rate because of the Federal Reserve Bank's accommodative monetary policy at the pandemic onset. These accommodative Federal Reserve Bank were designed to settle the economy and prevent a sharp economic contraction due to the pandemic.

2. The initial pandemic surge resulted in >25% of Hospital beds filled with COVID-19 patients, but the overall census became <55% of capacity, reduced from the pre-pandemic baseline census of >90% of hospital bed capacity due to plunging elective admissions for patients with illnesses other than COVID-19 infection. These two effects peaked in May 2020. To accommodate the surge of COVID-19-infected patients, the Hospital nearly ceased performing elective surgery or GI endoscopy; the number of surgeries declined by >90%, and the number of GI endoscopies declined by 96% at its nadir from the pre-pandemic baseline. Indeed, most hospital operating rooms from March to May 2020 were transformed into ICUs to accommodate the explosive growth of patients requiring ICU beds after undergoing endotracheal intubation and mechanical ventilation for COVID-19 pneumonia. The overall decrease in hospital admissions, surgeries, ambulatory procedures, and emergency room visits together with increased hospital expenses incurred from purchasing massive quantities of personal protective equipment (PPE), which rose sixfold in price during the COVID-19 pandemic onset, and increased purchases of mechanical ventilators abruptly caused a 278.4 million dollar deficit for the January to March 2020 quarter, compared with a profit of 129.1 million dollars during the same quarter in 2019.[6] In March and April 2020, the federal government granted the Hospital a COVID-19 stimulus package of 75 million

dollars, to partly compensate the Hospital for this loss. The cumulative deficit in the next several fiscal quarters climbed much higher to many hundred million dollars,[7,8] but the Hospital received altogether four extraordinary bonus payments from the federal government totaling about 500 million dollars via Medicare and Medicaid during the pandemic (March 2020 through early 2021).

Opinion: The pandemic's onset greatly affected hospital finances, as occurred in this Hospital.

3. Owing to this large Hospital deficit early in the pandemic, the Hospital on April 21, 2020, terminated 450 hospital employees and temporarily furloughed 2,500 (>7% of the employees, mostly hospital administrative staff, other employees not directly performing patient care, and employees whose clinical departments were temporarily closed due to the pandemic, such as cardiac rehabilitation.[9–11] Additionally, Beaumont Hospital at Wayne, which had been transformed in March 2020 into an exclusively COVID-19 patient hospital, closed indefinitely on April 24, 2020. Other hospitals in the Detroit metropolitan area also furloughed or terminated hospital staff.[12]

Opinion: The Hospital selectively terminated senior, older, highly accomplished, and distinguished academicians with outstanding reputations (approximately June 2021 to current), including the highest and most senior Hospital-employed physician who was a well-known and highly regarded academic researcher with an outstanding curriculum vitae. The Hospital abruptly terminated several other highly distinguished and senior clinical leaders without cause. The hospital replaced these highly accomplished leaders with attendings which had much inferior academic credentials and who earned significantly lower salaries.

4. Division permanently terminated one half-time divisional administrative secretary and temporarily furloughed one 0.4 full-time equivalents GI fellowship program manager/coordinator, who represented nearly all the support staff of the Division. The GI endoscopy unit furloughed seven (10% of) GI endoscopy nurses and terminated all but one of the GI endoscopy schedulers. Furloughs went into effect immediately. Furloughed employees lost their salaries for 60 days, but the hospital maintained their medical insurance during the furlough, and these employees were allowed to apply for and receive unemployment insurance during their furloughs. Furloughed employees were rehired by June 30, 2020. Other hospital systems in the greater metropolitan Detroit area, including Detroit Medical Center, Trinity Health Michigan, and the Henry Ford Health System, announced similar employee furloughs or terminations in April 2020 because of similar financial problems.[12]
5. In October 2019, just a few months before the pandemic began, the eight Beaumont Hospitals drastically reduced the number of employed librarians and library technicians. After the pandemic onset, all the remaining librarians/library technicians were furloughed without pay (March to September 1, 2020). During this period the hospital library at Royal Oak remained open to physicians and other health care professionals *sans* librarians. Librarian assistance was subsequently furnished virtually, which proved highly inconvenient and cumbersome for clinicians and researchers due to the lack of live, face-to-face interactions with librarians. The five remaining librarians returned physically to work in the Hospital library approximately in January 2021.

Opinion: This cost-cutting measure damaged the educational, clinical, and research missions of the Medical School and Hospital but saved little money due to the small costs of the librarians' salaries compared with the overall Hospital budget.

6. The Hospital administration expended considerable Hospital funds, normally expected to fund patient care, to prevent the unionization of Hospital nurses. This effort successfully blocked their unionization. The Hospital also campaigned hard to successfully block the unionization of house staff. Beginning in December 2020, the Hospital encountered severe difficulties in recruiting new endoscopy nurses to replace the endoscopy nurses who left during the pandemic surge.

Opinion: I believe this action against the unionization of nurses caused many GI endoscopy nurses to leave the Hospital which created a large shortfall in the GI endoscopy nursing staff that was required to maintain staffing for the GI endoscopy suite and contributed to long delays in scheduling GI endoscopies.

7. The Hospital administration terminated a longstanding (20-years-long) exclusive contract with a highly regarded academic anesthesiology group (December 31, 2020), and hired another, nonacademic anesthesiology group to save costs (effective January 1, 2021). However, about half of the affiliated anesthesiologists left when the anesthesiology group contract was terminated, which left the Hospital very short staffed with anesthesiologists during the pandemic crisis. Also, about half of the nurse-anesthetists employed by the Hospital left when the previous academic anesthesiology group left.

Opinion: This change in the anesthesiology group resulted in a sustained severe shortage of anesthesiologists required to provision anesthesia services for GI endoscopies that compelled frequent cancelations of GI endoscopies (January to April 2021). The anesthesiology group termination contributed to the successful unionization of nurse-anesthetists at the Hospital.

8. The income of GI practitioners in private practice abruptly plummeted due to greatly decreased volume of GI endoscopies (reduced at the nadir to only 4% of the pre-pandemic baseline) performed at the Hospital and decreasing GI office visits (April 2020). For example, my crude, oral survey of five GI colleagues in private practice affiliated with the Hospital revealed that their revenues declined by >80% during the pandemic peak in late April 2020. Similarly, in a poll conducted in April 2020, 97% of dentists reported that their offices were closed, except for dental emergencies, and reported that their monthly income plummeted by $\geq$ 95%.[13] GI specialists and dentists may share high risks of contracting COVID-19 infection from examining and working within oral cavities of COVID-19-infected patients during EGD or dental work, respectively, and contrariwise may share high risks of transmitting infection from themselves to their patients via close oral contact. The surge temporarily threatened the economic viability of GIs in private practice or employed by the Hospital as well as undermined GI training, education, and research due to the Hospital's financial crisis. Fortunately, the plunge in GI income slowly and gradually reversed starting July 2020, with a substantial resumption of GI endoscopy from <4% of the baseline rate to approximately 50% of the baseline rate by November 2020. Widespread vaccination of the American population against COVID-19 infection in 2021 is bringing recovery to the general American economy and to the GI market.
9. GI attendings in private practice received a bonus (March to May 2020) from the federal government amounting to several percent of their compensation in 2019 from Medicaid and Medicare, based on their individual 2019 tax returns. This bonus compensated GI physicians for their large losses in clinical income during the pandemic surge (March to May 2020).

10. During the pandemic in 2020, the Hospital network raised the minimum wage of employees to $15.00/h. This constituted a large raise for the lowest-paid hospital workers (custodial staff) who had previously earned only $11.00 per hour. The rationale for this raise was to compensate workers who worked under stress during the pandemic. This raise did not affect the salaries of clinical employees in the Division who already earned more than the new minimum wage.

Opinion: I believe this salary raise was motivated by market forces: the wages of the lowest-paid Hospital workers were raised due to the limited supply and increased demand for them during the pandemic. Similar raises occurred for the lowest-paid workers in many industries.

11. Hospital residents and fellows, including GI Fellows, successfully petitioned Hospital administration, with unanimous support from the institutional GME Committee administrators, to receive a modest bonus of $1,000.00 (in June 2020) per physician to compensate them for their extra clinical workload and increased health risks from the pandemic onset (March to May 2020). House staff requested this bonus because medical and GI attendings in private practice received several clinical bonuses from the federal government and the Hospital received several large clinical bonus packages from the federal government because of the pandemic. In November 2020, the Hospital administration granted another $1,000.00 bonus to all residents and fellows, including GI fellows, to recognize their continuing clinical work due to the on-going pandemic.[14] This time, the Hospital administration also granted a $1,000.00 clinical bonus to all full-time-employed, medical attendings for their extra work during the pandemic.

Opinion: Physicians employed full-time by the Hospital felt justified in receiving this symbolic bonus because they had worked extra hard under the stress of the pandemic and the Hospital had been awarded approximately 500 million dollars in cumulative bonuses by the federal government during the pandemic.

12. The Hospital administration provided all clinical employees one complementary lunch per week for four consecutive weeks in appreciation of their hard clinical work during the pandemic (April to May 2021).

Opinion: I believe this gesture was politically motivated because of the low morale of hospital employees due to rumors circulating that the hospital was being offered or sold to other medical institutions. The selling of the hospital became public a few months later and was subsequently consummated. This symbolic hospital gesture did not achieve its aim of improving the morale of hospital-employed physicians.

13. Hospital administration approved voluntary annual hospital contributions amounting to up to six thousand dollars per year per hospital-employed physician to their 401K retirement fund for 2020 and 2021. Most years the Hospital funded this voluntary contribution but in some years the Hospital did not fund this annual contribution due to budgetary shortfalls.

Opinion: This contribution in 2020 and 2021 likely reflected that the Hospital administration felt that the physicians deserved this voluntary contribution for their hard work during the pandemic.

Infection Control Measures with Particular Focus on Gastrointestinal Endoscopy

1. Cleaning solutions and cleansing regimens for GI endoscopy equipment between endoscopy cases changed early during the pandemic to provide longer cleaning

sessions with more intensely viricidal chemicals. This change lengthened turnover times between GI endoscopies and thereby diminished by 10% the maximal number of endoscopy cases that could be accommodated per endoscopy room per day (April 2020 to current). As aforementioned, the number of cases per day was much more severely decreased due to shortages of endoscopy nurses and anesthesiologists.

2. To reduce COVID-19 infections, the Hospital installed new soap dispensers containing viricidal chemicals designed to kill 99.9% of the COVID-19 virus, next to all sinks in hospital bathrooms, lavatory rooms, and kitchens (April 2020 to current).
3. Hospital changed the type of disposable gloves available in the endoscopy suite and other procedure rooms (such as the cardiac catheter laboratory) to thicker gloves to reduce the risk of COVID-19 virus transmission by hand contact to endoscopists or other proceduralists from patients. The Hospital also stocked the endoscopy suite and other interventional suites with disposable face masks and safety goggles to protect the eyes of endoscopists or other proceduralists from being contaminated by fluid spraying into their eyes during procedures.
4. From April to May 2020, hospital physicians were encouraged to change daily into freshly laundered surgical scrubs rather than wear their normal civilian attire within the hospital.

Opinion: This represented a radical shift in Hospital policywhich previously and explicitly forbade physicians from wearing surgical scrubs outside the operating room, endoscopy suite, cardiac catheter suite, or interventional radiology areas.

5. Soon after the pandemic onset, the hospital endoscopy suite transitioned from flimsy, single-use, disposable surgical gowns to thick, impermeable, plastic gowns for endoscopy personnel that were laundered after each use to reduce transmission of COVID-19 infection at endoscopy. On approximately April 1, 2021, the thick plastic gowns were replaced by cheap, flimsy, single-use, and disposable endoscopy aprons/gowns that did not completely cover the torso of endoscopy personnel during endoscopy, apparently as a cost-saving measure.

Opinion: This policy change was not discussed with me or other GI attendings performing GI endoscopy. We were unhappy about this policy change and that it was unfortunately effected without notifying GI attendings in advance.

6. The Hospital had an acute shortage of N95 masks at the pandemic onset requiring health care workers in the endoscopy suite to reuse face masks for an entire day after daily sterilization. This scarcity was partly relieved by substituting the much cheaper K95 masks, made in China, for N95 masks. With time, highly effective N95 face masks became widely available to Hospital physicians (June 2020 to current). In July 2020, all hospital patients and visitors were required to wear face masks to cover their mouths and nose while in the hospital. The Hospital supplied cheap complementary face masks to hospital patients and visitors.

Opinion: I believe the K95 masks were almost as effective as N95 masks and were much cheaper. The reuse of face masks after sterilization after one day of use was an abomination that was necessitated by an acute shortage of face masks during the pandemic onset that was later corrected.

7. The Hospital started offering employed house staff, including GI fellows and attendings, and affiliated medical attendings vaccination against COVID-19 infection, using the Pfizer-BioN-Tech vaccine starting on December 13, 2020, soon after emergency approval of the vaccine was obtained from the FDA (Food and Drug

Administration). I and all the GI fellows received our first vaccine dose by December 31, 2020, and our second dose by January 21, 2021. The public started receiving vaccines soon thereafter, with prioritization according to their risk factors, such as age >65 years. Everybody was offered booster shots soon thereafter. After a few months, the public was able to receive vaccines at walk-in clinics without scheduled appointments and with minimal waiting times.[15] Vaccines are now tailored for effectiveness against emerging mutant COVID-19 strains, such as the Omicron variant. Offering universal vaccination of adults for free was a wise governmental decision and public health measure that saved many lives.

Opinion: The manufacture and availability of a relatively effective vaccine constitutes a great accomplishment of modern medicine that saved many millions of lives in America and worldwide. Prioritization of vaccination of physicians appears justified because physicians willingly accepted increased risks of contracting COVID-19 infection, by voluntarily treating COVID-19-infected patients.

8. COVID-19 testing became progressively more available, faster, and more accurate (April 2020 to current).

Changes in Ancillary Hospital Services due to the Pandemic

1. Hospital cafeteria changed to offer disposable plastic utensils (including silverware, plates, and trays) during the pandemic to reduce risks of COVID-19 transmission (April 2020 to current).

Opinion: This represented a radical change in Hospital policy because the Hospital had previously instituted using metal utensils and discontinued using disposable plasticware to protect the environment. This reminds me of an old Jewish proverb, "man plans und der Heibishter *lacht*" (Yiddish for "and God laughs").

2. The Hospital cafeteria erected plastic (Lucite) barriers between cafeteria customers and food servers to reduce risks of COVID-19 virus transmission.
3. Patients were reluctant to present to the Hospital emergency department with diseases or disorders other than COVID-19 infection due to fears of contracting COVID-19 infection while in the Hospital for other reasons (March 2020 to current).

Opinion: This phenomenon was suspected of causing higher mortality of diseases unrelated to COVID-19 infection, such as ischemic cardiovascular disease and systemic hypertension during the pandemic due to the failure of patients to present for preventive cardiac care.[16,17]

4. Before the pandemic, the Hospital during normal business hours had one hospitality clerk and no security guards manning major hospital entrances (except for the emergency room entrance which always maintained tight security) and had no hospital personnel guarding minor hospital entrances. With the pandemic onset, the Hospital initially closed the main (East) entrance; closed minor, unguarded, entrances; and maintained enhanced security, with two hospitality clerks and four other personnel, mostly previously furloughed rehabilitation technicians, manning major entrances from March to June 2020. All hospital employees, including GI employees, had to sign a form upon entering the hospital daily for work declaring that they were healthy and free of suspected symptoms of COVID-19 infection. From March to July 2020 all patient visitors, whether visiting patients with COVID-19 infection or not, were barred entry to the hospital to reduce infection transmission. Subsequently, hospital clerks dispensed antiviral cleaning solutions to hospital employees and hospital visitors to clean and disinfect their hands upon entering the

Hospital. Enhanced security was gradually reduced starting in August 2020, with security eventually reduced to one or two clerks at all major entrances due to decreasing concern about morbidity and mortality from COVID-19 infection.

Opinion: Enhanced security was reasonable to protect Hospital patients and their visitors from contracting COVID-19 infection.

5. The Hospital added a module consisting of 12 slides (March to May 2021) on general medical knowledge about COVID-19 infection that was mandatory for all Hospital-affiliated physicians. The slides included COVID-19 infection symptoms, signs, laboratory abnormalities, epidemiology, diagnostic testing, treatment, and vaccination. This teaching module was presented virtually, by Internet, with slides and brief video presentations, and with post-module multiple choice questions graded automatically by computer by the Internet.

Opinion: This mandatory module was brief and appropriate in view of the importance of the pandemic.

Reduction of Gastrointestinal Physician Stress During the Pandemic

1. Medical house staff working at the Hospital contracted COVID-19 Infection at a moderately higher rate than the public experienced in the Detroit area (Marchto June 2020). House staff generally had asymptomatic or mild infections attributed to the relative youthfulness of house staff. The GI attendings and GI fellows had a similar rate of contracting COVID-19 infection (March to June 2020).
2. GI fellows were highly susceptible to emotional stress from risks of contracting COVID-19 infection from infected patients while working as medical attendings on medical wards exclusively treating COVID-19-infected patients (April-May 2020). Increased stress of health care workers due to the pandemic was documented for general physicians.[18,]

Opinion: As GI fellowship program director, I individually contacted all GI fellows twice weekly by telephone to discuss their emotional state and perceived workload burden to support their morale and psychological health (April and May 2020). Starting June 1, 2020, my intense engagement with GI fellows as program director reverted to baseline as the work rotations for GI fellows returned to baseline (without their functioning as supervisory medical attendings on exclusively COVID-19 wards). GI fellows, indeed, recommended one change in their workload schedule which I implemented without diminishing the quality of patient care. The original GI fellow schedule for April to May 2020 had one GI fellow on-call covering the GI service and another GI fellow on-call supervising a medical ward for COVID-19-infected patients. At the GI fellows' request, I modified the on-call schedule to have one GI fellow cover both of these on-call services. All the GI fellows were delighted to have one GI fellow working moderately hard covering the two services on-call, rather than having two GI fellows, each working less hard, cover only one on-call service. With gradually decreasing pandemic mortality and severity of infection,[19] GI fellows should experience substantially less psychological stress from the pandemic. .

3. To reduce work-related stress and risks to endoscopy staff during the COVID-19 surge, inpatient endoscopies for elective indications were postponed for at least several weeks to be performed as outpatients after patient discharge. Also, GI fellows performed mildly delayed GI consultations on COVID-19-infected patients due to their overwhelming clinical load. Medical attendings and house staff quickly complained in five cases about these two issues during the first twenty days of the

pandemic (March 2020). This rate of complaints was tenfold more than the baseline rate of about five complaints annually before the pandemic! Moreover, these complaints during the early pandemic were lodged to the Chair of Medicine or GME administrators rather than within the Division (chief of GI or GI fellowship program director), as had usually occurred previously.

Opinion: I advised GI fellows and GI attendings to proactively engage medical house staff and attendings when postponing GI endoscopies in patients with COVID-19 infection to prevent such complaints. I advised medical residents and medical attendings about the GI policy of postponing elective GI endoscopies. These two types of complaints rapidly abated; the high rate of complains during the first 20 days of the pandemic reverted to the baseline rate of about five complaints annually, thereafter. This reduction was attributed to less volume of COVID-19 patients as their rate hospitalization decreased and more understanding by medical attendings and house staff of the difficult circumstances encountered by GI fellows due to the pandemic.

Evaluation of Gastrointestinal Fellows

1. Supervisory GI attendings evaluate GI fellows monthly using a somewhat lengthy, comprehensive, computerized questionnaire involving seven medical competencies plus an overall performance evaluation. During the pandemic surge, I, as GI fellowship program director, replaced these time-consuming monthly GI attending evaluation forms with a highly abbreviated form asking only two questions requiring only yes or no answers and that took only a moment for a GI attending to complete per evaluation described under heading 2 below. I then contacted key faculty by telephone if they had problems about individual GI fellows. Monthly attending evaluation forms reverted to the traditional, somewhat lengthy, monthly evaluation forms starting June 1, 2020.

Opinion: No GI supervisory attendings completed the standard detailed monthly GI fellow evaluation forms on time during the pandemic surge (0 forms completed out of 18 submitted to me by the GI attendings fromMarch to May 2020) because the GI attendings were overwhelmed by their clinical work during the pandemic surge. After I retroactively revised the evaluation forms for March to May 2020 in June 2020, the GI attendings promptly completed and submitted the greatly abbreviated evaluation forms.

2. Normally the six key GI faculty met quarterly face-to-face to review the clinical and academic progress of the six GI fellows, but the April 2020 quarterly meeting was canceled and replaced by only two brief questions sent by email by me as program director to all the 6 key faculty (requiring only yes or no answers). The questions asked whether individual fellows had (1) experienced significant problems, and (2) had satisfactorily progressed toward promotion/graduation during the prior quarter. I then contacted key faculty by telephone if they had problems about individual GI fellows. Regularly scheduled face-to-face quarterly GI key faculty meetings resumed in June 2020, with about half of the GI faculty committee members present virtually and about half present physically at the meeting.

Opinion: I instituted the abbreviated and simplified quarterly key faculty evaluations (April 2020) as an emergency measure during the height of the pandemic surge.

3. Annual Accreditation Council for Graduate Medical Education (ACGME) and National Board of Medical Examiners annual evaluations of all six GI fellows maintained fully and on time without delays despite pandemic (June 2020). The

required evaluation forms were maintained complete and without abbreviation despite the pandemic to fully evaluate the GI fellows.

Opinion: I wholeheartedly agree with the decision to have these forms completed on time and in full to not delay promotions or graduations of GI fellows and not delay graduating GI fellows from eligibility to sit for the GI board examination, and to have such critical decisions about GI fellow graduations or promotions rendered on a complete and unabbreviated evaluation. Similar actions were designed to prevent medical students' graduation from being delayed for one year due to the pandemic (see Discussion).

4. The GI Division traditionally celebrates a graduation party to honor graduating GI fellows and their spouses (or significant others) attended by GI physician assistants, secretaries, program coordinator/manager, fellowship program director, Chief of GI, and voluntary and full-time GI attendings. From 2006 to 2019 the graduation party was always held at a local restaurant and the party costs were paid by a philanthropic grant donated to the Division. In June 2020, the graduation party was held virtually rather than physically. To simulate the traditional party experience, each graduating fellow ordered two fully catered takeout dinners which were delivered to their home from a local restaurant of their choice and were paid for by the Division. The party was held remotely with partygoers connected by telephone conference call. GI fellows, including the graduating GI fellows, key GI faculty, and the Program Director spoke at the virtual party via telephone conference calls. The day after the virtual party, the two graduating GI fellows received their diplomas and graduation gifts in person from the GI faculty. The annual GI graduation party (June 2021) was held physically at a local restaurant. Aside from the GI divisional party, the Hospital traditionally celebrated a hospital-wide graduation party and awards ceremony every June for all graduating house staff in all divisions and departments. This celebration was canceled in June 2020 because of the pandemic.

Opinion: Although everyone appreciated the virtual GI graduation party in 2020, especially the graduating GI fellows, it lacked the camaraderie, spontaneity, and emotional satisfaction of a “live” graduation party. Nevertheless, it was the best that could be accomplished under the pandemic circumstances.

5. For the last 15 years before the pandemic, the Division had celebrated a holiday party around the Christmas and New Year holidays at a local restaurant, with the party funded by the Division. In December 2020 the annual party did not formally occur because of the pandemic, but it was replaced by a small informal and unofficial gathering of some faculty and GI fellows to celebrate the Holidays (December 2020).
6. The medical school traditionally celebrated the following ceremonies or parties annually: a white coat party for medical students entering the clinical wards, a party on match day when fourth-year medical students are notified of their matches with residency programs, and a graduation convocation and party in which graduating medical students receive their diplomas and in which deserving medical students and faculty receive awards. All these celebrations were changed from physical to virtual in 2020 and 2021.

Opinion: All these ceremonies felt much less celebratory as virtual rather than live and face-to-face ceremonies but were the best that could be accomplished under the circumstances of the pandemic.

Graduate Medical Education, Gastrointestinal Research, and Gastrointestinal and Hepatology Professional Societies

1. During the pandemic surge (April to June 2020), committee meetings of Hospital GME administrators with program directors and representative house officers were changed from monthly to weekly to quickly adapt to the rapidly changing needs of residency and fellowship trainees and their patients due to the pandemic surge and were changed from face-to-face to virtual meetings to reduce pandemic exposure.

Opinion: This increased frequency of committee meetings was necessitated by the rapidly changing circumstances of patient care due to the pandemic.

2. The Hospital, in collaboration with the Medical School, traditionally held an education week annually in May to recognize house officers who present posters or brief podium talks based on their clinical research projects conducted during the prior academic year, to disseminate their research, and to compete for monetary prizes based on the clinical importance and quality of their research presentations. The education week also featured a nationally known visiting professor who presented several lectures on academic medicine, which were endowed by a philanthropic grant. Annual education week meetings were always held publicly, live, and face-to-face in conference rooms or assembly halls before the pandemic. The annual education week was extremely limited in May 2020 due to the pandemic, with only a few research posters, presented virtually via the Internet, to reduce pandemic exposure. Monetary prizes were not awarded in 2020 and podium talks and lectures by a visiting professor were canceled in 2020. The education week was, however, reinstituted fully in May 2021, including awarding prizes for the best research papers authored by residents and fellows. Research abstracts or talks were presented only virtually with no podium or other physical research talks, but the lectures by an invited visiting professor were fully reinstated and presented live and physically in an auditorium and also streamed live virtually by the Internet.

Opinion: It was good to see some recovery of the educational week activities as the pandemic crisis eased in 2021.

3. The Hospital in collaboration with the Medical School publishes annually a comprehensive compilation of scholarly activities, including publications (original articles, reviews, and case reports) published in peer-reviewed journals, articles in books, abstracts presented orally or as posters at national or international professional meetings, and invited talks or presentations at academic hospitals during the prior academic year for all residents, fellows, clinical attendings, and research faculty in all Divisions and Departments at all Beaumont Network Hospitals. The annual compilation of scholarly achievements for the academic year of 2019 was extremely delayed (until December 2020) and this compilation was only published virtually, without publication as a physical book, as had occurred in previous years. Publication of the annual 2020 scholarly achievements was published soon after the normally expected date (June 2021) with minor delays because of the declining pandemic impact and was disseminated virtually and was also not physically published.
4. The American Gastroenterology Association normally holds an annual in-service examination for GI fellows that evaluates their cognitive skills in GI and hepatology via a 3-h-long examination using multiple choice questions in the fields of hepatology, esophagus, stomach, small bowel, colon, hepatobiliary tree, pancreas, and GI

endoscopy. The grades of individual GI fellows are compared with that of their peers, stratified according to fellowship year of training. Normally a proctor is physically present in the room to proctor test-takers taking the test by computer. This annual examination provides GI fellows a valuable service by indicating how they compare with their peers in each individual subject to identify topics in which they are comparatively weak and may want to study further for the Board examination. The annual examination was not postponed but was changed from physical proctoring to remote proctoring of the computerized examinations due to the pandemic (March 2020 and March 2021). It was held virtually by computer by Internet, as in previous years, without any changes required because of the pandemic except for the remote proctoring.

5. The major annual GI national/international professional conventions in 2020 were all scheduled as physical events in specific cities, including Digestive Disease Week sponsored by the American Gastroenterology Association and American Society for Gastrointestinal Endoscopy scheduled for May 2020 in Chicago, Illinois; American College of Gastroenterology scheduled for October 2020 in Memphis, Tennessee; and American Association for the Study of Liver Diseases scheduled for November 2020 in Boston, Massachusetts. These conventions traditionally were massive affairs, sometimes exceeding 10,000 participants and involving hundreds of commercial exhibitors. These conventions were, however, all changed to virtual meetings conducted via the Internet in 2020 to reduce transmission of COVID-19 infection in crowded convention halls.

Opinion: The change to virtual meetings saved conventioneers time and money by avoiding the costs of round-trip flights to the host city and local lodging. The author, however, feels significant loss from the absence of physical meetings due to the loss of professional camaraderie and interactions between speakers, researchers, exhibitors, and physicians. In 2021, the Digestive Week Convention was also held entirely virtually, rather than as a physical meeting.[20]

6. Program managers, including the GI fellowship program manager, were furloughed (March to May 2020), and then instructed to work virtually from home (June 2020 to June 2021) to decrease their exposure to COVID-19 infection from the pandemic, and instructed to perform their duties by telephone or Internet.

Opinion: This policy change mildly decreased the program manager's efficiency but its effect was mitigated by program managers still coming to the hospital physically to occasionally attend critical meetings.

7. The ACGME and RRC normally comprehensively annually survey by Internet all six GI fellows at the Hospital with 30 questions about the academic and clinical quality of the fellowship program and annually survey all six key GI faculty at the Hospital with 30 similar questions to indicate the clinical and teaching quality of the program. Both surveys are detailed and relatively time-consuming. These surveys are normally mandatory. The ACGME and RRC emailed the annual surveys to GI fellows and to key GI faculty (March 2020) with a response due by April 2020. However, the ACGME abruptly canceled both surveys due to the pandemic (April 2020) and subsequently reinstituted the surveys on a voluntary basis in May to June 2020. The ACGME emailed the annual surveys for 2021 (March 2021) to both the GI fellows and key GI attendings. These surveys were completed electronically and returned by email by the key faculty and GI fellows (April 2021) despite the ongoing pandemic. The resulting survey evaluations were sent to program directors, together with extensive descriptive statistics comparing institutional performance

of the GI fellows with nationwide performance parameters in late April 2021. Descriptive evaluation statistics were sent anonymously, without revealing individual evaluators.

Opinion: The GI fellow and GI attending surveys were filled, compiled, analyzed, and sent to program directors in 2021 because all these actions were performed virtually by Internet.

8. The ACGME and RRC periodically perform physcial site visits of accredited residency and fellowship programs, with the physical site visit interval set according to program performance during the prior site visit. Site visits are prolonged affairs requiring one or two RRC surveyors to carefully survey the Hospital fellowship and residency programs. For example, two site visitors spent one week at the Hospital surveying the Department of Medicine at the last Hospital site visit. During a site visit, surveyors meet program directors, division chiefs, program managers, hospital administrators, medical residents, fellows, and the designated hospital GME official. Surveyors audit all divisions and departments to ascertain that all mandated paperwork from fellowship and residency program directors and program managers are complete, accurate, and up-to-date. Surveyors report their findings on quality of residency and fellowship programs to the relevant RRC committee based upon the surveyors' findings and the committee decides whether to grant programs continuing accreditation; sets the time interval for continuing accreditation; decides whether to impose citations or warnings that must be addressed by the institution, residency, or fellowship programs in a timely manner; and determines whether to place a program on probation or suspension. The ACGME cancelled all physical site visits for residency and fellowship programs during the pandemic surge (March to July 2020) and then resumed site visits (starting August 2020), while changing the site visit format from physical to virtual. Paperwork previously submitted during physical site visits were now submitted by Internet. For example, the Critical Care and Pulmonary Medicine training program at the Hospital had a virtual rather than physical site visit scheduled in October 2021. The ACGME initially planned a physical site visit for the Internal Medicine and the GI fellowship program at the Hospital in 2020 but canceled this physical site visit due to the pandemic and deferred this visit until at least 2022 or possibly later, because the pandemic delayed the entire ACGME work schedule.

Opinion: Physical site visits involve large expenditures by the RRC for surveyors to visit a hospital typically for about one week, incurring costs of airline flights, local lodging, and food expenses. Although virtual visits do not engender such expenses, virtual visits, do not provide the camaraderie and intimate conversations available at physical meetings that potentially provide informal informative discussions about the visited sites.

9. Significantly reduced GI research electives for GI fellows at the Hospital due to the pandemic (March to June 2020). The pandemic may lead to less resident and fellow research electives and less time dedicated to clinical research because of a greater clinical load. However, research on COVID-19 infection has blossomed. This is indicated by the more than 300,000 articles published in peer reviewed medical journals until November 2022 on this subject.[2] The pandemic provides physicians a once-in-a-lifetime opportunity to perform exciting, cutting-edge, research on COVID-19 that can potentially save lives. I encourage young medical researchers to consider focusing their research on COVID-19 infection.

Opinion: Catastrophes, including war, economic depression, famine, plague, and other natural disasters are the traditional enemies of medical research because of less financial resources available to devote to medical research. Despite my heavy clinical obligations during the pandemic, I took my own advice and devoted my research exclusively on GI manifestations of COVID-19 from the pandemic onset, starting with my first publishing an article on diarrhea with COVID-19 infection in April 2020[22] and I have so far published 10 articles in peer-reviewed journals on this subject and am currently editing this book on this subject.[21,23–25] Also, in my experience, decisions on acceptance of medical research papers submitted for publication normally take about two months or longer after submission for peer review, but I had a case report on a COVID-19-infected patient with diarrhea accepted within one week of submission and published virtually one week thereafter in a leading clinical GI journal.[22] I believe accelerated peer-review and publication in medical journals of papers on the pandemic[26] is justified by the overwhelming clinical need to disseminate new medical findings on the pandemic to save patient lives.

DISCUSSION

This work shows that the pandemic severely affected the American businesses climate and consumer behavior. The economy abruptly contracted at the pandemic onset by >30% in the first fiscal quarter of 2020. House sales plummeted at the pandemic onset due to home buyers unwillingness to expend large funds to purchase homes in the face of economic uncertainty engendered by the pandemic.

The Hospital, located at a pandemic epicenter in suburban Royal Oak near Detroit, was severely affected by the pandemic. During the pandemic surge, twenty-five percent of inpatients had COVID-19 infection. Hospital costs rose rapidly due to purchases of mechanical ventilators required to treat respiratory decompensation from COVID-19 pneumonia. Most operating rooms were converted to ICU beds to accommodate patients suffering from respiratory decompensation from COVID-19 pneumonia. As more patients were admitted with COVID-19 infection, revenue decreased from other admissions because much fewer patients than normal underwent elective ambulatory procedures or were admitted to short stay wards for procedures. Hospital occupancy plunged to approximately 55% of capacity from >90% of capacity before the pandemic. Moreover, the Hospital tended to lose money on patients admitted with respiratory decompensation from COVID-19 pneumonia due to their requirements for intense medical resources, such as ICU beds and mechanical ventilators, whereas patients did not come for elective short stays, minor surgeries, and ambulatory procedures, such as GI endoscopy, which all tended to be highly lucrative for the Hospital due to low resource utilization and relatively high insurance reimbursements. For example, the rate of GI endoscopy plummeted drastically to 4% of baseline during the initial pandemic onslaught. The Hospital faced several fiscal quarters of budgetary shortfalls.

This problem was exacerbated and compounded by Hospital mistakes. First and foremost, the Hospital paid a huge penalty to settle a long-standing claim, stemming from 2006-2012, against it by the Department of Justice for alleged Hospital violations of the Stark (antikickback) Law in paying eight cardiologists undeserved compensation (alleged kickbacks) for referring their private patients to the Hospital. This 84.5-million-dollar settlement was consummated at an exceedingly inopportune time for the Hospital just before the pandemic onset. This settlement also badly damaged the Hospital's reputation which decreased the willingness of patients to entrust their own or their families healthcare to the Hospital and lowered the morale of full-time

Hospital-employed and voluntarily affiliated physicians. Second, to cut costs, the Hospital terminated a 20-years-long exclusive contract with a highly respected anesthesiology group in favor of a low-cost anesthesiology group. This proved to be a disaster because the low-cost anesthesiology group could not provide an adequate number of anesthesiologists to staff the endoscopy suite rooms. About half of the endoscopy suite rooms were left idle due to the shortage of anesthesiologists. This caused the Hospital to absorb very significant unrealized (or lost opportunities) for revenues. Many already scheduled GI endoscopies (January-April 2021) were cancelled after the patient and the endoscopy attending came for the scheduled endoscopy because anesthesiologists were unavailable. Third, the nurse-anesthetists voted overwhelmingly, during the anesthesiology controversy, to unionize adding more expenses to run endoscopy rooms. Fourth, the Hospital won a pyrrhic victory against unionization of nurses because many nurses left the Hospital after being frustrated and demoralized by the failed unionization drive. The hospital had spent about two million dollars waging a campaign to discourage nurse unionization.[40] I wonder out loud whether such payments are permissible to a nonprofit institution or would have to be accounted by a for-profit branch of the institution (I do not know whether the appropriate accounting occurred or not). This loss of endoscopy nurses further exacerbated the shortage of professionals staffing the GI endoscopy unit and precipitated other fierce Hospital cost-cutting measures that caused other mistakes. Fifth, the Medical School (approximately half owned by the Hospital) furloughed 20% of its IT staff just when they would need them the most to implement virtual technology (for virtual medical school lectures and virtual meetings) because of the pandemic. This lack of IT support predictably resulted in six medical school lecture cancellations without warning for the GI and renal courses (or about 12% of the total clinical lectures in these two courses) because of computer gaffes made by clinical educators recording their lectures without IT guidance or supervision. One hundred and twenty-five medical students, who had paid an estimated $15,000 in tuition money (at about $125.00 per student per lecture x 125 students), were punished by coming to attend these lectures which were abruptly cancelled without warning. Seventh, the Hospital selectively abruptly terminated senior, older, highly accomplished, and distinguished academicians with outstanding reputations (approximately June 2021-on), including the Chief Medical Officer, the highest and most senior Hospital-employed physician who was a well-known and highly regarded academic researcher with an outstanding curriculum vitae,[41] and abruptly terminated several highly distinguished, and older Departmental Chairs without cause. The Chief Hospital Quality officer left to accept a position at another hospital. The Hospital replaced these highly accomplished leaders with physicians with much inferior academic credentials but who were paid much lower salaries. Eighth, the Hospital severely cut back librarian staff to cut costs. This saved negligible money due to the low salaries of the librarians compared to the overall Hospital budget, but negatively impacted the educational, clinical, and research missions of the Hospital as the primary teaching hospital of a medical school.

The government invested heavily in providing the Hospital four bonus payments totaling approximately 500 million dollars in 2020-2021 but even these payments could not create a financially healthy environment for the Hospital. Consequently, the Hospital offered itself as a suitor to one hundred hospital systems in proposed buyouts, mergers, or acquisitions.[45] During this time the Hospital announced two planned mergers or acquisitions, one by Advocate Aurora Health,[42] and another by Summa Health,[43] only to see both deals fail. Finally, the Hospital was either bought by or merged with Spectrum Health during the pandemic.[44]

The Hospital made several token gestures to employed physicians during the pandemic such as complementary lunches for four days; small $1,000 bonus payments to house staff or full-time attendings; and paying the annual voluntary employer matching contributions to employee retirement funds for 2019 and 2020. However, these gestures failed to achieve their objective of improving the morale of dispirited hospital-employed and voluntary physicians who were seeing the Hospital being offered to other medical institutions without their involvement.

The Hospital made an abrupt about face decision on several "pet" Hospital projects because of the pandemic. The Hospital stopped using metal non-disposable silverware (originally instituted to help the environment) and returned to using disposable plastic silverware to decrease pandemic exposure; and the Hospital reversed itself to permit physicians to wear surgical scrubs anywhere in the Hospital to decrease clothing contamination from its prior policy that strictly forbade physicians from wearing surgical scrubs outside operating room-like settings. This change reminds me of an old Jewish proverb, "man plans *und der Heibishter lacht*" (Yiddish for "and God laughs").

The Hospital and Medical School often used an opaque decision process without involving hospital-employed or voluntary physicians in the decisions. For example, endoscopy suite gowns were changed to substantially thinner and cheaper gowns during the pandemic (2021) without consulting or informing GI attendings. The academic anesthesiology group was terminated and replaced by a low-cost anesthesiology group during the pandemic without consulting GI attendings. The medical school course structure was substantially changed due to the pandemic without consulting the course codirectors and the course codirectors were only informed of these changes on short notice.

I created several minor innovations to ameliorate problems created by the pandemic. One, I called GI fellows weekly during the height of the raging pandemic to check on their psychological stresses while they worked as medical attendings on exclusively COVID-19 wards (April & May 2020). Two, I advised medical residents and medical attendings about the GI policy of postponing elective GI endoscopies on patients with active COVID-19 infection. This announcement greatly decreased the number of complaints by house staff and medical attendings about postponing GI endoscopies in such patients. Three, in response to GI attendings not completing the standard monthly GI fellow evaluations at the height of the pandemic, I greatly shortened the monthly evaluation forms. Four, I greatly abbreviated and simplified the quarterly key GI faculty evaluation (April 2020) as an emergency measure during the pandemic surge.

I wholeheartedly agree with the important medical school decision to graduate medical students on time in June 2020 and in June 2021 despite their missing small parts of the medical school curriculum[33] to avoid delaying medical school graduation for one year due to the pandemic.[34] To quote the show business motto, "the show must go on"!

This comprehensive work shows the pervasiveness of the changes at how one extremely large, academic, GI division, in an academic tertiary care hospital that is the primary teaching hospital of a medical school. The Hospital reorganized when facing massive clinical needs caused by a pandemic explosively spreading from zero patients to >one-fourth of all hospital patients within one month, for a total onslaught of >13,000 distinct infected patients treated over one year. This work shows the revolutionary (profound and abrupt) changes in both institutions engendered by the pandemic. The suddenness of the crisis in Detroit is partly due to its being a local pandemic epicenter, like New York City, and the Hospital serving as a tertiary referral center for COVID-19-infected patients. This Hospital is an unusual academic hospital in that most attendings are voluntary and in private practice, with 36 GI attendings in private practice (recently reduced to 29 voluntary GI attendings after several GI attendings voluntarily left the Hospital) and only three (recently reduced to two) hospital-employed GI attendings. This composition of GI attendings resembles that of Baylor Medical Center, in Houston, Texas, a large academic hospital with a similar attending composition. GI practitioners in private practice had to agree to Hospital practice changes made during the pandemic. This involved complicated negotiations between the GI division and GI attendings, such as assigning voluntary GI attendings for GI endoscopies on staff (ward) patients with COVID-19 infection.

Traditional "live" lectures were replaced by virtual lectures. The medical school first used "canned" lectures of audiovisual tapes which had been filmed "live" during the previous academic year. This policy had advantages in that it could be implemented quickly and without costs but faced mild drawbacks including (1) not incorporating into preexisting audiovisual tapes curriculum changes recommended during the ensuing year; (2) several lecturers dropped from the lecture roster due to weak teaching ability were perforce still delivering "canned" lectures; and (3) questions asked during prior year lectures could not be easily edited out of "canned" lectures. Medical school administrators minimized these drawbacks by authorizing a new set of taped audiovisual "virtual" lectures, presented by the newly scheduled lecturers.

Beyond the change from physical to virtual lectures, the medical school and Hospital changed numerous other educational and clinical activities from physical to virtual, which included: GI divisional conferences, annual education week lectures, committee meetings, GI fellowship applicant interviews, program manager communications with program directors, and divisional parties or graduation ceremonies.

Virtual activities lack spontaneity, camaraderie, and personal interactions between speakers and live audiences due to computerized communications. How can I compare watching a sports event on television to the excitement and intensity of watching the same event "live" and in person at a stadium?[21] I felt emotionally detached when delivering virtual lectures by videoconference to medical residents in June 2020 because of no visual feedback from my virtual audience while I lectured. Lecturers presenting virtually cannot gauge audience reactions since they are not physically in the same room. Other lecturers have expressed similar feelings. Likewise, audience may experience decreased attentiveness and less satisfaction during virtual lectures ("in a virtual lecture, the lights go out and the minds tune out"). Virtual parties and ceremonies lack the comradery and feelings experienced in physical parties. Videoconferencing created a need for more information technologists and upgrading computer equipment for videoconferencing. IT personnel should be readily available to help clinicians or educators set-up videoconferences because clinicians or educators typically lack sophistication in computer technology as forementioned. During the early change to videoconferencing from physical meetings, few hospital computers had cameras or software for transmitting videoconferences. My ancient hospital computer installed about ten years before the pandemic had to be upgraded to a new computer provisioned with a video camera and microphone to enable videoconferencing during the pandemic. Some conferences early during the pandemic, before the computer upgrades were accomplished, had to be conducted by conference calls via cell phones. Virtual instead of physical activities will likely become the standard in many situations due to lower costs and elimination of travel time, but the benefits of physical activities must be considered in the equation. Virtual meetings are not all-or-none and can include physical attendance for participants who can easily attend physical meetings and virtual attendance only for far away participants. A two-tiered system may emerge: virtual for low-priority activities and low-priority participants (e.g., liaison participants), and physical for high-priority activities and high-priority participants (e.g., team leaders). For example, GI clinic visits may be physical for sick patients and virtual for relatively stable patients. Physical visits have the advantage of physical examination which can be important in patient evaluation. Before the pandemic, GI clinic televisits were not performed and not billed because Medicare and Medicaid only instituted reimbursement for televisits during the pandemic.[36] The closest activity resembling televisits before the pandemic was telephone calls from physicians to patients or vice versa, for which I did not bill for until the ruling allowing such billing during the early pandemic. Simulators have been developed to train GI fellows in GI endoscopy but are still in their infancy.

The Hospital strongly recommended changing in-hospital GI consults of COVID-19-infected patients from physical to virtual to decrease transmitting infection to physicians during the pandemic from March 2020 to current. Patients without COVID-19 infection were mostly seen through traditional physical visits. This change received the imprimatur of the Centers for Medicare and Medicaid Services which approved insurance reimbursement for virtual patient visits in April 2020.[36]

The author salutes the American Healthcare system for investing heavily in developing relatively effective vaccines using novel mRNA technology against the coronavirus and offering the vaccines for free to the general adult population. This saved many millions of lives. The manufacture and availability of a relatively effective vaccine constitutes a landmark accomplishment of modern medicine.

I remember and will never forget my first forceful confrontation with the explosive pandemic surge upon entering the hospital observation unit in the windowless cavernous halls in the hospital basement at high noon, circa March 13, 2020.[21] I reconnoitered with three fellow soldiers, a medical attending in the medical observation unit, a physician's assistant assigned to working with me, and an EKG technician. The lurking insidious enemy was present but invisible and could shoot to kill from any perch if we just got too close – less than six feet away.[21] We palpated the risks in manning the trenches, just like in the Great World War (also known as the War to End all Wars).

Among the four of us, only the physician's assistant working with me was wearing a facemask. We were as edgy as the untried soldier in the Red Badge of Courage. We lacked effective tools, guidance, and marching orders. The EKG technician complained that she had already entered dozens of patient rooms that day to perform EKGs without facemask protection. The medical attending worried out loud about his risks in seeing new patients with unknown COVID-19 status. The physician's assistant advised me to get a facemask forthwith. I hunted for twenty minutes until I found the only remaining N95 facemask, after searching six supply rooms. I then saw my consults several of whom proved later to have COVID-19 infection and one of whom I reported as the first mortality in which severe dehydration and electrolyte abnormalities from COVID-19-associated-diarrhea largely contributed to the patient's death.[22]

There is true grit in a grunt just following orders on such fateful days. Physicians and nurses deserve immense credit for heroically managing the pandemic crisis professionally, by willingly risking their health and even their lives as part of their job to treat COVID-19-infected patients without receiving extra compensation. These healthcare workers received extraordinary public support and praise as expressed by emails posted by charitable organizations, grateful patients, and ordinary citizens; by posters cropping up on Hospital grounds stating "Beaumont healthcare workers are our heroes"; and by at least one giant billboard erected just 1 block from the Hospital stating, "THANK YOU! Health Care Heroes-Beaumont." On Friday April 17, 2020, a procession of >100 police cars, fire trucks, and ambulances, with several hundred participants in their vehicles drove around Beaumont Hospital, Royal Oak, to honor healthcare professionals working at the Hospital who risked their lives by treating patients with COVID-19 infection.[21]

This work has limitations. First, this work was written by one investigator. The investigator, however, claims expertise from a long history in hospital administration and medical school education as described in the Methods section. This study was prospectively compiled permitting a comprehensive review and analysis. Moreover, the author actively participated in parts of the reorganization which helps explain the comprehensiveness of this review and analysis. Single authorship might potentially introduce observer bias, but the author focused on objective data. The author did not withhold reporting on intitutional errors because such error analysis may be instructive to prevent error recurrence in the (predictable) next pandemic. Second, this author might be criticized for reporting nonclinical details outside the GI division, Hospital, or Medical School in a clinical GI journal. However, actions outside the GI division contributed greatly to the hospital atmosphere and work environment of GI attendings and GI fellows, and to the clinical experiences of hospitalized patients.[21] This report included all changes that I felt affected my clinical practice, my work as an employee, and my emotional state, as well as affecting other divisional employees, medical students, or patients. For example, enhanced hospital security might be considered irrelevant to academic GI departmental reorganization, but is relevant to increasing anxiety of GI faculty, house staff, and their patients. Many important details external to the division are previously unreported. Third, this paper may be criticized for lengthiness, but an unprecedented, reorganization of the GI Division, Hospital, Medical School and affiliated institutions by a historic pandemic merits comprehensive reporting. The length of these two papers reflects their thorough research and comprehensive reporting.

I conclude, by taking my own advice and devoting my research exclusively to GI manifestations of COVID-19 infection from the pandemic onset. My five previous articles on GI manifestations of COVID-19 and my current five articles on this subject in this monograph and the monograph itself, which I edited, are fruits of my exclusive focus on this subject. This work greatly supplements previously published data on the pandemic impact on the clinical and academic missions of GI divisions.[27–32] My current and previous work[21] on the reorganization is distinguished by its depth and comprehensiveness, including new, previously unreported data concerning the reorganization of a medical school and academic hospital, some of which might never have been otherwise reported.

ACKNOWLEDGMENTS

Dr M.S. Cappell initiated this article and wrote the entire manuscript. The Hospital Institutional Review Board (IRB) approved the previously published study on April 14, 2020.[21] The current work does not require IRB approval because it is solely a review article with no report of original patient data and only provides expert opinion based only on previously published data. Dr M.S. Cappell is employed as a gastroenterologist at the Aleda E. Lutz VA Hospital in Saginaw, Michigan. The Veteran's Administration Hospital in Saginaw and the federal government of the United States have no position or opinion on this publication. Dr. Cappell dedicates these two related special critical review articles to Dr. Anthony Fauci, the Head of Infectious Diseases at the National Institutes of Health, who has served selflessly in this capacity or other positions as a public servant at the National Institutes of Health over a long career, and who despite this dedicated service was the subject of vitriol because of advocating vaccination for the pandemic that has been proven to save millions of lives throughout the world.

On the occasion of the retirement of Dr. Anthony Fauci from the National Institutes of Health, Dr. Cappell dedicates this issue to Dr. Fauci for his distinguished, life-long governmental service especially for his role in championing vaccine development for COVID-19 infection in the face of vitriolic, political, and ad hominem attacks.

CONFLICT OF INTEREST

The author declares no conflict of interest. Dr M.S. Cappell, as a member of the United States Food and Drug Administration (FDA) Advisory Committee for Gastrointestinal Drugs, 2013 to 2018,[35] affirms that this paper does not discuss any proprietary, confidential, pharmaceutical data submitted to the FDA and reviewed by Dr M.S. Cappell. Dr M.S. Cappell was >4 years ago a member of the speaker's bureau for AstraZeneca and Daiichi Sankyo, co-marketers of Movantik. Dr M.S. Cappell had one-time consultancies for Mallinckrodt and Shire >3 years ago. This work does not discuss any drug manufactured or marketed by AstraZeneca, Daiichi Sankyo, Shire, or Mallinckrodt.

DISCLAIMER

M. S. Cappell is employed as a gastroenterologist at the Aleda E. Lutz Veterans Administration Hospital in Saginaw, MI and by the United States Government. These institutions do not have an opinion on the views expressed by Dr. Cappell herein.

REFERENCES

1. Federal response to COVID-19. This is how much was spent so far in response to COVID. Available at: https://www.usaspending.gov/disaster/covid-19?publicLaw=all. Accessed November 3, 2022.
2. NCBI SARS-CoV-2 resources. National Institute of Health, Library of Medicine, National Center for Biotechnology Information. SARS-CoV-2 Data. Available at: https://www.ncbi.nlm.nih.gov/sars-cov-2/. Accessed November 2, 2022.
3. Watson OJ, Barnsley G, Toor J, et al. Global impact of the first year of COVID-19 vaccination: a mathematical modelling study. Lancet Infect Dis 2022;22(9): 1293–302.
4. Savinkina A, Bilinski A, Fitzpatrick M, et al. Estimating deaths averted and cost per life saved by scaling up mRNA COVID-19 vaccination in low-income and lower-middle-income countries in the COVID-19 Omicron variant era: a modelling study. BMJ Open 2022;12(9):e061752.
5. Udalova, Victoria. Pandemic impact on mortality and economy varies across age groups and geographies. United States Census, March 8, 2021. Available at: www.census.gov/library/stories/2021/03/initial-impact-covid-19-on-united-states-economy-more-widespread-than-on-mortality.html. Accessed May 4, 2021.
6. Greene J. Beaumont drops $146.7 million loss, attributed to pandemic, reduction in elective surgeries. Crain's Detroit Business. Available at: www.crainsdetroit.com/health-care/beaumont-drops-1467-million-loss-attributed-pandemic-reduction-elective-surgeries.
7. Beaumont News Releases. COVID-19 pandemic affects Beaumont Health's year-end 2020 financial results. Available at: www.beaumont.org/healthwellness/

pressreleases/covid-19-pandemic-affects-beaumont-healths-year-end2020-financial-results.

8. Walsh D. Beaumont reports loss of nearly $100 million during first half of 2022. Crain's Detroit Business. Available at: www.crainsdetroit.com/health-care/beaumont-reports-loss-nearly-100- million-during-first-half-2022.
9. Anonymous. Beaumont Health temporarily laying off 2,475 employees, permanently eliminating 450 jobs. Fox 2, Detroit. Available at: www.fox2detroit.com/news/beaumont-health-temporarily-laying-off-2475-employees-permanently-eliminating-450jobs. Accessed April 22, 2020.
10. Livengood C. Beaumont lays off 2,475 employees, eliminates 450 jobs as major revenue streams dry up. Crain's Detroit Business News 2020. Available at: www.crainsdetroit.com/health-care/beaumont-la-2475-employees-eliminate-450-jobscut-executive-pay. Accessed April 23, 2020.
11. Cavitt M. Beaumont lays off 2,475 employees, eliminates 450 jobs as major revenue streams dry up. Available at: www.theoaklandpress.com/news/beaumont-lays-off-2-475-employees-eliminates-450-jobs-as-major-revenue-streams-dry-up/article_b5a5c8d2-83d0-11ea-a90e-efa0ffcac378.html. Oakland Press April 21, 2020. Accessed April 22, 2020.
12. LeBlanc B. Henry Ford Health to furlough 2,800 employees amid COVID-19 losses. Detroit News. April 22, 2020. Available at: https://www.detroitnews.com/story/news/local/michigan/2020/04/22/henry-ford-health-furlough-2800-employees-amid-pandemic-losses/3008570001/. Accessed April 23, 2020.
13. Carey M. Second week of HPI polling shows dentists' response toCOVID-19: Four in five dentists closed their practices except for emergencies. ADA (American Dental Association News). Available at: https://www.ada.org/en/publications/ada-news/2020-archive/april/second-week-of-hpi-polling-shows-dentists-response-tocovid-19. Accessed April 25, 2020.
14. Kovanis, George. Trying to retain health care workers in times of COVID-19, Beaumont gives $1,000 bonus. Detroit Free Press November 12, 2020. Available at: www.freep.com/story/news/local/michigan/2020/11/12/coronavirus-covid-19-beaumonthealth-employee-bonus/6266431002/. Accessed April 27, 2021.
15. Beaumont Health offering walk-in COVID-19 vaccine clinic Thursday in Southfield. WWJ Newsradio 950. Local news. April21. 2021. Available at: www.audacy.com/wwjnewsradio/news/local/beaumont-opens-walk-in-vaccine-clinic-thursday-in-southfield. Accessed May 4, 2021.
16. Napoli N. COVID-19 pandemic indirectly disrupted heart disease care. 2021. Available at: www.acc.org/aboutacc/press-releases/2021/01/11/16/40/covid19-pandemic-indirectly-disrupted-heart-disease-care. Accessed May 4, 2021.
17. Banerjee A, Chen S, Pasea L, et al. Excess deaths in people with cardiovascular diseases during theCOVID-19 pandemic. Eur J Prev Cardiol 2021;zwaa155. https://doi.org/10.1093/eurjpc/zwaa155. Available at:.
18. Jalandra RN, Shahul AS, Asfahan S, et al. Emotional distress among health professionals involved in care of inpatients with COVID-19: a survey based cross-sectional study. Adv Respir Med 2022. https://doi.org/10.5603/ARM.a2022.0026. published online ahead of print, 2022 Feb 24.
19. Centers for Disease Control and Prevention. COVID-19 Data Review: Update on COVID-19–Related Mortality. 2022. Available at: https://www.cdc.gov/coronavirus/2019-ncov/science/data-review/index.html. Accessed: December 12, 2022.
20. Available at: www.hpnonline.com/events/event/21202555/digestive-disease-week-ddw-virtual. Accessed April 27, 2021.

21. Cappell MS. Local COVID-19 epicenter in Detroit metropolitan area causing profound and pervasive reorganization of clinical, educational, research, and financial programs of a large academic gastroenterology division with a GI fellowship and primary medical school affiliation. Dig Dis Sci 2021;66(11):3635–58.
22. Cappell MS. Moderately severe diarrhea and impaired renal function with COVID-19 infection. Am J Gastroenterol 2020;115:947–8.
23. Cappell MS. Novel modifications for a virtual interview visit to simulate the traditional, live, site visit for GI fellowship applicants for an academic GI fellowship program due to the COVID-19 pandemic. Dig Dis Sci 2021;66:1370–1.
24. Gill I, Shaheen AA, Edhi AI, et al. Novel case report: A previously reported, but pathophysiologically unexplained, association between collagenous colitis and protein-losing enteropathy may be explained by an undetected link with collagenous duodenitis. Dig Dis Sci 2021;4:1–8.
25. Cappell MS. Problems for gastrointestinal patients with diarrheal disorders: Limited access to public bathrooms because previously open public bathrooms have closed due to COVID-19 pandemic and inadequate number of bathrooms in some endoscopy suites. Am J Gastroenterol 2021;116:1355–6.
26. Tingley K. Coronavirus Is forcing medical research to speed up. New York Times Magazine. April 21, 2020. Available at: https://www.nytimes.com/2020/04/21/magazine/coronavirus-scientific-journals-research.html. Accessed April 25, 2020.
27. Papaefthymiou A, Koffas A, Kountouras J, et al. The impact of COVID-19 pandemic on gastrointestinal diseases: a single-center cross-sectional study in central Greece. Ann Gastroenterol 2021;34:323–30.
28. Koo CS, Siah KTH, Koh CJ. Endoscopy training in COVID-19: Challenges and hope for a better age. J Gastroenterol Hepatol 2021. https://doi.org/10.1111/jgh.15524.
29. Li J, Li C, Wang X, et al. Considerations and perspectives on digestive diseases during the COVID-19 pandemic: a narrative review. Ann Palliat Med 2021;10:4858–67.
30. Tepper DL, Burger AP, Weissman MA. Hands down, COVID-19 will change medical practice. Am J Manag Care 2020;26:e274–5.
31. Crespo J, Fernández Carrillo C, Iruzubieta P, et al. Massive impact of corona virus disease 2019 pandemic on gastroenterology and hepatology departments and doctors in Spain. J Gastroenterol Hepatol 2020;36:1627–33.
32. Gross SA, Robbins DH, Greenwald DA, et al. Preparation in the Big Apple: New York City, A new epicenter of the COVID-19 pandemic. Am J Gastroenterol 2020 Jun;115:801–4.
33. Coronavirus outbreak forces OUWB medical students to embrace 'new normal' in learning. Oakland University William Beaumont School of Medicine, Mar 24, 2020. Available at: https://oakland.edu/medicine/news/auto-list-news/2020/Coronavirus-outbreak-forces-OUWB-medical-students-to. Accessed December 8,2022.
34. Oakland University William Beaumont School of Medicine. Getting across the finish line: How OUWB keeps next-gen physicians on track during pandemic. Friday, May 01, 2020. Available at: oakland.edu/medicine/news/auto-list-news/2020/Getting-acrossthe-finish-line-How-OUWB-keeps-next-gen-physicians-on-trackduring-pandemic. Accessed May 4, 2021.
35. Ambulatory Surgery Centers: Gastroenterologist Dr. Mitchell Cappell appointed to FDA GI Advisory Committee, Becker's Hospital Review. Thursday, September 20th, 2012. Available at: https://www.beckershospitalreview.com/asc/gastroenterologist-dr-mitchell-cappell-appointed-to-fda-gi-advisory-committee.html. Accessed December 8, 2022.

36. Centers for Medicare & Medicaid Services. President Trump expands telehealth benefits for Medicare beneficiaries during COVID-19 outbreak. CMS.gov. Mar 17, 2020. Available at: https://www.cms.gov/newsroom/press-releases/president-trump-expands-telehealth-benefits-medicare-beneficiaries-during-covid-19-outbreak. Accessed April 14, 2020.
37. Edbrooke DL, Minelli C, Mills GH, et al. Implications of ICU triage decisions on patient mortality: a cost-effectiveness analysis. Crit Care 2011;15(1):R56. https://doi.org/10.1186/cc10029.
38. Cappell MS. A critical review two-years thereafter of the effectiveness of the revolutionary changes in a gastroenterology division at a medical school teaching hospital in response to the initial COVID-19 pandemic: Medical school, medical residency and GI fellowship education; clinical practice of GI attendings, and GI endoscopy
39. Amadeo K., How COVID-19 has affected the US economy. The Balance, Available at: https://www.thebalance.com/how-covid-19-has-affected-the-useconomy-5092445 Accessed April 30, 2021.
40. Starkman E. Starkman: Beaumont Nurse Anesthetists At Royal Oak, Troy And Grosse Pointe Vote Overwhelmingly To Unionize. Deadline Detroit. March 29, 2021. Available at https://deadlinedetroit.com/articles/27683/starkman_beaumont_nurse_anesthetists_at_royal_oak_troy_and_grosse_pointe_vote_overwhelmingly_to_unionize.
41. Starkman E. Starkman: Bloodbath At Beaumont – COO Carolyn Wilson And Top Doctor Ousted; Chief Quality Officer Resigns Deadline Detroit July 22, 2021. Available at https://renaissance.deadlinedetroit.com/articles/28438/starkman_bloodbath_at_beaumont_coo_carolyn_wilson_and_top_doctor_ousted_chief_quality_officer_resigns. Accessed December 25, 2022
42. Beaumont. Advocate Aurora Health, Beaumont Health Exploring Partnership. June 17, 2020. Available at https://www.beaumont.org/health-wellness/press-releases/advocate-aurora-health-beaumont-health-exploring-partnership. Accessed December 25, 2022.
43. Greene J. Beaumont makes deal to acquire Ohio's Summa Health. Modern Healthcare. July 9, 2019. Available at https://www.modernhealthcare.com/mergers-acquisitions/beaumont-makes-deal-acquire-ohios-summa-health. Accessed December 25, 2022.
44. Reindl JC. Newly merged Beaumont Spectrum health system rebrands as Corewell Health. Detroit Free Press. October 11, 2022. Available at https://news.yahoo.com/newly-merged-beaumont-spectrum-health-153656641.html. Accessed December 25, 2022.
45. Starkman E. Starkman: Beaumont's Woes Prove CEO Tina Freese Decker Unfit To Run Michigan's Biggest Hospital System. August 19, 2022. Available at https://www.deadlinedetroit.com/articles/31125/starkman_beaumont_s_woes_prove_ceo_tina_freese_decker_unfit_to_run_michigan_s_biggest_hospital_system

9780443182167